Kidney Transplantatior
of Kidney Transplant R

MW01258376

JoeL
Thanks For
All the support
+ wisdom!.
Steve

Dianne B. McKay · Steven M. Steinberg
Editors

Kidney Transplantation: A Guide to the Care of Kidney Transplant Recipients

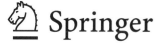
Springer

Editors
Dianne B. McKay
The Scripps Research Institute
10550 N. Torrey Pines Rd.
La Jolla CA 92037
USA
dmckay@scripps.edu
and
Sharp Memorial Hospital
Division of Transplantation
7910 Frost Street
San Diego, CA 92123

Steven M. Steinberg
Sharp Memorial Hospital
Division of Transplantation
7910 Frost Street
San Diego CA 92123
USA
ssteinberg@bnmg.org

ISBN 978-1-4419-1689-1   e-ISBN 978-1-4419-1690-7
DOI 10.1007/978-1-4419-1690-7
Springer New York Dordrecht Heidelberg London

Library of Congress Control Number: 2010922485

© Springer Science+Business Media, LLC 2010
All rights reserved. This work may not be translated or copied in whole or in part without the written permission of the publisher (Springer Science+Business Media, LLC, 233 Spring Street, New York, NY 10013, USA), except for brief excerpts in connection with reviews or scholarly analysis. Use in connection with any form of information storage and retrieval, electronic adaptation, computer software, or by similar or dissimilar methodology now known or hereafter developed is forbidden.
The use in this publication of trade names, trademarks, service marks, and similar terms, even if they are not identified as such, is not to be taken as an expression of opinion as to whether or not they are subject to proprietary rights.
While the advice and information in this book are believed to be true and accurate at the date of going to press, neither the authors nor the editors nor the publisher can accept any legal responsibility for any errors or omissions that may be made. The publisher makes no warranty, express or implied, with respect to the material contained herein.

Printed on acid-free paper

Springer is part of Springer Science+Business Media (www.springer.com)

To my father Barry, who inspired my journey into the world of medicine and to Andy and our children Liam, Nora and Danny who inspire life's endless possibilities.

Dianne B. McKay, M.D.

To Stephanie and the kids, who make me want to be a better man.

Steven M. Steinberg, M.D.

Preface

Kidney transplantation improves the length and quality of life for many patients with end-stage renal disease. Successful transplantation is ensured by specialists trained to recognize and manage both the immediate pre- and post-transplant issues and the initial decisions regarding immunosuppression. Of course, early expert medical and surgical care is paramount to the successes of transplantation.

Immediately after the transplant, particularly trained specialists at the medical center manage the post-transplant care. However, after discharge from the transplant center, long-term care of the transplant recipient often falls on the shoulders of the community nephrologist or the general internist, who may or may not be experienced with transplant care. This guide to the care of the kidney transplant recipient aims to provide practical guidelines for management of the post-transplant recipient and is targeted at community nephrologists and general internists who care for the patient with a kidney transplant.

Although this book outlines many aspects of transplant specialty care, it is not intended to replace textbooks directed at transplant physicians. The aim is to provide practical advice for the continuation of long-term care of the patient after they leave the transplant center. Our ultimate goal is to provide informed, consistent, and multidisciplinary care guidelines for recipients of kidney transplants. We hope that this text contributes to that process.

Dianne B. McKay
Steven M. Steinberg

Contents

Contributors

Patricia L. Adams, MD Section on Nephrology, WFU School of Medicine, Wake Forest University Baptist Medical Center, Medical Center Boulevard, NC Baptist Hospital, Winston-Salem, NC, USA

Roy D. Bloom, MD Kidney Transplant Program, Hospital of the University of Pennsylvania, Philadelphia, PA, USA

Daniel C. Brennan, MD Renal Division, Department of Internal Medicine, Washington University School of Medicine, St. Louis, MO, USA

Barry J. Browne, MD, MS, FACS Abdominal Transplantation, Transplant Surgery, Sharp Memorial Hospital, San Diego, CA, USA

Mary Beth Callahan, ACSW/LCSW, MSSW Dallas Transplant Institute, Dallas, TX, USA

Peter Chung-Wen Chang, MD Division of Nephrology and Hypertension, Department of Medicine, University Hospitals Case Medical Center, Cleveland, OH, USA

James E. Cooper, MD Department of Nephrology, University of Colorado, Aurora, CO, USA

Gabriel M. Danovitch, MD Division of Nephrology, Department of Medicine, Kidney and Pancreas Transplant Program, David Geffen School of Medicine at UCLA, Los Angeles, CA, USA

Connie L. Davis, MD Department of Medicine, University of Washington, Seattle, WA, USA

Francis L. Delmonico, MD The Transplantation Society, World Health Organization, Massachusetts General Hospital Transplant Center, Newton, MA, USA

Fabienne Dobbels, PhD Center for Health Services and Nursing Research, Katholieke Universiteit Leuven, Leuven, Belgium

Alden M. Doyle, MD, MS, MPH Renal, Electrolyte and Hypertension Division, Hospital of the University of Pennsylvania, Philadelphia, PA, USA

Richard N. Fine, MD Stony Brook University Medical Center, Stony Brook, NY, USA

Robert S. Gaston, MD Kidney and Pancreas Transplantation, Division of Nephrology, Department of Medicine, University of Alabama at Birmingham, Birmingham, AL, USA

Walter K. Graham, JD United Network for Organ Sharing, Richmond, VA, USA

Indira Guleria, PhD Renal Division, HLA Laboratory, Harvard Medical School, Brigham and Women's Hospital, Boston, MA, USA

Susan Gunderson, MHA LifeSource, St. Paul, MN, USA

Ruthanne L. Hanto, RN, MPH New England Organ Bank, New England Program for Kidney Exchange, Organ Procurement Organization, Newton, MA, USA

Donald E. Hricik, MD Division of Nephrology and Hypertension, Department of Medicine, University Hospitals Case Medical Center, Cleveland, OH, USA

Elizabeth Ingulli, MD Renal Transplant Program, UCSD and Rady Children's Hospital, Pediatrics, San Diego, CA, USA

Michelle A. Josephson, MD Department of Medicine, University of Chicago, Chicago, IL, USA

Roslyn B. Mannon, MD, FASN Division of Nephrology, Department of Medicine, University of Alabama at Birmingham, Birmingham, AL, USA

Arturo Martinez, MD, FACS Transplant, Laparoscopic and Robotic Surgeon, Department of Urology, The Permanente Medical Group, San Francisco, CA, USA

Dianne B. McKay, MD Department of Immunology and Microbial Sciences, The Scripps Research Institute, La Jolla, CA, USA; Sharp Memorial Hospital, San Diego, CA, USA

Edgar L. Milford, MD Renal Division, Tissue Typing Laboratory, Department of Medicine, Harvard Medical School, Brigham and Women's Hospital, Boston, MA, USA

Ken Park, MD Department of Family and Preventative Medicine, University of California San Diego, San Diego, CA, USA

Martha Pavlakis, MD Kidney and Pancreas Transplantation, Beth Israel Deaconess Medical Center, Transplant, Boston, MA, USA

David Perkins, MD, PhD Department of Medicine and Surgery, University of California San Diego, Medicine and Surgery, La Jolla, CA, USA

Phuong-Anh T. Pham, MD, FACC Mercy General Hospital, Heart and Vascular Institute, Cardiovascular Diseases, Sacramento, CA, USA

Phuong-Chi T. Pham, MD Division of Nephrology, Department of Medicine, Olive View-UCLA Medical Center David Geffen School of Medicine at UCLA, Sylmar, CA, USA

Phuong-Mai T. Pham, MD David Geffen School of Medicine at UCLA, Sepulveda VAMC, Internal Medicine, North Hills, CA, USA

Phuong-Thu T. Pham, MD Division of Nephrology, Department of Medicine, Kidney and Pancreas Transplant Program, David Geffen School of Medicine at UCLA, Los Angeles, CA, USA

Mary B. Prendergast, MB BCh BAO MRCP Division of Nephrology, Department of Medicine, University of Alabama at Birmingham, Birmingham, AL, USA

Alvin E. Roth, PhD Department of Economics, Harvard Business School, Harvard University, Boston, MA, USA

Milagros D. Samaniego, MD Departments of Medicine and Surgery, University of Wisconsin Hospital and Clinics, Madison, WI, USA

Carlos A.Q. Santos, MD Division of Infectious Diseases, Department of Medicine, Washington University/Barnes-Jewish Hospital/St. Louis Children's Hospital Consortium, St. Louis, MO, USA

Carmen Slavov, MD Division of Nephrology, Department of Medicine, Kidney and Pancreas Transplant Program, David Geffen School of Medicine at UCLA, Ronald Reagan UCLA Medical Center, Los Angeles, CA, USA

Stuart M. Sprague, DO Division of Nephrology and Hypertension, North Shore University Health System, Northwestern University Feinberg School of Medicine, Evanston, IL, USA

Steven M. Steinberg, MD, FACP Kidney Pancreas Transplant, Division of Transplantation, Sharp Memorial Hospital, San Diego, CA, USA

Robert Steiner, MD University of California at San Diego Medical Center, San Diego, CA, USA

Jose R. Torrealba, MD, FCAP, FRCPC Pathology and Laboratory Medicine, University of Wisconsin Hospital and Clinics, Madison, WI, USA

M. Utku Ünver, PhD Department of Economics, Boston College, Chestnut Hill, MA, USA

Bradford Lee West, MD, FACP Department of Nephrology, University of Chicago Medical Center, Chicago, IL, USA

Alan H. Wilkinson, MD, FRCP Division of Nephrology, Department of Medicine, Kidney and Pancreas Transplant Programs, David Geffen School of Medicine at UCLA, Los Angeles, CA, USA

Alexander C. Wiseman, MD Kidney and Pancreas Transplant Program, Department of Nephrology, University of Colorado, Aurora, CO, USA

Chapter 1
Ten Things Not to Do

Dianne B. McKay and Steven M. Steinberg

Introduction

The purpose of this *Guide to the Kidney Care of Transplant Recipients* is to provide practical up-to-date information for practitioners who care for transplant recipients. This guide is also helpful for the transplant physician, including physicians in training, who through this guide will obtain an appreciation for the complexities of caring for the transplant recipient outside of the transplant center. While much of this guide focuses on specific medical and surgical topics, we would like to begin with a brief chapter of some of the "takeaway" messages of this guide. These messages rely on the art of medicine, as well as the science, and it is hoped that the reader will indulge us in this pursuit. The following "Ten Things Not to Do" are mostly directed at the community nephrologist and the internist who, although not the primary caregiver at the time of transplant, soon becomes the major caregiver of these patients, often with limited guidelines for assistance.

1. Do NOT forget to refer your ESRD patients for transplantation early, encourage them to find a living donor and pay attention to the pretransplant workup.

Encourage your ESRD patients to present to the transplant center before they begin dialysis and get eligible patients listed for a deceased donor organ or worked up for a preemptive transplant as soon as possible. Renal transplantation is the treatment modality of choice for nearly all suitable candidates with end-stage renal disease. Transplantation improves both patient survival and quality of life. The longer the patients are on dialysis the poorer their overall health.

For many reasons, a live donor is preferable to a deceased donor. Encourage your patients to speak to family members, friends, and altruistic donors. If the patient feels uncomfortable advocating for himself/herself, enlist a family member

D.B. McKay (✉)
Department of Immunology and Microbial Sciences, The Scripps Research Institute, La Jolla, USA
e-mail: dmckay@scripps.edu

D.B. McKay, S.M. Steinberg (eds.), *Kidney Transplantation: A Guide to the Care of Kidney Transplant Recipients*, DOI 10.1007/978-1-4419-1690-7_1,
© Springer Science+Business Media, LLC 2010

or friend to speak to others on behalf of the patient. Do not encourage your patient to participate in transplant tourism, for it is illegal and often results in bad outcomes. Do encourage your patient to consider a paired donor swap if a blood type mismatch is preventing a willing donor from donating to your patient.

If the patient has no donor, encourage him/her to quickly fulfill the requirements of the pretransplant evaluation so that they can be listed as soon as possible. The waiting times are lengthy and many patients fall ill and become ineligible for transplantation during the lengthy waiting process. Encourage the patient to ask about listing for expanded donor (ECD) or donation after cardiac death (DCD) kidneys if they are older, have diabetes mellitus, or have poor general health and need to shorten their waiting time.

The pretransplant workup will likely identify issues that need clarification before the patient can be listed for transplantation. Be sure to address all requests promptly to avoid excessive downtime before your patient is placed on the deceased donor transplant waiting list. Be sure to administer all needed vaccinations before transplantation because post-transplant immunosuppression prevents adequate antibody responses to vaccines. Live virus vaccinations are contraindicated after transplantation.

The following chapters detail important information specific to these take-home points:

Chapter 5 – describes how donor organs are allocated
Chapter 6 – describes the live donor workup
Chapter 8 – describes the paired donor-swap program
Chapter 13 – describes the pretransplant workup
Chapter 15 – details the survival advantage offered by transplantation over dialysis
Chapter 16 – details information regarding vaccinations in transplant recipients

2. Do NOT underestimate the clinical clues provided in the transplant center report! Be sure that a full report accompanies the patient on return to your office.

Request a summary from the transplant center that summarizes the transplant surgery, perioperative surgical and medical events, the hospital course, and the first few post-transplant months. Transplant centers vary in length of acute post-transplant follow-up, from a month at some centers to over a year at others. As you might have a lot of information to synthesize regarding the acute post-transplant course of your patient, schedule plenty of time to go through the transplant center report! Table 1.1 summarizes the information that you need to know about the transplant surgery, hospitalization, and acute post-transplant follow-up.

If you do not understand the peritransplant events or the therapeutic rationale prescribed by the transplant center you cannot adequately care for the transplant recipient. If the information you need is not available you must speak to the transplant physician who took care of your patient. The transplant coordinator provides an excellent, additional source of information. Communication with the transplant center is KEY!

Table 1.1 Information to be obtained from the transplant center

1. *Donor information*
    a. Type of donor: live donor, deceased donor

    - Live donor organs generally last long longer than deceased donor organs
    - Live donor organs might be less immunogenic

    b. Size incompatibility

    - Small kidneys transplanted into a large person may result in hyperfiltration and might benefit from ACEI or ARB therapy

2. *Hospitalization information*
    a. Length of hospitalization

    - You need to know if the transplanted kidney had delayed graft function or prolonged ATN

    b. Ureteral stent

    - Make sure you know when the ureteral stent should be removed if it was not already removed at the transplant center

    c. Post-transplant biopsy/biopsies

    - You need to know all post-transplant biopsy results to help guide the immunosuppressive therapy
    - Early rejection places the patient at high immunologic risk for another later rejection
    - Your patient might need surveillance for development of anti-DSA antibodies

    d. Hospital readmissions

    - Why was the patient readmitted – rejection, surgical complications, etc.

    e. Naidir creatinine and baseline creatinine

    - You need to know what the transplant center thinks is the BEST creatinine the patient will have.

3. *Immunologic information*
    a. Information that suggests your patient is at *high* immunologic risk (high risk of rejection)

    - Elevated pretransplant antibody titers (PRAs)
    - Development of donor-specific antibodies (DSAs)
    - Multiple HLA mismatches
    - Early acute rejection
    - Prior transplantation (second, third, etc.)

    b. Information that suggests your patient is at *low* immunologic risk (low risk of rejection)

    - Zero HLA donor/recipient antigen mismatch

4. *Immunosuppressive medication information:*
    a. What is the prescribed combination of maintenance immunosuppressive medications?

    - What are the target doses and target therapeutic blood levels?
    - How often should you measure immunosuppressive drug levels?

    b. Is the patient on an experimental drug protocol and what is it?

    - You need to know the protocol drugs and the requirements of the protocol if any

Table 1.1 (continued)

c. Induction therapy (especially Thymoglobulin)

- Increases risk for infections (e.g., CMV) and possibly malignancies [post-transplant lymphoproliferative disease (PTLD)]

5. *Information about infectious risks*
   a. CMV status of the donor and recipient

   - CMV positive donor places the patient at high risk of CMV disease
   - Be sure the patient is receiving adequate CMV prophylaxis

   b. EBV status of the recipient

   - EBV negative recipient should be monitored for seroconversion
   - Seroconversion increases risk for PTLD

   c. History of TB exposure (+PPD or + QuantiFERON-TB)

   - Find out if patient was treated before transplant if not start empiric therapy

   d. Received a HBV+ or HCV+ kidney

   - Higher risk of cirrhosis and hepatocellular carcinoma
   - Follow LFTs q 3 months, consider annual liver ultrasound and alpha-fetoprotein level

   e. Prior graft loss associated with BK virus

   - Check BKV-DNA by PCR q months x 6 months then at 9 months, 12 months, and yearly.

   f. Prophylaxis for Candida, *Pneumocystis jiroveci*, CMV, herpes, EBV, etc.

   - Know when you should stop these agents

6. *Information about malignancy risks*
   a. Did your patient have any pretransplant malignancy or premalignant lesions?

   - All transplant recipients have increased lifetime risk of malignancy
   - Be sure to follow closely for common post-transplant malignancies, e.g., non-melanoma skin cancer, cervical cancer, Kaposi's sarcoma, non-Hodgkin lymphoma, kidney cancer, thyroid cancer, and others

7. *Other essential issues*
   a. New proteinuria

   - Suggests recurrent disease (especially FSGS)
   - Might need to avoid sirolimus conversion

   b. Post-transplant specialty consults

   - Gives clues about peritransplant morbidities (e.g., CVD)

The following chapters detail important information specific to these take-home points:

Chapter 2 – describes the surgical procedure
Chapter 5 – describes how donor organs are allocated
Chapter 7 – describes laparoscopic donation
Chapter 14 – describes the acute post-transplant care

3. Try NOT to do more than you can at the local level. Do not get in over your head!

Physicians should NOT be optimistic with transplant patients. Usually what can go wrong will go wrong. Treating an unknown illness, new unexplained elevation in serum creatinine, new proteinuria, and so on without the input of the transplant center can be unwise. Admitting a newly transplanted patient to a hospital not affiliated with the transplant center usually leads to a compounding of delay in diagnosis and to a critical delay in treatment, especially if the patient eventually has to be transferred.

We recommend that organ transplant recipients with anything more than the simplest of illnesses be referred to a transplant center experienced in their care. This is nearly mandatory in patients with surgical issues, as many community surgeons have almost no experience with operating on organ transplant recipients. This is especially true for combined kidney–pancreas recipients.

Do not treat or admit a patient with newly altered renal function to a place where a transplant surgeon or a transplant biopsy is not available!

The following chapters detail important information specific to these take-home points:

4. Do NOT underestimate nonadherence – it is a common and REAL PROBLEM!!

Nonadherence is defined as "any deviation from the prescribed medication regimen sufficient to influence adversely the regimen's intended effect." Nonadherence is very common in both adult and pediatric kidney transplant recipients. In adults, 25% of graft losses are due to nonadherence and in pediatric recipients it is even higher (44%). There are many reasons for nonadherence, including socioeconomic, patient and disease and treatment-related factors, as well as health-care team-related factors. You MUST have high suspicion and maintain vigilance to avoid graft loss due to nonadherence!

There are several important clues that should raise your suspicion of nonadherence:

1. Missed office appointments or blood draws
2. Fluctuating drug levels (especially CNI levels)
3. Age: especially teenagers and young adults

4. Preemptive LRD, never before on dialysis
5. Late acute rejection (>6 months post-transplant)

It is difficult to be a transplant patient and the physician and staff must be cheerleaders and coaches for their patients. Would you let a dialysis patient miss appointments without some type of intervention and follow-up by the dialysis team? Members of the staff – nurses and medical assistants – are the primary effectors of this strategy and must be trained in the importance of insuring follow-up.

Medication drug levels provide an important clue to nonadherence, but they do not necessarily need to be low for a patient to be nonadherent. There is a unique type of "white coat syndrome" in which patients prepare for the MD visit by taking their medications correctly for a few days so as to have good drug levels, but are nonadherent in the interim. Some pharmacies offer compliance tracking programs and these should be utilized if available.

A particularly risky time for nonadherence is the time of transition from the pediatric to the adult transplant clinic. During this time, the teenager/young adult is at risk of losing medical insurance coverage. Usually their coverage stops at age 23, although it can stop before if they are not a full-time student. If they receive Medicare benefits only because of renal disease, their medical coverage will cease 3 years after transplantation. Patient assistance programs will pay for medications, but usually not laboratory work, office visits, and procedural examinations. You need to prepare ahead. You need to enlist the social worker to formulate a plan for these young, vulnerable patients. Teenagers and young adults are a particularly difficult group for other reasons. They may have altered sleep patterns (e.g., stay up late at night, sleep in and miss their AM medications), and they are concerned with cosmetic side effects and the effect of the medications on their body image and their sexuality. Be careful with pregnancy in female transplant recipients (not necessarily related to nonadherence).

Preemptive live donor recipients do not know what it is like to be on dialysis and might be prone to think that if they reject they can just get another transplant if they want one. As they have not experienced dialysis they see the medications, not the disease, as the problem.

Rejection rates in the 6 months immediately post-transplant are 5–10% at most centers. Why would someone reject at 6 months or later? Please investigate for partial adherence or full nonadherence in these patients. These patients often do not admit to nonadherence despite rejection episodes or undetectable levels of CNI.

The following chapters detail important information specific to these take-home points:

Chapter 20 – describes sexuality and reproductive issues in transplant recipients
Chapter 21 – describes socioeconomic issues in transplant recipients
Chapter 22 – describes nonadherence in the transplant recipients
Chapter 23 – describes the difficult period of transition from pediatric to adult clinic for the young transplant recipient

5. Do NOT change immunosuppressive medications without talking to the transplant center and seriously considering that you might precipitate either acute or chronic rejection. Respect the recipient's immune system!

When medication side effects or toxicities occur, you will likely be pressured to reduce or change immunosuppressive dosing. Do not make major changes to immunosuppressive medications without talking to the transplant center! Only clinicians familiar with the patient's immune history should be manipulating the immunosuppressive therapy.

Immunosuppressive drug levels can be falsely high, falsely low, or falsely normal in the case of nonadherence, unexpected drug interactions, or food–drug interactions (e.g., grapefruit juice). Drug levels may also be erroneous due to laboratory errors or sample timing.

If the immunosuppressive medication level is low, e.g., in the case of calcineurin inhibitors ACT ON IT!! Do not have the patient come back in a week or so to repeat serum creatinine and CNI levels, they need to come back immediately! Ineffective immunosuppression will precipitate rejection and the development of anti-DSA antibodies. DSA antibodies can appear anytime after transplantation when immuno-suppressive medication levels have been allowed to remain low. You can also count on the fact that you may not detect rejection right away – there may be a slow rise in creatinine that is easy to miss (see creatinine creep below).

Just because a patient has intolerable side effects/toxicity from an immuno-suppressive agent does not mean that they need less of it to prevent rejection. Toxicity and efficacy are two different and often unrelated properties. Over the years, many physicians continuously decrease immunosuppression based on their patient's request and perceived side effects without regard to immunological need.

A good example is prolonged reduction of mycophenolate mofetil (MMF) in patients for gastrointestinal symptoms who later demonstrate evidence of under-immunosuppression (i.e., acute or chronic rejection or development of donor-specific antibodies). If you must reduce a dose of one medication, increase the dose of another unless toxicities prevent this maneuver. If you reduce the dose of a medication you must have the patient return to your office for repeat laboratory evaluations, within at least 2 weeks, if not sooner. The sooner you catch a rise in creatinine, the better. Ask the transplant center for advice if considering individual tailoring of immunosuppressive medications.

Withdrawing steroids late, in our opinion, is NOT advisable. Actually, even for early steroid avoidance, it is not clear if steroid withdrawal is safe for all, is safe for the long term, or if it is associated with more chronic fibrosis in the transplant. Late withdrawal of steroids is not without risk of acute or chronic rejection and is of no clear benefit.

The following chapters detail important information specific to these take-home points:

Chapter 3 – describes the basics of transplantation immunology
Chapter 4 – describes tissue typing and HLA matching

Chapter 9 – describes immunosuppressive medications, dosing, and their side effects
Chapter 10 – describes minimization strategies for immunosuppressive medications

6. Do NOT delay the diagnosis or treatment of creatinine creep. There may be many reasons for a slow decline in renal allograft function.

Creatinine creep is the descriptive term for the slow, insidious rise in serum creatinine that occurs in some patients after transplantation. While most nephrologists are appropriately alarmed by a sudden and rapid decline in renal function, creatinine creep is often undertreated and certainly underinvestigated.

With the elevation of the serum creatinine in a transplant patient, the default or fallback strategy is often to lower the calcineurin inhibitor (CNI) without much diagnostic evaluation in order to see what happens. This is especially true in practices where a renal biopsy is difficult to obtain or the local pathologist has limited experience in renal transplantation.

Certainly, the creatinine may go down initially after the CNI dose is reduced, but this is often just the effect of less renal vasoconstriction, and then it frequently will rise again. Time lost in the delay in diagnosis cannot be recovered. Often this dose lowering "guess" is paired with the other errors of omission including reordering the labs, waiting, and hoping that the creatinine elevation is a laboratory error. There are numerous reasons for an elevation in creatinine and a full serologic, radiologic, and pathologic interpretation is mandatory.

Unfortunately, the optimal therapy for a slowly rising creatinine is not defined. If the transplant ultrasound shows new obstruction, a urologic consultation should be obtained and BK virus DNA should be measured in the blood; BK nephropathy can present as a late ureteral obstruction. Be careful interpreting the transplant ultrasound as mild to moderate calyceal distention can be normal in transplanted kidneys; you need to make a comparison to the baseline post-transplant renal transplant ultrasounds.

If the transplant biopsy shows acute rejection, IMMEDIATELY consult the transplant center for advice on optimal treatment! After acute rejection is treated, intensify the baseline immunosuppression, and address nonadherence. A frequent finding in the biopsy of a transplanted kidney with a slowly rising creatinine is interstitial fibrosis and hyaline arteriolopathy. It is difficult to distinguish CNI toxicity from chronic alloimmune injury of the kidney allograft and therefore clinical judgment needs to be applied to interpretation of the biopsy findings (e.g., if the CNI levels are chronically low you probably have rejection rather than CNI toxicity). The capability for C4d (to detect BK virus) and SV-40 (to detect humoral rejection) staining is essential.

Do not forget that there are other causes of allograft dysfunction besides rejection. Transplant biopsies done greater than 6–12 months post-operatively should include immunofluorescence and electron microscopy due to the possibility of recurrent disease. Failure to remember this may lead to a second biopsy. Other late causes of allograft dysfunction include transplant artery stenosis, often associated with difficult to control hypertension, and sometimes with a bruit over the transplant artery. Ureteral stenosis, especially in those patients with a history of previous acute rejection, urine leak, or BK virus nephritis are other late causes of allograft dysfunction.

The following chapters detail important information specific to these take-home points:

Chapter 11 – describes evaluation of renal function in transplant recipients
Chapter 12 – describes the pathologic findings of kidney transplant biopsy
Chapter 14 – describes the acute care of the transplant recipient

7. Do NOT drop your vigilance regarding drug interactions. Be careful of generic immunosuppressive medications!

There are important interactions between immunosuppressive drugs and other medications that might be prescribed to your patient. Vigilance is needed to avoid serious drug interactions! A common example is the interaction between calcineurin inhibitors (CNIs) and drugs that regulate the cytochrome P450 3A enzyme system located in the liver and gastrointestinal tract. Non-dihydropyridine calcium channel blockers (CCB) (diltiazem and verapamil) increase CNI levels and therefore you need to monitor CNI levels with any CCB dose change; some transplant programs prescribe CCBs to purposely lower the required dose of CNIs and decrease patient expense. There are many drugs that alter the P450 system and common interactions with immunosuppressive medications are described in later text. Your patients should be told that only their nephrologist should modify the dose of medications that might influence immunosuppressive drug levels.

Generic immunosuppressive medications may not have the same bioavailability as the parent drug due to differences in the manufacturing process. Of particular concern with regard to immunosuppressive medications is that immunosuppressive drugs have a narrow therapeutic range. Be sure to know if your patient's pharmacy has substituted a generic immunosuppressive medication, and if so realize that you will need to perform more frequent immunological monitoring. It is important to also realize that not all generic medications have the same bioavailability and there might be significant variability in effective immunosuppression. If your patient is taking a generic substitute you will need to follow the patient closely because there are serious consequences to overdosing or underdosing. If you permit their use, you will need to consider generic drugs as an important variable in the management of your patient's immunosuppressive medications.

The following chapters detail important information specific to these take-home points:

Chapter 9 – describes immunosuppressive medications and their side effects
Chapter 14 – describes acute care of the transplant recipient

8. Do NOT forget your patients are living in the real world.

Transplantation is the gift of life and with that gift comes the opportunity to resume active, productive lives. An active life usually involves employment, lifting of dietary restrictions, and renewed sexuality.

Employment is the key to your patient's economic viability and probably a major factor in their ability to adhere to post-transplant medical advice. Patients who have been under the umbrella of a relatively secure medical system (Medicare) while on dialysis are suddenly faced with economic challenges after transplantation (e.g., co-pays for immunosuppressive medications, office visits). If a person has Medicare only based on kidney disease, coverage will end 3 years after transplantation. You need to plan ahead so that your patients do not find themselves at serious financial risk. Ask for help from your social worker or other patient advocate. Be sure you do not let your patient's insurance coverage lapse!

After transplantation, dietary restrictions are lifted and patients become hungry. A healthy lifestyle should be encouraged, including a healthy diet and regular exercise. Up to 29% of transplant recipients have a BMI > 30 kg/m^2 and even more are overweight (BMI > 25 kg/m^2). Overweight patients often become obese after transplantation and so you need to plan ahead by recommending a formal dietary program and a diet support group. Steroid reduction for obesity must be carefully weighed against the risk of allograft rejection and loss. Do not use pharmacologic medications to reduce weight, do consider gastric bypass in morbidly obese patients. An exercise program is mandatory and might involve referral to a physical therapist to initiate a safe exercise regimen.

Most ESRD patients are sexually inactive. That changes after transplantation! Women of reproductive age can easily become pregnant. You need to be sure that your female transplant patients are using effective contraception, e.g., oral contraceptives, not barrier methods. Be sure if your female transplant recipient wants to become pregnant that she is not taking CellCept or Myfortic or sirolimus. If so, you need to send her back to the transplant center to change her immunosuppressives. Male transplant recipients wishing to father a child should not be placed on sirolimus as there is an increased risk for infertility with sirolimus.

Please also remember that your patients have families that might also be affected by your patient's illness. The transplant social worker and other patient advocates are an excellent source for help.

The following chapters detail important information specific to these take-home points:

9. Do NOT forget the general medical problems of the transplant recipient – some of these are accelerated by the transplant medications. The most common cause of graft loss is death with a functioning graft!

All transplant recipients have comorbidities, many of which are compounded by immunosuppressive medications. Common comorbidities include hypertension, hyperlipidemia, anemia, new-onset diabetes, cardiovascular disease, and bone disease. Detailed information on each of these conditions is found in the text, but we will briefly describe some of the "take-home lessons."

Hypertension is common and blood pressures should be measured at every office visit. The goal is to reduce blood pressure to <130/80, but in proteinuric renal transplant recipients, the goal is less than 125/75 mmHg. There is no contraindication to any type of antihypertensive agent – even ACEI or ARBs. The CCBs diltiazem and verapamil increase CNI levels and therefore must be used with caution and CNI levels followed closely.

Hyperlipidemia is common and needs to be aggressively managed after the first six post-transplant months. Most patients will require pharmacotherapy. Be careful with the dose of statins because they interact with CNIs; CNIs cause a several-fold increase in statin blood level and increase the risk for myopathy and rhabdomyolysis. If statins do not work or cannot be tolerated try fibrates. Target low-density lipoprotein (LDL) concentrations should be less than 100 mg/dl (optimal <70 mg/dl), high-density lipoproteins (HDLs) >40 mg/dl for men and >50 mg/dl for women. A fasting lipid profile should be measured at least annually.

Anemia is commonly associated with azathioprine, mycophenolate, sirolimus, and ACEIs and ARBs. The goal for anemia correction, based on the KDOQI guidelines, is to achieve hemoglobin levels in the 11–12 g/dl. Erythropoiesis-stimulating agents are often used in transplant recipients to treat anemia. Be sure to evaluate for other causes of anemia though, such as PTLD. Erythrocytosis is also common and can be treated with angiotensin blockade and phlebotomy.

Cardiovascular disease is the norm in renal transplant recipients. Cardiovascular risk reduction strategies such as stopping smoking, losing weight, controlling blood pressure, and dyslipidemia are a mainstay of treatment. Proteinuria is an independent risk factor for CVD and so ACEI or ARBs should be considered in patients with microalbuminuria or proteinuria. Annual cardiac stress testing is recommended for high-risk patients (e.g., those with a history of MI, diabetes mellitus, known or symptomatic coronary artery disease).

New-onset diabetes after transplantation (NODAT) is common; it occurs in as many as 30% of post-transplant patients. The criteria for diagnosis follow the World Health Organization and American Diabetes Association Guidelines of a plasma glucose ≥200 mg/dl, fasting plasma glucose ≥126 mg/dl, or 2 h glucose tolerance test (after a 75 g glucose load) of ≥200 mg/dl. There are several risk factors, including family history of DM, obesity/metabolic syndrome, HCV, and pretransplant impaired glucose tolerance testing. If the patient develops NODAT the management should follow the conventional approach for patients with type 2 diabetes mellitus.

Bone disease is common in patients before and after kidney transplantation. During the first 6 months after the transplant, most patients experience a rapid decline in bone mineral density due to immunosuppressive medications and immobilization. Fall risk is also increased and fracture rates are high. Screening for bone disease is imperfect, but until better screening tools are available, bone mineral density screening should be performed within the first 3 months after transplantation if the GFR > 30 and if the patient is taking corticosteroids or has other risk factors for bone loss. Assessments should also be made for 25-hydroxy vitamin D deficiencies and treatment instituted if necessary.

The following chapters detail important information specific to these take-home points:

Chapter 15 – describes cardiovascular disease in renal allograft recipients
Chapter 16 – describes new-onset diabetes mellitus in renal allograft recipients
Chapter 19 – describes bone disease in renal allograft recipients

10. Do NOT forget that kidney transplantation is a temporary treatment for ESRD (not a cure) and that even the most successful kidney transplant recipient does not have normal glomerular filtration rate and has CKD.

Transplant patients should be classified with a "T" after the chronic kidney disease (CKD) as CKDT 2-3-4. Please bear in mind that your patient should be managed like a CKD patient, with all their associated comorbidities. CKDT tend to have a slower progression toward ESRD but a longer burden of cardiovascular risk due to the patient's previous history of advanced CKD, with or without accumulated dialysis time. Consider the cumulative vasculopathy including cerebral and peripheral vascular disease. Many successful transplants experience limb loss post-operatively. Not surprisingly, this is especially problematic in diabetics.

As you would monitor a patient with CKD, you should monitor renal allograft function at each office visit by measuring serum creatinine. Also screen for urinary protein and albumin excretion. Proteinuria is an early and sensitive marker of kidney damage in renal allograft recipients and persistent proteinuria is an important predictor of outcomes. Causes include allograft rejection and drug toxicity and also de novo and recurrent glomerular diseases (e.g., membranous glomerulonephritis, diabetic nephropathy, focal glomerulosclerosis). An allograft biopsy may be indicated to differentiate treatable causes of proteinuria. Albuminuria is increasingly being recognized as an indicator of poor renal allograft outcomes. Timed renal allograft biopsies are still outside the standard of care.

The following chapters detail important information specific to these take-home points:

Chapter 11 – describes evaluation of renal function in transplant recipients
Chapter 12 – describes the pathologic findings of kidney transplant biopsy
Chapter 14 – describes the post-transplant care of transplant recipients

A final consideration on the care of the kidney transplant patient is that it is easy to fall into the cognitive trap of trying to save the current allograft at all costs. All transplanted kidneys will eventually be lost to poorly defined processes that involve variable contributions from immunologic and nonimmunologic factors. Therefore, most patients will require multiple modalities for treatment of their ESRD. They may be on dialysis and then transplanted, return to dialysis and then receive a second transplant. The options are multiple and may be very unpredictable in any one patient.

In this spirit, it is preferred to minimize blood transfusions in order to decrease HLA sensitization, protect veins for AV fistula creation, and avoid excessive immunosuppression with repeated rejection therapies that increase malignancy and infection risk. For the patient it is sometimes better to "let the chronically diseased kidney allograft go" in the short term to protect their overall health for the long term and allow them to return to dialysis and later retransplantation. Of course this does not mean to discard a kidney that can be saved. But, if there is marginal kidney allograft function, you should not rely on heroics that might ultimately harm the patient.

There are many more things "not to do", which the reader will appreciate from the chapters in this guide. Hopefully, this introductory list will help the practitioner avoid common pitfalls and develop an overall strategy for the long-term care of the renal transplant recipient.

Chapter 2
The Transplant Procedure: Surgical Techniques and Complications

Barry J. Browne

Renal Transplantation

Introduction

Contrary to the way transplant surgery is portrayed on popular television shows, transplantation in the real world is less glamorous, less exciting, and when done correctly, quite routine. While the success or failure of the surgical procedure rests primarily on the shoulders of the transplant surgeon, the ingredients necessary to create a positive outcome rely on a team of specialists from a variety of fields. Matching the right patient with the right organ is an art developed by years of experience. The decisions involved in offering kidneys to patients, while highly regulated, are influenced greatly by nephrologists, surgeons, transplant coordinators, and social workers. Organ allocation is more fully discussed in Chapter 5.

There are four options for patients who reach end-stage renal disease (ESRD): death, peritoneal dialysis, hemodialysis, and transplantation. It is the responsibility of each nephrologist to discuss these options with each patient so that the correct path is chosen. Although we sometimes tend to look at care options as a single decision, many patients will bounce from modality to modality as their health and outlook change. This reality complicates the surgical care of patients with ESRD since each operation along the pathway from renal failure to eventual death can affect the next operation required.

The simplest surgical pathway involves pre-emptive living donor transplantation (LD). In this scenario, the list of pre-transplant operations is minimized and the operative choices are maximized. The transplant team has the opportunity to "tune up" the patient and best prepare him/her for a safe procedure. The anatomy and the quality of the donor's organ is well known before beginning and a positive outcome, while not assured, is expected. On the other hand, a patient with superior vena cava

B.J. Browne (✉)
Transplant Surgery, Sharp Memorial Hospital, San Diego, CA, USA
e-mail: bbrowne@bnmg.org

D.B. McKay, S.M. Steinberg (eds.), *Kidney Transplantation: A Guide to the Care of Kidney Transplant Recipients*, DOI 10.1007/978-1-4419-1690-7_2, © Springer Science+Business Media, LLC 2010

syndrome who dialyzes through a femoral AV graft being transplanted in the middle of the night with a cadaveric organ (CAD) procured by unknown surgeons in another state presents quite a different set of circumstances and may call for a different approach to have the best chance for success. It is the ability to predict, adapt, and modify both the medical and surgical approach to these complex patients that often separates good surgical outcomes from bad. In this chapter, I will address the most common scenarios encountered in the operating room and explain the surgical approaches that can be used to give the patients their best chance for long-term survival.

History

Alexis Carrel[1] and C.C. Guthrie[2] developed the surgical techniques required for organ transplantation at the turn of the twentieth century. The modern era of renal transplantation began with a series of unsuccessful CAD and LD kidney transplants carried out in Europe,[3-5] which were doomed due to poorly understood immunologic barriers. These obstacles were circumvented in the 1950s through the use of identical twin donors and led to the first successful kidney transplant at the Peter Bent Brigham Hospital in Boston in 1954.[6] Introduction of the antimetabolite azathioprine by Roy Calne[7] and Joseph Murray[8] coupled with the empirical addition of corticosteroids by Goodwin[9] in the early 1960s ushered in the era of widespread clinical transplantation. While surgical techniques have undergone refinement over the years, the basic procedure has changed little over the last 50 years.

Building on Carrel's descriptions of vascular anastomotic techniques Ullman[10] and Unger[11] first described experimental autotransplantation and allotransplantation of kidneys in dogs over 100 years ago. By 1914, technical progress in animal models was so successful that Carrel boasted that little work remained to perfect transplantation techniques.[12] The Ukrainian surgeon, Yu Yu Voronoy, transplanted six patients between 1933[13] and 1946[14] but without a good understanding of immunology, all of the grafts were lost and he abandoned clinical transplantation. Prior to Murray's historic transplant in 1954, the closest anyone came to clinical success was David Hume in 1945. While serving as a surgical resident at the Brigham, he sewed a CAD kidney at bedside to the brachial vessels of a woman with acute post-partum renal failure. Although this brief treatment likely played little role in the patient's recovery and the results were never published, it nonetheless kindled the interest of many surgeons[15] and ultimately led to the creation of the clinical transplant program at the Brigham. The modern technique of placement of the kidney in the pelvis with vascular anastomoses to the iliac vessels and ureteral drainage into the bladder was first described by Kuss.[16] Murray's team modified this procedure slightly by changing from Kuss' intraperitoneal approach to the preperitoneal approach used today for most kidney transplants.[17]

Living Donors

Every effort should be undertaken to identify willing living donors. Not only does this decrease the time that the recipient must wait for an organ, it also converts the procedure from an emergency to an elective basis. As mentioned earlier, the LD facilitates pre-emptive transplantation and eliminates the need for dialysis. There are three medical advantages to the use of LDs: (1) decreased risk of acute tubular necrosis (ATN) due to the shortened cold ischemia time, (2) increased potential for HLA matching, and (3) opportunity to initiate and optimize immunosuppressive therapy pre-operatively, thereby reducing risk of early acute rejection episodes. However, living donor nephrectomy subjects a healthy volunteer to a potentially lethal operation with no physical benefit to the donor. Thus it is the transplant center's responsibility to insure that (a) the physical risks of the procedure are acceptably low and (b) the donor has exerted informed consent of his/her own volition. The evaluation of living donors is described by Dr. Steiner in Chapter 6 while the technical aspects of donor nephrectomy are described by Dr. Martinez in Chapter 8.

Although the functional quality of LD kidneys is generally superior to CAD kidneys, this is no longer universal due to the shift over the last 10 years toward minimally invasive surgery for the donors. While delayed graft function (DGF) was rare in the past, it has become more common since the advent of laparoscopic nephrectomy for a number of reasons. First, the pneumoperitoneum required for laparoscopy decreases renal blood flow. Second, manipulation of the kidney often causes the renal artery to go into spasm. Third, removal of the kidney through a small incision can result in mechanical trauma to the organ. And finally, technical delays in extracting the kidney from the abdomen can result in prolonged warm ischemia time. In the most extensive single center review to date from the University of Maryland, laparoscopic nephrectomy was associated with an increase in DGF and a decrease in long-term outcome.[18] A recent meta-analysis, however, showed no difference in long-term outcome[19], so each center must continuously evaluate its outcomes to assure that transplant strategies are being optimized.

LD kidneys can also present technical problems for the surgeon during implantation. Because the donor's safety is paramount, the lengths of the renal arteries and veins are shorter in kidneys procured from LDs. In patients with multiple renal arteries, backtable reconstruction can be quite challenging and time consuming. In some cases, surgeons have resorted to using recipient saphenous vein grafts in order to simplify transplantation although I have not yet found this to be necessary in my practice.

Cadaver Kidneys

Kidneys from donors between the ages of 1 and 80 years may be acceptable under the right circumstances although special care should be taken at each end of the age spectrum. Following pronouncement of brain death and authorization for organ donation, the care of the donor is transferred to the organ procurement coordinator whose goal is maintenance of adequate renal perfusion up until the time the donor is taken to the operating room. In the early days of transplantation, the procuring team and transplanting team were one and the same. Today, however, it is most common to have different teams procure and implant the organs. Since most CAD procurements involve the removal of extra-renal organs, the kidneys are usually removed by the surgical team responsible for removal of the liver. In situations where kidneys are the only solid organs being procured, the procuring team may consist of transplant surgeons, transplant urologists, or even local surgeons recruited at the last moment to help out.

There are many variables that affect the quality of the organ which ultimately arrives in a sterile container packed in ice. The single most important factor is the baseline condition of the kidneys prior to the event leading to the donor's presentation to the hospital. The old adage that you cannot make a silk purse from a sow's ear is never more true. Older patients presenting with elevated creatinines rarely go on to successful donation. Conversely, young adults with normal creatinines who go on to become donors usually yield high-quality organs, despite transient, reversible events which often occur during the hospitalization in failed attempts to save their lives. Following the declaration of brain death and obtaining consent to donation, the care of the donor is transferred to the organ procurement organization. Its coordinators endeavor to optimize perfusion to the kidneys, liver, and other transplantable organs prior to proceeding into the operating room for procurement.)

Once in the operating room, the surgical team's job is to remove the organs in a timely fashion after they have been flushed with chilled perfusion solution and then package them for distribution. Although there have been many attempts to standardize procurement techniques, every procurement is different. In the situation where the kidneys are the only organs being procured, the operation is straightforward and quick. If extra-renal organs are being procured, the kidneys are always removed last. Unless care is taken to keep ice on the kidneys while the heart, lungs, liver, and pancreas are removed, the quality of the kidneys can be compromised by what effectively becomes warm ischemia time. Additionally, it is not uncommon to receive kidneys obtained during multiorgan procurements with surgical damage to either the renal artery or vein. For this reason, I always examine kidneys sent to me from unknown surgeons before beginning the recipient operation.

Organ Implantation

The operative procedure can be divided into five separate parts: preparation, exposure, vascular anastomoses, ureteral anastomosis, and closing. A schematic representation of the completed implantation is shown in Fig. 2.1.

Preparation

Although regional anesthesia can be used, nearly all patients today undergo general anesthesia. If not begun pre-operatively, this is a good time for the surgeon to discuss

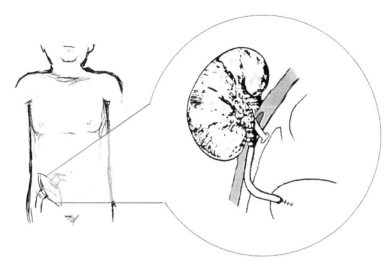

Fig. 2.1 Most common technique of heterotopic renal transplantation. Kidney is lying in the *right* iliac fossa in the retroperitoneal space. Patch of aorta containing renal artery applied directly to side of external iliac artery and external (Lich) ureteroneocystostomy. Venous anastomosis is end renal to side external iliac. Veins are *shaded* while arteries and graft ureter are not

intra-operative management with the anesthetist and prepare for anything special the surgeon might request. I nearly always ask for a central line as this is the most reliable way to assess fluid status and it also simplifies post-operative care. Most patients are given a steroid bolus at this time followed by an induction agent if warranted. I take this opportunity to discuss blood pressure parameters, depth of anesthesia, and other medications that I will ask for later in the operation. I confirm that the peri-operative antibiotic has been given and participate in the mandatory "time out" to assure that we are operating on the correct patient and have the correct kidney in the room. A Foley catheter is placed. Clot retention can complicate post-operative management so it is best to place the largest catheter possible. I prefer to use a 22F catheter unless restricted by a small urethral opening. Antibiotic solution can be instilled into the bladder at this time or just before beginning the ureteral anastomosis. This maneuver facilitates rapid identification of the bladder within the pelvis and in some circumstances gives the surgeon a nudge toward utilizing uretero-ureterostomy when the bladder appears hostile to intra-operative manipulation.

Exposure

After prepping and draping the patient, an incision is made in either the right or left lower quadrant of the abdomen. The site of implantation is chosen based on the degree of peripheral vascular disease. In general, the right iliac fossa is preferred because the external iliac vein tends to have a more superficial and direct course and the sigmoid colon does not interfere with exposure of the bladder. Tissues are divided and the retroperitoneal cavity is converted from a potential space into a workable cavity. The epigastric vessels are divided between ties because attempts to spare them are not uncommonly associated with undetected injury and delayed hemorrhage. In cases of multiple renal arteries, a healthy epigastric artery can be mobilized for later use as one of the inflow conduits. The round ligament may be safely divided in women while the spermatic cord is best retracted medially. Lymphatic tissues overlying the iliac artery and vein are divided between ties in order to reduce the risk of post-operative lymphocele formation. Historically, the preferred inflow vessel was the internal iliac artery because this minimized the risk of ischemia to the ipsilateral leg. Most surgeons today, however, use the external iliac artery because it is easier and safer to dissect. The internal iliac is also more commonly diseased due to an aging recipient population and increased incidence of diabetes. The external iliac vein is nearly always used for venous return. The hypogastric veins can be sacrificed if necessary in order to mobilize the iliac vein and simplify the venous anastomosis. If the iliac vein is absent, thrombosed, or very small, any suitably sized vein in the area can be utilized.

Vascular Anastomoses

In a straightforward operation, the venous anastomosis is usually completed first and the arterial anastomosis done last. This is due to the geometry of the vessels in the pelvis, in that the vein lies posterior to the artery. During this part of the operation, care is taken to keep the kidney chilled and topical ice is used liberally. Once the venous portion of the operation is complete, a small clamp can be placed across the renal vein and the clamps removed from the iliac vein. This releases the venous congestion in the leg and may lessen the risk of deep venous thrombosis. The arterial anastomosis is then rapidly accomplished, being careful to choose a site on the recipient artery as free of plaque as possible because endarterectomy carries the risk of raising a distal flap that may compromise flow to the leg. During the anastomoses, I usually ask the anesthetist to give 12.5 g albumin, 25 g mannitol, and 80 mg furosemide to promote immediate diuresis. Mottling of the graft surface due to arterial spasm is not uncommon, but generally resolves within 30 min as long as there is adequate perfusion pressure. Following reperfusion of the graft, meticulous hemostasis is achieved as manipulation of the kidney becomes more difficult once the ureteral anastomosis is complete. In patients given systemic heparin due to a known hypercoagulable state, protamine can now be safely administered.

Ureteral Anastomosis

Ureteroneocystostomy is the preferred method to establish urologic continuity. Both transvesicle (Politano and Leadbetter[20]) and extra-vesicle (Lich[21]) anastomotic techniques yield excellent results. Although the merits of various techniques will continue to be argued by their evangelical supporters, there does not appear to be any one superior or inferior method. Provided that a ureteral stent is used and an adequate blood supply to the ureter has been preserved, nearly all techniques connecting the ureter to the bladder are successful. A tunneled segment under the detrusor muscle is integral to all techniques as this provides a check-valve mechanism upon voiding and decreases the risk of hydronephrosis. In situations where the bladder capacity is severely diminished or access to the bladder is treacherous due to prior pelvic surgery, uretero-ureterostomy or ureteropylostomy can be performed with acceptable results.

Closing

Closing the wound is sometimes considered an afterthought but long-term problems often occur due to lapses during this step. The first part of closing involves checking for hemostasis. Any residual bleeding left unchecked will slowly dissect out the entire retroperitoneum resulting in a large retroperitoneal hematoma and may require transfusion or re-exploration. Drains are generally ineffective in the retroperitoneum and are not usually required. Prior to closing the abdominal wall, the kidney is sometimes placed in a pocket over the psoas muscle in an attempt to keep the kidney from rotating into a position that might kink the artery or the vein. Interestingly, short veins and long arteries seem to be most prone to kinking. This explains why most surgeons prefer to use the left kidney when given the option. While positioning the kidney prior to closing may reduce the risk of thrombosis, it is probably the relative positioning of the anastomoses that puts some kidneys at risk. The abdominal wall may be closed in layers or en masse. I prefer to use absorbable sutures since the knots from permanent sutures can lead to stitch abscesses or chronic pain, particularly in thin women. Because high-dose steroids are still routinely used during the peri-operative period, close attention should be paid to the skin closure since technical or infectious problems can lead to a prolonged open wound and significant morbidity.

Complications

The most common complication following kidney transplantation is oliguria due to ATN. While nearly all LD kidneys and most CAD organs start making urine in the operating room, up to 30% of transplants result in either DGF requiring dialysis or slow graft function requiring careful fluid management. A kidney is expected to make at least 100 cc/h urine within a few hours after transplantation. If this does not happen, it is critical to determine the cause. The differential diagnosis for post-transplant renal failure follows the same algorithm as any other type of acute renal failure. Pre-renal and post-renal causes must be quickly ruled out before defaulting to a presumptive diagnosis of ATN. A CVP > 10 mmHg combined with mean perfusion pressure of 100 mmHg should result in adequate blood delivery. A color flow Doppler (CFD) or renal scan is obtained to rule out vascular compromise which requires an emergent trip back to the operating room. I prefer CFD because it is usually quicker, cheaper, and can be done in the recovery room. The only advantage of renal scan is the ability to pick up urine leaks, but these are usually of little importance if a ureteral stent and Foley catheter are in place. Clot retention in the bladder obstructing the catheter is the most common cause of post-renal oliguria and can be addressed with gentle irrigation through the Foley catheter.

The most common cause of post-operative oliguria is ATN due to the ischemia–reperfusion. This self-limited insult generally recovers without treatment but can be prolonged by post-operative fluid mismanagement and some commonly used drugs, most notably the immunosuppressant sirolimus. Definitive diagnosis is confirmed by biopsy which most recommend at 1 week if improvement is not seen. Rejection is highly unlikely during the first 48 h after transplant. Hyperacute rejection is usually recognized within minutes after reperfusion leading to immediate graft failure and explantation. Early rejection at 2–3 days post-transplant implies presensitization to the donor while de novo acute cellular rejection requires 4–5 days to become apparent. In each case, aggressive use of percutaneous needle biopsy is generally safe and helps to unravel clinical uncertainties.

Other peri-operative complications are similar to those encountered after vascular surgery in the pelvis – bleeding, infection, hernia, and pain. Nearly all patients develop some degree of perigraft hematoma and some may require transfusion. Reoperation for bleeding is rare and, in my experience, occurs when intra-operative hypotension is followed by post-operative hypertension. Remarkably, wound infection is only a significant problem in obese patients undergoing transplantation. The most common infection following kidney transplantation is urinary tract infection which is readily treated by antibiotics but may require removal of the ureteral stent and Foley catheter to prevent recurrence. Incisional hernia is rarely seen in the early post-operative period but is impressive when it does occur as it can be accompanied by evisceration of both bowel and the transplanted kidney. Rapid return to the operating room is required to prevent vascular compromise to the graft. Pain or numbness along the inner thigh can occur due to inadvertent damage to the ilioinguinal or genitofemoral nerves. These are generally self-limited but may require intervention in some cases. A more serious nerve injury can occur to the femoral nerve due to errant placement of a retractor during the initial operation. This entirely preventable complication can result in transient, and sometimes permanent, leg weakness requiring extensive physical therapy to overcome.

Summary

The demographics of an aging population combined with the end results of a sedentary lifestyle and a poor diet have produced a growing cohort of patients with ESRD. Patients unable to produce living donors are waiting longer and longer for CAD donors just as the number of high-quality CAD donors is decreasing. This has resulted in surgeons pushing the envelope – with more marginal organs being placed in older, more complex recipients. Although conceptually simple, the technical aspects of renal transplantation can be formidable in today's high-risk patients with ESRD. In this chapter, I have described the most common techniques involved in transplantation. In order to be successful today, the transplant surgeon must deal with a plethora of pre-operative, intra-operative, and post-operative challenges which are outside the realm of what can be described in a single chapter. I hope I have provided a taste of what is involved in the operative care of kidney transplantation and refer those wishing to pursue this area further to the excellent multimedia surgical *Atlas of Organ Transplantation.*[22]

References

1. Carrel A. La technique operatoire des anastomoses vasculires, et la transplantation des visceres. *Lyon Med* 1902; 98: 859.
2. Guthrie CC. Blood Vessel Surgery and Its Application. Longmans Green, New York, 1912
3. Kuss R, Teinturier J, Milliez P. Quelques essais de greffe de rein chez l'homme. *Mem Acad Chir* 1951; 77: 755.
4. Servelle M, Soulie P, Rougeulle J et al. La greffe du rein. *Rev Chir* 1951; 70: 186.
5. Dubost C, Oeconomos N, Nenna A, Milliez P. Resultats d'une tentative de greffe renale. *Bull Soc Med Hop Paris* 1951; 67: 1372.
6. Merrill JP, Murray JE, Harrison JH et al. Successful homotransplantation of the human kidney between identical twins. *J Am Med Assoc* 1956; 160: 277.
7. Calne RY, Alexandre GP, Murray JE. A study of the effects of drugs in prolonged survival of homologous renal transplants in dogs. *Ann NY Acad Sci* 1962; 99: 743.
8. Murray JE, Merrill JP, Harrison JH et al. Prolonged survival of human-kidney homografts by immunosuppressive drug therapy. *N Eng J Med* 1963; 268: 1315.
9. Goodwin WE, Mims MM, Kaufmann JJ. Human renal transplantation: III. Technical problems encountered in six cases of kidney homotransplantation. *Trans Am Assoc Genitourin Surg* 1962; 54: 116.
10. Ullman E. Experimentelle Nierentransplantation. *Wien Klin Wochenschr* 1902; 15: 281.
11. Unger E. Nierentransplantation. *Berlin Klin Wochenschr* 1910; 47: 573.
12. Carrel A. The transplantation of organs. *NY Med J* 1914; 99: 839.
13. Voronoy Y. Sobre et bloqueo del aparato reticuloendotelial del hombre en algunas formas de intodicacion por el sublimado y sobre la transplacion del rinon cadaverico como metodo de tratamiento de al unuria consecutiva a aquella intodicacion. *El Siglio Med* 1936; 97: 296.
14. Hamilton DNH, Reid WA. Yu Yu Voronoy and the first human kidney allograft. *Surg Gynecol Obstet* 1984; 159: 289.
15. Murray JE. Les Prix Nobel. The Nobel Foundation, Stockholm, Sweeden, 1990, p. 207
16. Kuss R, Teinturier J, Milliez P. Quelques essais de greffe de rein chez l'homme. *Mem Acad Chir* 1951; 77: 755.
17. Murray JE, Lang S, Miller BJ et al. Prolonged functional survival of renal autografts in the dog. *Surg Gynecol Obstet* 1956; 103: 15.
18. Nogueira JM, Haririan A, Jacobs SC et al. The detrimental effects of poor early graft function after laparoscopic live donor nephrectomy on graft outcomes. *Am J Transplant* 2009; 9(2): 337–347.
19. Nanidis TG, Antcliffe D, Kokkinos C, Borysiewicz CA, Darzi AW, Tekkis PP, Papalois VE. Laparoscopic versus open live donor nephrectomy in renal transplantation: a meta-analysis. *Ann Surg* 2008 Oct; 248(4): 691–692.
20. Politano VA, Leadbetter WF. An operative technique for the correction of vesicoureteral reflux. *J Urol* 1958; 79: 932.
21. Lich R Jr, Howerton LW, Davis LA. Recurrent urosepsis in children. *J Urol* 1961; 86: 554.
22. Humar A, Matas AJ, Payne WD. Atlas of Organ Transplantation. Springer Publishing, New York, 2009

Chapter 3
What Is Transplant Immunology and Why Are Allografts Rejected?

Dianne B. McKay, Ken Park, and David Perkins

Chapter Overview

This chapter focuses on how a transplanted organ is recognized by the recipient's immune system and how an allograft is rejected. It is important to understand fundamentals of immunology in order to better apply immunosuppressive strategies. Understanding how the recipient immune system recognizes the donor organ will also make it apparent to the reader that there are "holes" in our current immunosuppressive therapy. Many basic science laboratories are working to fill the "holes" and new immunosuppressive approaches are likely to be available in the future. While the focus of this chapter is on kidney transplant rejection, basic immunologic mechanisms of rejection are similar between all transplanted organs. Chapter 9 describes the optimal prescription of immunosuppressive medications.

The immunologic events relevant to solid organ transplantation are described in a temporal manner sequentially following the processes of donor harvest, anastomosis of the donor and recipient vessels, and the recipient immune response to the transplanted organ. Long-term immunologic responses that correlate with chronic rejection are also described, as is the concept of immunologic tolerance. Illustrations are provided that correlate with the processes described in the text.

Donor Harvest

The Donor Kidney Is Comprised of Immune Cells That Are Activated by Ischemia

The process of donor harvest involves a highly skilled team of professionals assembled to optimally remove organs from either a deceased or a living donor and pass on

D.B. McKay (✉)
Department of Immunology and Microbial Sciences, The Scripps Research Institute, La Jolla, CA, USA
e-mail: dmckay@scripps.edu

D.B. McKay, S.M. Steinberg (eds.), *Kidney Transplantation: A Guide to the Care of Kidney Transplant Recipients*, DOI 10.1007/978-1-4419-1690-7_3,
© Springer Science+Business Media, LLC 2010

the "gift of life." The harvest team works with vigorous attention to surgical detail (as described in Chapter 2 and 7), a key to subsequent organ function. Another key for excellent graft function involves attention to the immunologic events that initiate during the process of donor kidney harvest and transplantation.

The donor kidney is comprised not only of glomeruli, tubular cells, mesangium, and endothelium but also of resident immune cells such as dendritic cells,[1] as seen in the schematic in Fig. 3.1. Dendritic cells are specialized phagocytes found in the interstitial spaces of most tissues of the body that are easily activated to engulf fragments of damaged tissue and pathogens. Resident dendritic cells are usually dormant, but they acquire phagocytic ability and mobility upon the slightest injury to the kidney, even before the donor organ is transplanted into the recipient.[2,3]

One of the major ways resident dendritic cells become activated is through low blood flow to the kidney. In the case of a deceased donor, brain death plays a major role because it is characterized by rapid swings in blood pressure; an early hypertensive phase is followed by a hypotensive phase.[4] The rapid swings in blood

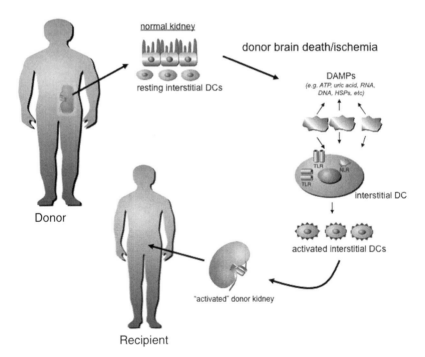

Fig. 3.1 Immunologic events within the donor kidney at the time of donor harvest. In response to ischemia/anoxia, cells within the donor kidney die and spill their intracellular contents into the tissue milieu. Included in the spilled contents are danger-activated molecules (DAMPs). DAMPs activate interstitial resident dendritic cells by binding to innate immune receptors on their cell surface (toll-like receptors, TLRs) or within the cytoplasm (TLRs and non-toll-like receptors, NLRs). By the time the donor kidney is transplanted into the recipient it is highly activated

pressure result from a catecholamine-induced autonomic storm. In animal models, brain death is accompanied by a massive cytokine storm that activates not only immune cells in the kidney but also parenchymal cells such as endothelium and tubular epithelial cells.[5] The donor kidney is thus highly "activated" even before removal of the deceased donor graft. Making the situation worse, the process of removing the kidney, from either a live or a deceased donor, unavoidably involves interruption of the organ's blood supply and frank anoxia of the organ, heightening the "activated" state of the donor organ.

Ischemia/Anoxia-Induced Death of Kidney Cells Results in the Release of Intracellular Contents and Activation of Donor Innate Immune Cells

The immune events associated with transplantation begin with ischemia/anoxia-induced death of donor kidney cells (Fig. 3.1). Ischemic cells spill their intracellular contents into the tissue milieu. The intracellular contents that are released from dead and dying cells contain immunologically active molecules called damage-activated molecular patterns (DAMPs).[6] The name "molecular patterns" refers to the fact that the molecules have structural similarity; it is the common molecular structure that defines the DAMPs. Examples of DAMPs are heat-shock proteins, ATP, uric acid, RNA, DNA, as well as proteins derived from the extracellular matrix including hyaluronan fragments and heparin sulfate proteoglycans.

Epithelial, mesenchymal, and endothelial cells within the donor kidney contain receptors for DAMPs. The DAMP receptors are located either on cell surfaces or within the cytoplasm of most cell types and provide a means for cells to rapidly respond to "danger" in their environment. Several families of these receptors have been identified including toll-like receptors (TLRs) and nucleotide-binding oligomerization domain-like receptors (NLRs).[7-9]

It is important to mention TLRs and NLRs because they are thought to trigger the immune events that cause acute rejection. Ligation of the TLRs or NLRs sets off a biochemical signaling pathway that induces inflammatory signals (cytokines/chemokines), cell death pathways, upregulation of costimulatory molecules, and upregulation of other cellular molecules that trigger cell activation.[10] The inflammatory cytokines and chemokines that are produced from the DAMP/TLR/NLR interactions are very strong attractants for recipient inflammatory cells. Thus, the greater the ischemic damage to the donor organ, the more the DAMP/TLR/NLR signaling, the more inflammatory signals are presented to the recipient at the time of transplantation, and the greater the activation of the recipient's immune system. Precise identification of putative DAMPs and understanding how they are regulated under conditions of ischemia is a major focus of investigation in basic science laboratories and within the pharmaceutical industry. It is likely that blockade of DAMP molecules or their receptors (TLRs and/or NLRs) will provide a significant new direction for preemptive immune suppression.

Over the past few years it has become clear that rejection of a transplanted organ involves not only T cells and B cells but also an entire system of immunologic defense that is rapidly activated and distinguished from cellular acute rejection. This newly identified *Innate Immune System* plays an essential role in the earliest events associated with rejection. Cells of the mammalian innate immune system are exquisitely sensitive to molecules released from injured tissue and microbial products. In the case of a transplanted organ, the innate immune system triggers the adaptive immune system leading to cellular rejection.[11] Our current immunosuppressive medications are targeted to cells of the adaptive immune system. As yet, we have no therapies that specifically target the innate immune system. Table 3.1 shows basic differences between the innate and the adaptive immune systems.

Table 3.1 Innate vs. adaptive immune systems

Components	Innate	Adaptive
Physical components	Skin, mucosa, epithelium (e.g., urinary tract epithelium, respiratory epithelium)	None
Cellular components	Dendritic cells, macrophages, neutrophils, mast cells, natural killer cells	T cells B cells
Activation stimulus	"Nonspecific stimuli" molecules (e.g., DAMPs, PAMPs)	"Specific stimuli" (e.g., alloantigen)
Response Time	**Hours** ⟶	**Days**

Anastomosis of Donor and Recipient Vessels

Activation of the Recipient's Adaptive Immune Response Begins with Anastomosis of the Donor and Recipient Vessels

As soon as the donor and recipient blood vessels are connected, several important things occur. First, the recipient is exposed to a torrent of DAMPs/cytokines/chemokines derived from the ischemic donor organ. In response, the recipient's innate immune cells (such as neutrophils, natural killer cells, and macrophages) vigorously infiltrate the donor tissue and add to the ischemia-induced tissue injury.[12,13] Another thing that happens, almost simultaneously, is that activated donor dendritic cells migrate out of the graft to T-cell-rich regions of recipient lymph nodes where they encounter naive recipient T cells.[14,15] Dendritic cells and T cells are highly motile and, within lymph nodes, interact with each other in a dynamic, hectic, panoply.[16,17] The lymph node is comprised of multiple filaments that provide scaffolding for dendritic cells and T cells and structural stability for their interactions. The encounter between donor dendritic cells and recipient T cells is the key initiating event of cellular rejection. A schematic of these events is shown in Fig. 3.2.

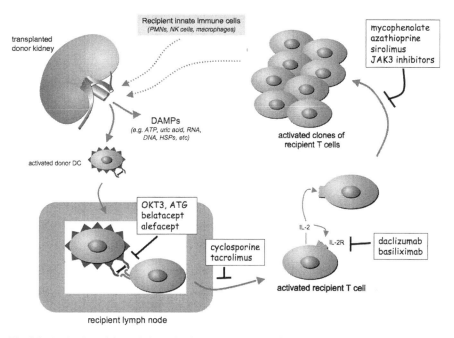

Fig. 3.2 Activation of the recipient adaptive immune system following transplantation. The recipient's immune system is activated rapidly following anastomosis of donor and recipient vessels. As soon as the vessels are connected, DAMPs/cytokines/chemokines as well as activated dendritic cells from the donor organ infuse into the recipient circulation. In response recipient innate immune cells are attracted to the donor organ and vigorously infiltrate the graft, worsening the damage induced by ischemia/anoxia. Donor dendritic cells migrate from the allograft to recipient lymph nodes, where they encounter recipient T cells. Engagement of donor dendritic cells with recipient T cells results in activation of the T cells, leading to their maturation. The activated T cells express IL-2 receptors on their surface and secrete IL-2. IL-2 then acts on the IL-2Rs to cause the T cells to undergo division and produce clones of T cells that participate in the rejection response. The process is blocked at several stages by immunosuppressive medications, as indicated. Corticosteroids act at multiple sites in the cascade as well as on innate immune responses

Interaction of Donor Dendritic Cells with T Cells – How the Recipient Becomes Aware of the Foreign Donor Kidney

Donor dendritic cells and recipient T cells contact each other within lymph nodes. The two cell types engage each other using cell surface receptors – the human leukocyte antigen (HLA) molecule on the dendritic cell and T-cell receptor (TCR) of the T cell. Each of these receptors is a sophisticated molecular complex.

The T-cell receptor (TCR) is comprised of two chains (an alpha chain and a beta chain) and several associated molecules called the CD3 chains.[18] The CD3 chains are the target for OKT3, an antibody that has been used in the past to prevent rejection and to treat severe episodes of rejection.

The HLA molecules are highly polymorphic, allowing presentation of a diverse number of "foreign" peptides. The foreign peptides are derived from the allograft. Each cell simultaneously expresses many different HLA molecule/foreign peptide complexes, which provide great complexity to the system. As described in Chapter 4, two kinds of HLA molecules are important in transplantation, HLA class I and class II molecules. HLA class I molecules can be found on all nucleated cells in the body, whereas HLA class II molecules are found on antigen-presenting cells (such as dendritic cells, macrophages, B cells, endothelial cells, and even some epithelial cells).

Foreign proteins can be presented by HLA molecules to either CD4 T cells or CD8 T cells. If the foreign protein is adjoined to HLA class II molecules it will be presented to CD4 T cells. On the other hand, if adjoined to HLA class I molecules, it will be presented to CD8 T cells. Both CD4 and CD8 T cells participate in the rejection process. The T cells discriminate between "self" (antigens of the recipient) and "nonself" (antigens of the donor) based on the "foreignness" of the HLA/peptide complex that is presented to them.[19]

Recipient Immune Response to Transplanted Organ

Formation of the Immunologic Synapse – Target of Costimulatory and Adhesion Molecule Blockers (Belatacept and Alefacept)

As soon as the dendritic cell HLA/peptide complex engages the T-cell receptor, several cell surface molecules coalesce at the junction between the two cell types and form what is called an "immunologic synapse"[20] (shown schematically in Fig. 3.3). Included in the synapse are the juxtaposed T cell (TCR and associated CD3 molecules) and dendritic cell (HLA/peptide complex). Additional molecules coalesce in the synapse, including costimulatory and adhesion molecules. These molecules bind with their complementary ligand (one on the T cell and one on the dendritic cell) and provide important "go" signals to the T cell. The immunologic synapse needs to be formed in order for the T cell to receive the proper combination of activation signals.

Within minutes of immunologic synapse assembly, profound biochemical signaling events are initiated within the T cell.[21] The biochemical events are "tuned" by the length of time the T cell stays in contact with the HLA/peptide complex. If a greater disparity exists between the HLA molecules of the donor and the HLA molecules of the recipient (e.g., a complete HLA mismatch between the donor and the recipient) then the cells stay in contact for a longer period of time. This longer contact time results in more robust signaling within the T cell. Two new immunosuppressive agents in clinical trials in transplant recipients are aimed at disrupting the normal signaling events that occur with this contact – belatacept (CTLA$_4$Ig fusion protein)[22,23] and alefacept (anti-CD2 antibody).[24]

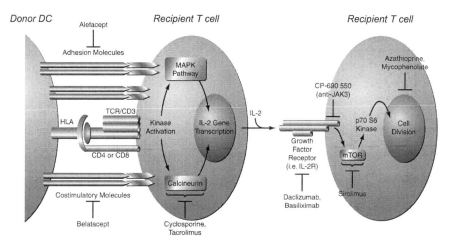

Fig. 3.3 T-cell signaling events that occur upon engagement of the donor dendritic cells. Upon donor dendritic cell/recipient T-cell engagement the immunologic synapse is formed, which consists of donor HLA molecules, recipient TCR and CD4 or CD8 molecules, costimulatory molecules, and adhesion molecules. Following immunologic synapse formation, the T cell is activated through two intracellular signaling pathways. One pathway leads to activation of calcineurin and the other to activation of mitogen-activated protein kinases (MAPKs). The end result is IL-2 gene transcription. Cyclosporine and tacrolimus block one limb of the activation, the calcineurin pathway. The MAPK pathway is not completely blocked by either cyclosporine or tacrolimus and therefore T-cell signaling still occurs. IL-2 acts on IL-2R on T cells causing the activation of mTOR, allowing the cell to progress through the cell cycle, ultimately promoting cell division. Sirolimus blocks mTOR, thereby interfering with cell division

T-Cell Receptor-Mediated Signaling Events – Target of Calcineurin Inhibitors (Cyclosporine and Tacrolimus)

Within seconds of immunological synapse assembly, several molecules are brought into close proximity on the surface of the T cell. This "closeness" results in the activation of cytoplasmic enzymes called kinases that transfer phosphate groups between adjacent molecules. The transfer of phosphate groups sets off a chain reaction that results in the sequential activation of molecules within the cytoplasm of the T cell.[25] The activated cytoplasmic molecules comprise defined molecular cascades that lead to transmission of the signal from the cell surface to the nucleus. Once the signal reaches the nucleus, genes are transcribed that lead to the secretion of cytokines, such as interleukin 2, and trigger entry of the T cell into cell cycle, causing it to divide. The T cell that divides in response to the donor DC is highly specific to the donor HLA/peptide complex, and so when the T cell divides it produces clones of T cells with specificity to the donor DC peptide. Current immunosuppressive strategies are designed to block the biochemical events in T cells before this stage. Failure to block this stage is akin to allowing the formation of massive numbers of ballistic missiles directed to a unified target. Once the button is pushed, it is very hard to stop the destructive salvo.

Several immunosuppressive medications have been developed that target early stages of T-cell activation (Fig. 3.2). Most potent are the calcineurin inhibitors, cyclosporine and tacrolimus.[26] These molecules bind to a carrier protein that is present in many tissues and therefore calcineurin inhibitors affect not only T cells but also many other cells in the body. Cyclosporine binds to cytoplasmic carrier proteins called cyclophilins and tacrolimus binds to cytoplasmic FK-binding proteins (FKBPs). There are several isoforms of both cyclophilins and FKBPs; their relative amounts vary between tissues and account for the tissue-specific toxicities. The relative toxicities and efficacy of these two types of calcineurin inhibitors are discussed in Chapter 9. A new strategy is to target protein kinase C isoforms with small molecule inhibitors. AEB071 or sotrastaurin is one such PKC inhibitor in clinical trials in renal transplant recipients.

T-Cell Activation: Cytokine Production – Target of Anti-IL-2 Receptor Blockers [Daclizumab (Zenapax®) and Basiliximab (Simulect®)] and the JAK3 Inhibitor CP-690 550

Once the T cell is activated through the T-cell receptor it manufacturers and secretes cytokines, such as interleukin 2 (IL-2) (Fig. 3.3). Once secreted, the cytokines act on receptors that are present on their own T cells (autocrine stimulation) as well as other T cells (paracrine stimulation). Interleukin-2 is a prototype for the cytokine-induced signaling of T cells. After secretion, IL-2 binds to a receptor (called the IL-2R) on the surface of T cells and activates three different cytoplasmic signaling cascades: the mitogen-activated protein (MAP) kinase pathway, the phosphoinositide 3-kinase (PI3K) pathway, and the Janus kinase/signal transducers and activators of transcription protein pathway (JAK/STAT).[27] These three pathways regulate various functions of the cells, such as gene transcription, cell division, cell survival, and cell death. A pharmacologic approach to inhibiting one limb of this pathway (the JAK/STAT pathway) is currently in clinical trials in transplantation using the JAK3 inhibitor CP-690 550.[24] Another strategy to block the cytokine signaling pathway has been to prevent the cytokine (IL-2) from interacting with its receptor. Two monoclonal antibodies have been widely used for this purpose – daclizumab and basiliximab.[28]

T-Cell Division: Target of Azathioprine, Mycophenolate, and Sirolimus

Once the T cell receives a "go" signal, through cytokine receptor-mediated signaling, it begins to make the proteins needed to undergo DNA replication. The biochemical signaling events that culminate in cell cycle progression are complex and are induced by many different signals besides IL-2. One of the steps common to many of the stimuli that induce the T cell to divide is a molecule called mTOR (mammalian target of rapamycin). This molecule is blocked by sirolimus, which is a potent immunosuppressive medication now commonly used for maintenance immunosuppression.[29] Sirolimus binds to a cytoplasmic carrier protein called FKBP12 that is similar to the carrier protein for FK506 (tacrolimus) and is also present in many cell types. Since blockade of cell cycling is so potent, several other mTOR inhibitors have been developed and are either approved for therapeutic use or are currently in clinical studies, including Everolimus, Temsirolimus, and Zotarolimus. Temsirolimus is used for treatment of renal cell carcinoma,[30] while the others are approved for organ transplant rejection and coronary artery restenosis. Since cell division is so dependent on mTOR, the use of mTOR inhibitors in pregnant women is probably contraindicated due to concerns regarding their effect on the developing fetus.[31]

Azathioprine and mycophenolate mofetil also target the cell cycle, but at a later stage than sirolimus.[32] Azathioprine is a purine synthesis inhibitor. Purines are biochemically significant components of RNA, DNA, ATP, GTP, AMP, NADH, and coenzyme A. Mycophenolic acid is available as the prodrug mycophenolate mofetil (CellCept) or mycophenolate sodium (Myfortic). The way that mycophenolate works is that it inhibits inosine monophosphate dehydrogenase, the enzyme that controls the rate of synthesis of guanine monophosphate, a nucleotide important to synthesis of RNA. Since azathioprine and mycophenolate mofetil effectively block cell division, they have been a mainstay of maintenance immunosuppressive regimens for many years.

Corticosteroids also have several anti-inflammatory effects and therefore it is difficult to attribute a single effect to their efficacy. Steroids affect both innate and adaptive immune responses by altering the trafficking of neutrophils, decreasing phagocytosis by macrophages and dendritic cells, and directly affecting T-cell proliferation, activation, and differentiation.[33] Therefore, withdrawal of steroids might be risky because steroids play such an important role in suppressing multiple limbs of the immune response.

Effectors of Rejection – The Adaptive Immune System

The traditional cells that we associate with acute rejection (T cells and B cells) are part of the *Adaptive Immune System*, and to clarify nomenclature they will be described below.

T cells

T cells are white blood cells produced in the thymus (thus the designation "T") that divide rapidly and play a primary role in the cellular immune response seen in acute cellular rejection. T cells have a specialized cell surface receptor that is a highly sophisticated molecular complex called the T-cell receptor (TCR).

There are different types of T cells, such as T helper cells (also called CD4 T cells), T cytotoxic cells (also called CD8 T cells), memory T cells, and gamma delta T cells. The CD4 or CD8 molecules are coreceptor molecules that strengthen the contact between CD4 T cells with HLA class II molecules or CD8 T cells with HLA class I molecules. HLA molecules are discussed briefly above and also in Chapter 4. The following is a brief description of the basic types of T cells:

T helper cells: T helper cells (CD4 T cells) rapidly divide upon exposure to foreign proteins into various subsets (Th1, Th2, Th3, Th17, ThF) that secrete different cytokines.[34] Cytokines are messengers of the immune response and, in the case of graft rejection, they function to recruit the army of recipient immune cells aimed at destruction of the foreign allograft.

Cytotoxic T cells: Cytotoxic T cells (CD8 T cells) also divide rapidly upon exposure to foreign proteins. When activated, cytotoxic T cells directly destroy target cells by releasing cytotoxins such as perforin and granzyme. Perforins form pores in the target cell membranes and granzymes enter the target cell and destroy the cell from within.[35] Cytotoxic T cells play a role in graft rejection as well as destruction of virally infected tissue.

Memory T cells: Memory T cells are either helper T cells or cytotoxic T cells and they respond rapidly to foreign antigens. Whether memory T cells differentiate linearly or in parallel with the helper and cytotoxic T cells is not yet known. Nevertheless, memory T cells survive in an inactive state in the host for long periods of time after the initial exposure to foreign antigen. If the host is reexposed to the same foreign proteins, memory T cells will quickly expand and mount an aggressive response. This phenomenon is the basis for immunologic memory and it is the reason that prior exposure to transplanted organs or multiple blood transfusions (which also exposes the recipient T cells to foreign antigen) results in an enhanced immune response that is difficult to control.[36]

Regulatory T cells: Regulatory T cells are also seen in the helper and cytotoxic T cell lineages and they play an important role in the immune response to a transplanted organ. Formerly known as suppressor T cells, these specialized T cells function to shut down cell-mediated immunity toward the end of an immune response.[37] Experimental strategies in rodents have shown that expanding regulatory T cells during the rejection response can control allograft rejection, although reliable clinical strategies in humans to expand regulatory T cells are not yet available.[38]

Gamma delta T cells: Gamma delta T cells are a specialized type of T cell, with a unique type of T-cell receptor that does not play a direct role in graft rejection. These cells are found in the gut mucosa and skin and are important for wound healing.[39] Their effective suppression by sirolimus might be a reason that there is a high incidence of wound healing defects with the use of sirolimus.[40]

B Cells

B cells are another type of leukocyte, which produces antibodies in response to foreign proteins. B cells are formed in the bone marrow and play a primary role in the humoral immune response. The primary role of B cells is to produce antibodies in response to antigens, to act as antigen-presenting cells, and to develop into memory B cells. Like T cells, B cells have a functional cell surface receptor (called the B-cell receptor, or BCR) that allows them to "recognize" foreign antigens.[41] Unlike T cells they do not have to have the antigen "presented" to them in a processed form, but rather they can recognize foreign antigens in a soluble form in the blood or lymph. To become fully functional B cells need signals from T helper cells that direct them to either become a plasma cell capable of producing antibodies or a memory cell capable of a vigorous response upon re-exposure to foreign antigens.[41]

Donor-Specific Antibodies (DSAs)

Plasma cells can produce antibodies against HLA antigens and nonHLA antigens that may or may not be specific to the donor [endothelial antigens such as MHC class I polypeptide-related sequence A or B (MICA and MICB) antigens, smooth muscle cell antigens such as vimentin, and cell surface receptors such as the type 1 angiotensin II receptor (AT1R)].[42–45] It is difficult to detect these antibodies before transplantation as they often develop against antigens that are only expressed with tissue injury. DSAs are now measured in the clinic to detect reactivity of the recipient B cells against the donor antigens. If the titer of specific DSAs rises, it suggests inadequate immunosuppression and several therapeutic options, including plasmaphaersis, thymogoblulin, intravenous immune globulin (IVIG), and anti-CD20 antibody (rixtuximab), can be attempted.[46] Emerging therapies include proteosome inhibitors such as bortezomib.[47,48] It is important to address donor-specific antibodies because antibody deposition results in complement fixation, which triggers lysis of donor kidney cells through the membrane attack complex as well as by NK cells and macrophages. Several studies have suggested that antibodies to recipient HLA antigens and to endothelial antigens may be a driver of not only acute antibody-mediated rejection (AMR) but also chronic rejection.[49,50]

Acute Cellular vs. Humoral Rejection

Older concepts of acute rejection have considered T cells to be responsible for acute cellular rejection and B cells responsible for humoral rejection, but this is a simplistic view as both cell types as well as cells (e.g., neutrophils, NK cells, macrophages, and dendritic cells) and molecules (e.g., DAMPs) of the innate immune system harmonize in a unified quest to reject the foreign tissue. The pathologic features of acute cellular and humoral rejection are discussed in Chapter 12.

After Transplantation: The Later Phase Months to Years Later

Chronic Allograft Dysfunction, Chronic Allograft Nephropathy

All allografts are eventually lost to a process that involves variable contributions from immunologic and nonimmunologic factors. Several theories have evolved to explain the immunology of chronic allograft dysfunction/nephropathy.[51] One theory is that there is an insidious recipient immune response to the antigens of the donor, manifest as a slow decline in allograft function over time. The immunologic response can come from recipient dendritic cells engulfing and processing donor peptides and presenting these to recipient T cells (indirect presentation), from chronic recipient B-cell activation (producing antidonor-specific antibodies), as well as by endothelial activation and vascular fibrosis. Additional contributions likely come from direct medication toxicities (e.g., calcineurin inhibitors) or chronic viral infections (e.g., BK virus). Clinical data have clearly shown that we have not yet solved the problem of chronic rejection. Whether chronic immune activation plays a major role is unknown at this time. Several pharmacologic strategies have been employed, including minimization of calcineurin inhibitors and use of alternative medications such as sirolimus, in lieu of calcineurin inhibitors.

The Concept of Immunological Tolerance

The goal of tolerance is the holy grail of transplantation. Tolerance is strictly defined as immunologic unresponsiveness to a particular antigen, while retaining the ability to respond to another antigen. Immunologic tolerance is demonstrated by immunologic unresponsiveness to a transplanted organ of one donor, followed by adequate immunologic responses to a second genetically unrelated donor. Usually the test of "true tolerance" involves transplantation of second graft from the original donor and a third-party graft onto the recipient to demonstrate that the second graft is not rejected, while the third-party graft is rejected. Tolerance is obviously difficult to test for in humans, but it has been achieved and validated in animal models. At this time there are no clinically acceptable methods to induce acceptance of the donor graft by the recipient without the continued use of immunosuppressive medications. Two clinical studies have suggested that the recipient's immune system can be taught to accept the transplanted organ as its own using extensive initial induction therapy and a bone marrow transplant.[52,53]

At this time, tolerance has not yet been reliably achieved clinically and therefore it is important to maintain adequate immunosuppression. Even a brief lapse in immunosuppressive medication dosing allows the recipient's immune response to become active and to respond again to donor antigens. The donor antigens do not change, they are always there, and the recipient's immune response always needs to be suppressed to prevent a reaction to the antigens (see the discussion of nonadherence in Chapter 22). The recipients' immune response will never accept the allograft as its own and there will forever be a simmering battle that can easily expand when there is a lapse in immunosuppressive medications.

References

1. Soos TJ, Sims TN, Barisoni L, Lin K, Littman DR, Dustin ML, Nelson PJ. CX(3)CR1(+) interstitial dendritic cells form a contiguous network throughout the entire kidney. *Kidney Int* 2006; 70:591–596.
2. Randolph GJ. Dendritic cell migration to lymph nodes: cytokines, chemokines, and lipid mediators. *Semin Immunol* 2001; 13:267–274.
3. John R, Nelson PJ. Dendritic cells in the kidney. *J Am Soc Nephrol* 2007; 18:2628–2635.
4. van Der Hoeven JA, Ter Horst GJ, Molema G, de Vos P, Girbes AR, Postema F, Freund RL, Wiersema J, van Schilfgaarde R, Ploeg RJ. Effects of brain death and hemodynamic status on function and immunologic activation of the potential donor liver in the rat. *Ann Surg* 2000; 232:804–813.
5. Kusaka M, Pratschke J, Wilhelm MJ, Ziai F, Zandi-Nejad K, Mackenzie HS, Hancock WW, Tilney NL. Early and late inflammatory changes occurring in rat renal isografts from brain dead donors. *Transplant Proc* 2001; 33:867–868.
6. Bianchi ME. DAMPs, PAMPs and alarmins: all we need to know about danger. *J Leukoc Biol* 2007; 81:1–5.
7. Beutler B, Hoffmann J. Innate immunity. *Curr Opin Immunol* 2004; 16:1–3.
8. Ting JP, Lovering RC, Alnemri ES, Bertin J, Boss JM, Davis BK, Flavell RA, Girardin SE, Godzik A, Harton JA, Hoffman HM, Hugot JP, Inohara N, Mackenzie A, Maltais LJ, Nunez G, Ogura Y, Otten LA, Philpott D, Reed JC, Reith W, Schreiber S, Steimle V, Ward PA. The NLR gene family: a standard nomenclature. *Immunity* 2008; 28:285–287.
9. Rosenstiel P, Till A, Schreiber S. NOD-like receptors and human diseases. *Microbes Infect* 2007; 9:648–657.
10. Kawai T, Akira S. The roles of TLRs, RLRs and NLRs in pathogen recognition. *Int Immunol* 2009; 21:317–337.
11. Land WG. Injury to allografts: innate immune pathways to acute and chronic rejection. *Saudi J Kidney Dis Transpl* 2005; 16:520–539.
12. Kinsey GR, Li L, Okusa MD. Inflammation in acute kidney injury. *Nephron Exp Nephrol* 2008; 109:e102–e107.
13. Kim BS, Lim SW, Li C, Kim JS, Sun BK, Ahn KO, Han SW, Kim J, Yang CW. Ischemia-reperfusion injury activates innate immunity in rat kidneys. *Transplantation* 2005; 79: 1370–1377.
14. Austyn JM, Larsen CP. Migration pattern of dendritic leukocytes: implications for transplantation. *Transplantation* 1990; 49:1–7.
15. Jenkins MK, Khoruts A, Ingulli E, Mueller DL, McSorley SJ, Reinhardt RL, Itano A, Pape KA. In vivo activation of antigen-specific CD4 T cells. *Annu Rev Immunol* 2001; 19: 23–45.
16. Negulescu PA, Krasieva TB, Khan A, Kerschbaum HH, Cahalan MD. Polarity of T cell shape, motility and sensitivity to antigen. *Immunity* 1996; 4:421–430.
17. Wei SH, Miller MJ, Cahalan MD, Parker I. Two-photon imaging in intact lymphoid tissue. *Adv Exp Med Biol* 2002; 512:203–208.

18. Blackman M, Kappler J, Marrack P. The role of the T cell receptor in positive and negative selection of developing T cells. *Science* 1990; 248:1335–1341.
19. Cohn M. The common sense of the self-nonself discrimination. *Springer Semin Immunopathol* 2005; 27:3–17.
20. Bromley SK, Burack WR, Johnson KG, Somersalo K, Sims TN, Sumen C, Davis MM, Shaw AS, Allen PM, Dustin ML. The immunological synapse. *Annu Rev Immunol* 2001; 19: 375–396.
21. Grakoui A, Bromley SK, Sumen C, Davis MM, Shaw AS, Allen PM, Dustin ML. The immunological synapse: a molecular machine controlling T cell activation. *Science* 1999; 285:221–227.
22. Emamaullee J, Toso C, Merani S, Shapiro AM. Costimulatory blockade with belatacept in clinical and experimental transplantation – a review. *Expert Opin Biol Ther* 2009; 9:789–796.
23. Latek R, Fleener C, Lamian V, Kulbokas E 3rd, Davis PM, Suchard SJ, Curran M, Vincenti F, Townsend R. Assessment of belatacept-mediated costimulation blockade through evaluation of CD80/86-receptor saturation. *Transplantation* 2009; 87:926–933.
24. Vincenti F, Kirk AD. What's next in the pipeline. *Am J Transplant* 2008; 8:1972–1981.
25. Smith-Garvin JE, Koretzky GA, Jordan MS. T cell activation. *Annu Rev Immunol* 2009; 27:591–619.
26. Schreiber SL, Crabtree GR. The mechanism of action of cyclosporin A and FK506. *Immunol Today* 1992; 13:136–142.
27. Taniguchi T, Minami Y. The IL-2/IL-2 receptor system: a current overview. *Cell* 1993; 73:5–8.
28. Vincenti F, de Andres A, Becker T, Choukroun G, Cole E, Gonzalez-Posada JM, Kumar MA, Moore R, Nadalin S, Nashan B, Rostaing L, Saito K, Yoshimura N. Interleukin-2 receptor antagonist induction in modern immunosuppression regimens for renal transplant recipients. *Transpl Int* 2006; 19:446–457.
29. Sehgal SN. Rapamune (Sirolimus, rapamycin): an overview and mechanism of action. *Ther Drug Monit* 1995; 17:660–665.
30. Kapoor A, Figlin RA. Targeted inhibition of mammalian target of rapamycin for the treatment of advanced renal cell carcinoma. *Cancer* 2009; 115(16):3618–3630.
31. McKay DB, Josephson MA. Pregnancy in recipients of solid organs – effects on mother and child. *N Engl J Med* 2006; 354:1281–1293.
32. Suthanthiran M, Morris RE, Strom TB. Immunosuppressants: cellular and molecular mechanisms of action. *Am J Kidney Dis* 1996; 28:159–172.
33. Perretti M, D'Acquisto F. Annexin A1 and glucocorticoids as effectors of the resolution of inflammation. *Nat Rev Immunol* 2009; 9:62–70.
34. Boniface K, Blom B, Liu YJ, de Waal Malefyt R. From interleukin-23 to T-helper 17 cells: human T-helper cell differentiation revisited. *Immunol Rev* 2008; 226:132–146.
35. Clayberger C. Cytolytic molecules in rejection. *Curr Opin Organ Transplant* 2009; 14:30–33.
36. Woodland DL. Immunologic memory. *Viral Immunol* 2007; 20:229–230.
37. Feng G, Chan T, Wood KJ, Bushell A. Donor reactive regulatory T cells. *Curr Opin Organ Transplant* 2009; 14(4):432–438.
38. Khattar M, Chen W, Stepkowski SM. Expanding and converting regulatory T cells: a horizon for immunotherapy. *Arch Immunol Ther Exp (Warsz)* 2009; 57(3):199–204.
39. Hayday AC. [gamma][delta] cells: a right time and a right place for a conserved third way of protection. *Annu Rev Immunol* 2000; 18:975–1026.
40. Mills RE, Taylor KR, Podshivalova K, McKay DB, Jameson JM. Defects in skin gamma delta T cell function contribute to delayed wound repair in rapamycin-treated mice. *J Immunol* 2008; 181:3974–3983.
41. Parker DC. T cell-dependent B cell activation. *Annu Rev Immunol* 1993; 11:331–360.
42. Tinckam KJ, Chandraker A. Mechanisms and role of HLA and non-HLA alloantibodies. *Clin J Am Soc Nephrol* 2006; 1:404–414.
43. Stastny P, Zou Y, Fan Y, Qin Z, Lavingia B. The emerging issue of MICA antibodies: antibodies to MICA and other antigens of endothelial cells. *Contrib Nephrol* 2009; 162:99–106.

44. Briggs D, Zehnder D, Higgins RM. Development of non-donor-specific HLA antibodies after kidney transplantation: frequency and clinical implications. *Contrib Nephrol* 2009; 162: 107–116.
45. Ansari MJ, Tinckam K, Chandraker A. Angiotensin II type 1-receptor activating antibodies in renal-allograft rejection. *N Engl J Med* 2005; 352:2027–2028; author reply 2027–2028.
46. Vo AA, Lukovsky M, Toyoda M, Wang J, Reinsmoen NL, Lai CH, Peng A, Villicana R, Jordan SC. Rituximab and intravenous immune globulin for desensitization during renal transplantation. *N Engl J Med* 2008; 359:242–251.
47. Trivedi HL, Terasaki PI, Feroz A, Everly MJ, Vanikar AV, Shankar V, Trivedi VB, Kaneku H, Idica AK, Modi PR, Khemchandani SI, Dave SD. Abrogation of anti-HLA antibodies via proteasome inhibition. *Transplantation* 2009; 87:1555–1561.
48. Everly MJ, Everly JJ, Susskind B, Brailey P, Arend LJ, Alloway RR, Roy-Chaudhury P, Govil A, Mogilishetty G, Rike AH, Cardi M, Wadih G, Brown E, Tevar A, Woodle ES. Proteasome inhibition reduces donor-specific antibody levels. *Transplant Proc* 2009; 41:105–107.
49. Piazza A, Poggi E, Ozzella G, Borrelli L, Scornajenghi A, Iaria G, Tisone G, Adorno D. Post-transplant donor-specific antibody production and graft outcome in kidney transplantation: results of sixteen-year monitoring by flow cytometry. *Clin Transpl* 2006; 323–336.
50. Lachmann N, Terasaki PI, Schonemann C. Donor-specific HLA antibodies in chronic renal allograft rejection: a prospective trial with a four-year follow-up. *Clin Transpl* 2006; 171–199.
51. Nankivell BJ, Chapman JR. Chronic allograft nephropathy: current concepts and future directions. *Transplantation* 2006; 81:643–654.
52. Scandling JD, Busque S, Dejbakhsh-Jones S, Benike C, Millan MT, Shizuru JA, Hoppe RT, Lowsky R, Engleman EG, Strober S. Tolerance and chimerism after renal and hematopoietic-cell transplantation. *N Engl J Med* 2008; 358:362–368.
53. Kawai T, Cosimi AB, Spitzer TR, Tolkoff-Rubin N, Suthanthiran M, Saidman SL, Shaffer J, Preffer FI, Ding R, Sharma V, Fishman JA, Dey B, Ko DS, Hertl M, Goes NB, Wong W, Williams WW Jr, Colvin RB, Sykes M, Sachs DH. HLA-mismatched renal transplantation without maintenance immunosuppression. *N Engl J Med* 2008; 358:353–361.

Chapter 4
What Is Histocompatibility Testing and How Is It Done?

Edgar L. Milford and Indira Guleria

Introduction

The purpose of immunogenetic testing in kidney transplantation is to minimize post-transplant acute rejection episodes and to decrease the intensity of chronic rejection. To the degree that the kidney donor is mismatched with the recipient there will be an increased number of targets for both the cellular and humoral immune responses. To the degree that the recipient has been sensitized against donor antigens, there will be greater risk for rejection episodes. This chapter is an exposition of what histocompatibility testing is and how it is done.

HLA Antigens

The predominant antigens that form the targets for the immune response in the context of kidney transplantation are the "HLA" antigens. Homologous antigen systems are found in vertebrate species including mouse (H-2), rat (RT1), dog (DLA), and swine (SLA) where they also are the major targets of the transplant immune response. Because of the dominant role they play in rejection, the HLA antigens are also called "major histocompatibility antigens" or MHC antigens.

Genetics of the HLA Region

Human major histocompatibility antigens (MHC, HLA) are encoded by a number of loci within a short span on the short arm of human chromosome 6. Some of these loci are monomorphic or have limited polymorphism, while other loci contain a large number of allelic variants within the population, which in turn lead to a host

E.L. Milford (✉)
Renal Division, Tissue Typing Laboratory, Department of Medicine, Harvard Medical School,
Brigham and Women's Hospital, Boston, MA, USA
e-mail: emilford@rics.bwh.harvard.edu

D.B. McKay, S.M. Steinberg (eds.), *Kidney Transplantation: A Guide to the Care of Kidney Transplant Recipients*, DOI 10.1007/978-1-4419-1690-7_4,
© Springer Science+Business Media, LLC 2010

of different expressed HLA variants at the protein level. The HLA genetic loci are named with the prefix "HLA" followed by "-" and then an alphanumeric designator for the specific locus whose letter code indicates the class of HLA gene to which the locus belongs. Specific genetic variants, or alleles, at a particular locus are named according to World Health Organization convention by placing an asterisk after the locus name and then a unique numeric designator for the allele. There are alphabetic suffixes added to some alleles to indicate if they are variants that do not cause a change in amino acid sequence or if they are "null alleles" that are not expressed.[1] The HLA genes are among the most polymorphic loci known in vertebrates. Much of the polymorphism is concentrated within short sequences of nucleotides in exons of the HLA genes that encode protein domains that are most distal from the cell and which play an antigen presentation role. Many of the alleles appear to be a consequence of intragenic recombination of "cassettes" or short, highly variable DNA sequences which are shared with other alleles.

Classes of HLA: Class I

HLA genes and antigens fall into two classes based on DNA, protein, and structural homology. These are designated "class I" and "class II" (Fig. 4.1). The class I HLA genes encode molecules that consist of a single polypeptide chain. The class I molecule is anchored in the cell membrane with a short intracytoplasmic tail and has three extracellular domains. The two most distal domains of the molecule form opposing helices which form a "groove" that can noncovalently bind a variety of peptides and constitutes a target for T-cell recognition. The extracellular domains

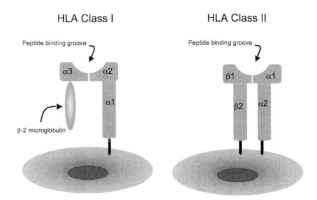

Fig. 4.1 Structure of class I and class II MHC proteins. *HLA class I*: (1) α1, α2, and α3 domains of heavy chain (α1 and α2 form peptide-binding groove; amino acid differences account for polymorphism and antigen specificity); (2) β2 – microglobulin (invariant but essential). *HLA class II*: (1) Composed of one α and one β chain; (2) α1 and β1 domains comprise the peptide-binding site. Again, amino acid differences account for polymorphism and antigen specificity. α2 and β2 domains are constant

of the HLA class I molecules are stabilized by noncovalent interaction with beta-2 microglobulin. Class I molecules are codominantly expressed, that is, both maternal and paternal inherited copies of a given HLA class I locus are expressed on the same cell. The HLA-A, HLA-B, and HLA-C gene products are ubiquitously expressed on all nucleated cells in the body as well as platelets.

Classes of HLA: Class II

Class II HLA genes share some structural features with class I, but also have some fundamentally different properties. Class II genes encode heterodimer proteins on the cell surface, unlike class I genes that contain just one MHC encoded chain. The molecules which are expressed products of the class II genes, and which play a role in kidney transplantation, are called HLA-DR and HLA-DQ. The class II antigens also have opposing helices in the distal-most domains, but two different chains that are noncovalently associated with each other, the alpha chain and the beta chain, encode these helices. Each class II molecule has both an alpha and a beta chain encoded by a different class II locus (Fig. 4.1). For HLA-DR, the alpha chain is monomorphic and is encoded by a gene designated HLA-DRA. The DR beta chain is encoded by a HLA-DRB locus. There is added complexity in that different inherited haplotypes can contain more than one HLA-DRB locus. All haplotypes contain the HLA-DRB1 locus, which encodes most of the more important HLA-DR antigens for kidney transplantation. The HLA-DRB3 and HLA-DRB4 loci encode beta chains which pair with the same monomorphic alpha chain encoded by HLA-DRA, forming a second DR molecule inherited on a single parental haplotype. Yet another set of class II molecules are encoded by the HLA-DQ genes. They too are alpha–beta heterodimers; however, in the case of HLA-DQ, both the HLA-DQA1 and HLA-DQB1 loci are polymorphic in contrast to the monomorphic HLA-DRA locus and its product. Class II molecules (HLA-DR and HLA-DQ) are expressed on a limited subset of lymphoid and non-lymphoid tissues. Class II is highly expressed on B lymphocytes, dendritic cells, monocytes, and macrophages. It has lower expression on endothelial cells and renal proximal tubular cells. Resting T lymphocytes have no class II antigen; however, some class II can be induced with T-cell activation.

Role of HLA Molecules in Normal Immunity

Although HLA antigens form robust targets for kidney transplant rejection, the role for these proteins in the natural setting is to present antigenic peptides from exogenous pathogens or neoantigens from tumors to the immune system so that the cells that harbor them can be destroyed. "Foreign" proteins are broken down into peptides within cells. Those peptides can then bind to the grooves of the HLA class I or HLA class II proteins as these proteins are transported to the cell surface. While T lymphocytes are programmed during ontogeny not to respond to strictly "self"-HLA, they are actually positively programmed to respond vigorously to "self "-HLA that has been slightly modified, as in the case of bound peptide in the groove. Indeed, most T lymphocytes will not respond to a protein antigen unless it is presented in this HLA context. In a non-transplant setting the HLA molecules that present antigens are always self-HLA on autologous antigen-presenting cells or somatic cells.

HLA Molecules as Antigens

When a kidney transplant recipient receives an organ from a donor that bears one or more non-self-HLA antigens, those mismatched donor HLA molecules can serve as antigens and targets of the immune response. There are two possible mechanisms for recognition of mismatched HLA antigens called "direct" and "indirect" recognition[2] (Fig. 4.2). Direct recognition of mismatched HLA molecules involves T lymphocytes that are activated by the donor HLA antigens on transplanted donor cells. In this context, the donor HLA appear as altered self-HLA and stimulate the immune response. Indirect recognition of mismatched HLA molecules requires processing of donor HLA molecules by recipient antigen-presenting cells and presentation of donor HLA antigenic epitopes in the context of recipient HLA.

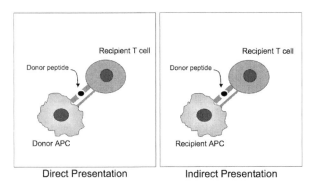

Fig. 4.2 Types of allorecognition (direct and indirect)

Class II HLA molecules (HLA-DR) selectively stimulate T lymphocytes that bear the CD4 antigen to become activated, to proliferate, and to secrete cytokines that are largely pro-inflammatory "helper" cells. Some subsets of CD4-positive lymphocytes are also capable of then regulating the immune response. Indeed the T cell CD4 molecule has binding affinity for an epitope on the HLA-DR molecule that is distinct from the epitope that engages the antigen-specific T-cell receptor (CD3).

Class I HLA molecules (HLA-A, B, C) selectively stimulate T lymphocytes that bear the CD8 differentiation antigen. Many of these CD8-positive T cells are cytotoxic lymphocyte precursors, which mature into active cytotoxic effector cells on antigen stimulation. The CD8 molecule has proven affinity for an epitope on the

HLA class I molecule that is monomorphic and distinct from the antigen-presenting domain of class I.

Serologic Definition of HLA Antigens

In the era before DNA-based molecular testing, HLA antigens were only defined by their reactivity with human sera obtained from multiparous women or patients sensitized through blood transfusion or transplantation.[3,4] Random panels of individuals from the population were tested with individual sera, using methods ranging from leukoagglutination to microcytotoxicity, and each panel member was scored as either positive or negative with a given serum. Patterns of reactivity of multiple sera were correlated with each other, and a statistical inference was drawn that sera with similar patterns of reactivity are likely to have antibodies directed against the same antigen(s) expressed on the panel cells. The antigens were given arbitrary names and panel members labeled as bearing those antigens defined by the sera. Family studies showed evident autosomal codominant inheritance of specific "series" of these antigens and enabled the definition of loci and calculation of linkage and recombination rates. Large international workshops, in which many thousands of panel members were tested against thousands of sera submitted by hundreds of laboratories around the world, led to a common nomenclature of the serologically defined HLA antigens (Table 4.4). The World Health Organization Nomenclature updates the list of serologically defined antigens on a regular basis.

The workshops have led to an understanding of the serological complexity of the HLA antigens and have led to important concepts about the natural humoral immune response to the HLA antigens. A case in point is the HLA-A9, A23, and A24 antigens. A9 was initially defined as an antigen because many multiparous sera reacted in the same manner with a subset of individuals who were said to have the HLA-A9 antigen.[5] Analysis of a much larger number of sera revealed that there were two additional sets of sera that reacted with mutually exclusive subsets of individuals who bore the HLA-A9 antigen. These were arbitrarily labeled HLA-A23 and HLA-A24.[6] It was clear that HLA-A9 was no longer a distinct molecule and that those individuals previously labeled as A9 were either A23 or A24. The sheer number of anti-A9 sera, however, was not likely to be a consequence of those sera containing a mixture of anti-A23 and anti-A24 antibodies. Indeed elution and absorption studies revealed that the A23 and A24 molecules must have both a "private" domain, or antibody-binding epitope which uniquely defines them as 23 or 24, and a "public" domain which is the target of anti-A9 antibodies. An individual who is challenged by blood transfusion or transplantation with HLA-A23, can therefore make an antibody against only A23 or may make an antibody against the shared A9 epitope too, thereby making the serum cross react against A24 as well. Some public epitopes are shared among a wide range of individual HLA antigens. The implication of this is that a patient can be exposed (through transfusion, pregnancy or failed transplant) to a limited number of individual HLA antigens and yet mount a humoral immune response that can cross react with a large fraction of the general population.

Serologic Typing for HLA

Individuals are serologically typed for their HLA phenotype using a microcytotoxicity assay. The result of the typing is a list of HLA specificities that the individual carries. A normal individual would usually bear two specificities at each locus (maternal and paternal inherited) unless they are homozygous at that locus and have by chance inherited the same specificity from the mother and father. The microcytotoxicity assay uses a large set of reference reagents consisting of extensively quality-controlled human sera, usually from multiparous women who have mounted a narrow antigen-specific immune response against just one or two HLA antigens. A different HLA-specific reference serum is pre-loaded into each well of a 96-well plastic microtiter tray. Lymphocytes from the individual to be typed are added to each well and the tray incubated to give the antibodies the opportunity to bind to the cells if the cells bear the target antigens. A source of complement (usually from rabbit) is added and the tray is further incubated so that cells in wells where the antibody binds are killed and remain alive in wells where antibody does not bind. Cell death in each well can be determined in a number of alternative ways, from inspection under polarized light to use of fluorescent dyes that selectively stain live or dead cells. A semiquantitative score is given to the degree of cell death in each well and a threshold is used to determine positivity in each well.[7–9]

The reagents used in serologic HLA typing usually are derived from multiparous women and have been quality controlled as either monospecific for a single World Health Organization defined HLA antigen or against a specific set of HLA antigens. A typical set of typing trays will include two or three sera against a given antigen so that the sensitivity and specificity of the kit are sufficiently high.

Typing for HLA-A, B, and C antigens is done using purified T lymphocytes derived from patient blood or, in the case of deceased donors, other lymphoid tissues. Typing for HLA-DR and DQ antigens is done using purified B lymphocytes as targets on typing trays that contain a set of reference reagents against class II antigens.

Phenotyping, Genotyping, and Haplotyping

The result of an HLA test is an HLA phenotype, a simple list of the HLA antigens that are positively detected on the subject. Because HLA antigens are codominantly expressed, the HLA type is directly reflective of the MHC genotype at a particular locus. With a set of reagent sera that cover all of the WHO HLA specificities, individuals who have just one HLA antigen at a given locus can be presumed to be homozygous for that antigen, though not necessarily at the level of inherited alleles.

Each individual inherits a haplotype from one of his/her two parents. Because the HLA genes are located within a relatively small region on the 6th chromosome, the HLA-A, B, C, DRA, DRB1, DRB3 or DRB4, DQA, and DQB genes are usually inherited en bloc, with only a 2% probability of recombination within the HLA genetic region. Although the HLA testing results for an individual simply produce an unordered list of the inherited antigens, it is possible to infer inheritance if one has access to the phenotyping on parents and/or multiple siblings. The specific A, B, C, DR, and DQ antigens inherited from a parent are called a "haplotype" and are for practical purposes the unit of inheritance for HLA, given the infrequent recombination between HLA loci. A biological child therefore shares one haplotype with each parent. Siblings can share 0, 1, or 2 haplotypes with their component HLA antigens. The probability of a 0-haplotype or 2-haplotype match between siblings is 25%, while 50% of siblings are 1-haplotype matched. Matching for a haplotype is of a much stronger degree than simply matching for the WHO serological antigens that comprise that haplotype. This is because haplotypes are identical by inheritance and therefore are identical at the molecular level, not simply the serological level.

Crossmatch

In order to determine whether a patient has antibody directed against a potential donor a crossmatch is done. There are several different methods for doing a crossmatch, each of which provides somewhat different information to the clinician (Table 4.1).

Table 4.1   Crossmatch methods and characteristics*

Crossmatch name	Methods	Characteristics
1. "Amos" crossmatch	Recipient serum mixed with donor cells Complement added	Standard crossmatch (if negative should not get hyperacute rejection)
2. "Anti-globulin" crossmatch ("anti-kappa" crossmatch)	Donor cells mixed with recipient serum Anti-human Ig potentiating reagent added Complement added	Potentiated crossmatch Amplifies reaction Fewer accelerated rejections Detects weaker antibody Detects non-complement-binding antibody
3. Flow crossmatch	Donor cells mixed with recipient serum Fluorescent anti-human Ig reagent added Assessed with flow cytometer	Potentiated crossmatch Amplifies reaction Fewer accelerated rejections Quantitative readout

*Reactivity with T and B cells identified by these crossmatch methods

The "Amos" cytotoxic crossmatch uses recipient serum and donor peripheral blood lymphocytes because lymphocytes bear the donor HLA antigens that are important in kidney transplantation. Peripheral blood provides a source for donor lymphocytes. Alternative rich sources of lymphocytes in deceased donors are lymph nodes or spleen. HLA class I antigens (HLA-A, B, and C) are found on both T and B lymphocytes. B lymphocytes also prominently express HLA class II antigens (HLA-DR, DQ). Pure populations of donor T cells or B cells can be obtained from mixed lymphoid suspensions by any one of several fractionation methods.

The cytotoxic crossmatch is performed by mixing a measured quantity of recipient serum with a known number of donor lymphoid cells and incubating for a specified period of time to allow any anti-donor antibody present in the serum to bind to the antigens on the donor cells. The cells are then thoroughly washed to remove any unbound antibody and then complement is added to the cells. If recipient antibody is on the cells, added complement will kill the cells. The cell kill is usually evaluated through use of fluorescent dyes that identify live and dead cells. A semiquantitative score is given to the results in each reaction well, depending on the percent cell kill in the well (Table 4.2). Two to six replicate wells are read in order to minimize variance. The assay is often performed with several serial twofold dilutions of the patient serum to assess the quantity of anti-donor antibody.

Table 4.2 Interpretation of cytotoxic crossmatch scores

Score	Condition	Interpretation
0	Few cells in well	"NOT READABLE"
1	0–10% cell death	"NEGATIVE"
2	11–20%	"DOUBTFUL NEGATIVE"
4	21–50%	"WEAK POSITIVE"
6	51–80%	"POSITIVE"
8	81–100%	"STRONGLY POSITIVE"

Antibodies directed against class I will result in a positive cytotoxic crossmatch with both T and B cells, whereas antibodies directed against class II will only cause a positive crossmatch with B lymphocytes (Table 4.3). In some cases, a very weak anti-class I antibody can also give a selective positive cytotoxic crossmatch against B cells depending on the source of complement and incubation conditions for the B-cell crossmatch that can render it more sensitive for detection of anti-class I antibodies (Table 4.3, line 3). A positive crossmatch against T cells is an indication of anti-class I antibody in the patient, whereas a positive crossmatch with B cells could

Table 4.3 Patterns of crossmatch on T and B lymphocytes

Serum with	Crossmatch on T lymphocytes	Crossmatch on B lymphocytes
1. Anti-class I HLA-A, B, or C antibody	+++	+++
2. Anti-class II HLA-DR or DQ antibody	–	+++
3. Weak anti-class I	–	+
4. Weak anti-class I (platelet absorbed)	–	–
5. Anti-class I + class II	+++	+++
6. Anti-class I + class II (platelet absorbed)	–	+++

be caused by either anti-class I or anti-class II antibody. In the presence of anti-class I antibody it is therefore impossible to determine, by simple crossmatch alone, whether there is also anti-class II antibody in the patient. One strategy which had historically been used to solve this dilemma was to absorb such a serum with pooled platelets from a large number of individuals. Pooled platelets are available and contain only class I antigen. Absorption of a serum that contains both anti-class I and anti-class II antibodies therefore removes the class I antibody and leaves behind the class II antibody (Table 4.3, line 6).

On occasion, a crossmatch will be negative with undiluted serum and positive when the serum is diluted 1:2 or more. This phenomenon, called "prozone," is thought to occur when there are weak anti-complementary substances in the serum which can be diluted before the anti-donor antibody is diluted.

There are a number of characteristics of antibodies detected in the crossmatch assay which are important for the clinician to be aware of. Antibodies can have autoreactivity (autoantibody), can have reactivity against the donor (alloantibody), can be of the IgG or IgM isotype, and can be directed against HLA antigens or non-HLA antigens expressed on target lymphocytes (Table 4.4).

Table 4.4   Types of recipient antibody in crossmatch

	Auto Antibody	Auto Isotype	Allo Antibody	Allo Isotype	Anti-HLA
1. Anti-HLA IgM alloantibody	–	–	+	IgM	+
2. Anti-HLA IgG alloantibody	–	–	+	IgG	+
3. No antibody against recipient or donor	–	–	–	–	–
4. Non-HLA IgM against recipient and donor	+	IgM	+	IgM	–
5. Non-HLA IgG against recipient and donor	+	IgG	+	IgG	–
6. Non-HLA IgM autoantibody only	+	IgM	–	–	–
7. Non-HLA IgG autoantibody only	+	IgG	–	–	–
8. Non-HLA IgM alloantibody only	–		+	IgM	–
9. Non-HLA IgG alloantibody only	–		+	IgG	–

The standard cytotoxic crossmatch is the so-called Amos crossmatch in which recipient serum and donor cells are incubated, followed by a wash and addition of complement. Even if there is anti-donor antibody in the recipient serum, those antibodies must be able to bind and activate complement in order for the assay to give a positive result. Complement activation requires that the isotype of the antibody is capable of engaging complement, and furthermore that the density of antibody binding allows crosslinking of at least two immunoglobulin molecules. Antibodies that are not complement activating can still play a role in kidney transplant rejection, however. Non-complement-binding antibodies can still target donor cells for destruction through other mechanisms such as "antibody dependent-cell mediated cytotoxicity" or ADCC.[10,11] ADCC effector cells bear receptors for the Fc portion of immunoglobulin and have a cytotoxic mechanism that is similar to that of "killer cells." The ADCC effector cells recognize donor cells to which antibody is bound (even some non-complement-binding antibodies) and kills those donor cells.

There is a potentiated cytotoxic crossmatch, called "anti-globulin" or "anti-kappa," which increases the sensitivity of the standard "Amos" crossmatch through use of a complement-binding anti-human Ig or antibody against the kappa chain component of human immunoglobulin. The flow cytometric crossmatch is more sensitive than complement-mediated crossmatches, although its significance is still unknown.

Autoantibody

Patients with autoimmune diseases such as systemic lupus erythematosus and individuals who have been treated with certain medications including hydralazine, alpha-methyl DOPA, and quinidine will sometimes produce autoantibody. These antibodies are usually directed against the recipient's own non-HLA proteins, glycoproteins, or glycolipids, but can also serve as "alloantibodies" in that the target antigens may be shared with donor cells and render the recipient anti-donor crossmatch positive. These autoimmune or medication-induced antibodies are not important in the setting of kidney transplantation and do not indicate greater susceptibility to humoral rejection post-transplant. Autoantibodies are virtually never directed against HLA. Many of them are of the IgM isotype and are persistent, i.e., do not switch from IgM to IgG, however, because this is not consistently the case IgM antibody should not be equated with autoantibody (Table 4.4).

IgM and IgG Antibody in Crossmatch

Exposure to HLA antigens through transfusion, pregnancy, or transplantation causes a classical humoral immune response. There is an initial IgM antibody response, followed within 2 weeks by a switch to the IgG isotype. Reexposure to the same HLA antigen can cause another transient spike in IgM production, followed by a faster and more profound IgG response that can persist for years. Human IgM is a potent cytotoxic antibody, though the initial IgM immune response often produces antibody of low affinity. This means that IgM antibodies can sometimes be dissociated from the cell by thermal energy alone and bind more tightly at lower temperatures. This has resulted in the observation that "cold antibodies," that is, antibodies that cause a positive crossmatch when incubated with cells at 4°F but not at 37°F are more likely to be of the IgM isotype. Another method for determining whether a cytotoxic antibody is IgM or not is to do the crossmatch prior to and after treatment of the recipient serum with dithiothreitol (DTT) or dithioerythritol (DTE).[12, 13] These chemicals are potent reducing agents which when properly used will cleave the disulfide bonds of IgM while leaving IgG intact. If a positive crossmatch turns negative after treatment with DTT or DTE, one can conclude that the antibody responsible for the positive crossmatch was an IgM isotype. Autoantibodies and non-HLA alloantibodies are frequently of the IgM isotype, and unlike anti-HLA antibodies, they often fail to switch from IgM to IgG with time. Nevertheless, presence of an IgM antibody cannot be taken as proof that the antibody is non-HLA. IgM anti-HLA antibodies, usually produced within a week or two of an immunological challenge, can cause severe humoral rejection, so it is important to demonstrate whether or not the antibody is directed against HLA antigens of the donor.

Screening of Recipient Serum

The crossmatch only gives the clinician the information that there is a recipient antibody that binds to donor cells and, in the case of the cytotoxic crossmatch, one that activates complement. The clinically significant anti-donor antibodies are predominantly directed against HLA. In order to fully interpret the importance of a crossmatch, it is helpful to have more complete information about the nature of the antibody that causes the positive crossmatch. Kidney transplant candidates routinely have their serum screened for presence of antibody. There are two types of information that are obtained from screening.

The first screening information obtained is the "panel reactive antibody" or PRA, an indication of whether there is any alloantibody at all in the candidate serum and, if so, how broadly the antibody reacts with the general population. This is done by testing (screening) the candidate serum against a panel of individuals sampled from the general population.[14, 15] The sample used can either be random, chosen to reflect the population of likely deceased donors, or chosen to represent as many HLA antigens specificities as possible. Most laboratories use panels of between 30 and 50 subjects in order to represent as many different HLA types as practical. Lymphocytes from each of the panel members are crossmatched with the serum of a given patient and scored as either "positive" or "negative." The proportion of panel members with a positive crossmatch with a given serum is taken as the %PRA, which ranges from 0 to 100%. A 0% PRA indicates that the patient has no antibody against the general population of which the panel is a representative sample, while a 50% PRA suggests that the patient will have a positive crossmatch against about 50% of individuals in the population. The PRA is used by clinicians to estimate the likelihood that a kidney transplant candidate will have a permissive (negative) crossmatch against an average donor. This is used to advise patients about how long they are likely to wait to receive a deceased donor transplant. It is also used by the UNOS national network or organ sharing to award extra allocation points to sensitized patients because of the lower likelihood of an acceptable donor being found.

If a patient is sensitized, the second type of information that can be inferred from the screening is a list of specific anti-HLA antibodies that account for the patient's PRA. This is done by using an HLA-typed panel for the screening and analyzing the pattern of positive and negative reactions with individual panel members by computer. For example, if a patient serum shows 20% reactivity with a panel, one may want to know what accounts for that 20% reactivity. If all the 20% of the panel members with positive reactions bear the HLA antigen A2, and none of the panel members with negative reactions bear the A2 antigen, then there is a 100% correlation of the reactivity pattern with HLA-A2, and we might conclude that the antibody that explains the reactivity is an anti-HLA A2. This analysis is iterated to find more anti-HLA antibodies that might account for residual reactivity.

HLA-Specific Screening Using Purified Antigen Targets

Screening of kidney transplant candidate sera using a panel of HLA-typed individuals by the cytotoxic method has a number of difficulties. Because of the extreme variation of HLA phenotypes in the population, no two laboratories use identical panels. Panel size can vary depending on the resources of the lab. Panel composition will determine both the PRA of a given serum as well as how many anti-HLA antibodies can be detected in a single patient serum. If a patient has three or four antibodies directed against commonly found HLA antigens, the PRA may exceed 90% and it will be impossible to determine if there are other HLA antibodies in the serum using the panel as there will not be a sufficient number of remaining panel members to analyze. Another difficulty with cytotoxic panel screening is that candidates with non-HLA antibody that reacts with lymphocytes will score as positive with the assay and give a PRA, but it may be impossible to define any anti-HLA specificities.

Because anti-HLA antibodies are clearly the most important predictors of post-transplant antibody-mediated rejection, assays that are more selective for HLA as well as more sensitive for detection of weak antibody have been developed. The assays use purified HLA antigens derived from human cell lines as targets. The HLA antigens are covalently affixed to a solid substrate such as a plastic enzyme-linked immunosorbent assay (ELISA) well or plastic bead. Serum from a patient is incubated with the fixed antigen, unbound antibody washed away, and an indicator anti-human immunoglobulin reagent used to detect any bound anti-HLA antibody. The readout for a given serum with an individual HLA antigen is a numerical fluorescent intensity that is converted into a semiquantitative score based on the intensity of negative and positive controls.[16,17] This is usually reported to the clinician as a list of anti-HLA antibodies that were found in the tested serum. It is possible to automate and miniaturize the assay. The HLA substrate used can be consistent. Unlike the cellular screening assay, the solid state assays can determine the presence or absence of antibodies against a large number of individual HLA antigens without "masking" by non-HLA antibodies or exhausting the panel. Based on the list of anti-HLA antibodies present in a given serum, one can calculate a "PRA" for any given population of target individuals based on the phenotype distribution in that population. This is the so-called cPRA or calculated PRA and can be a more standardized measure than the PRA determined with an arbitrary and rather small panel of target cells. There is not a perfect correlation between the predictions yielded by solid state screening results and the cytotoxic crossmatch. For example, one may have an anti-A2 antibody detected in a serum sample and that serum may be negative by cytotoxic crossmatch against a cell that has the HLA-A2 antigen on it. While this might be considered a "false-positive" screening, it is in fact a simple consequence of the greater sensitivity of the solid state assay for detection of antibody. The clinical significance of positive anti-donor antibody by the solid state binding assay in the presence of a negative cytotoxic or flow crossmatch against the donor is not yet determined and will probably depend on a number of other factors such as immunosuppressive protocol. Conversely, one might have no detectable anti-HLA antibody by solid state screening and yet have a positive crossmatch against a donor. This can occur if the candidate has non-HLA antibody that reacts with donor lymphocytes or in rare cases if the patient has an IgM antibody that has not yet switched to IgG.

Post-transplant Monitoring

In the post-transplant period, recipients may develop de novo antibody against donor HLA antigens and suffer antibody-mediated rejection. This is characterized by acute renal transplant dysfunction with "endothelitis" and C4d deposition in peritubular and/or glomerular capillaries on kidney biopsy. In current clinical practice it is common to obtain solid state, HLA antigen-specific screening on the recipient to determine if there is circulating anti-HLA antibody in the circulation. This is done in order to document that there is a specific antibody that might be responsible for the humoral rejection. The results are often used to decide whether removal of antibody by plasmapheresis is indicated. The results are also useful as a baseline that can be compared with a post-pheresis serum sample to determine if removal was successful.

Emerging Field of Non-HLA Antigens and Antibodies

Antibodies develop in transplant candidates and recipients that are not directed against HLA. Characterization of these antibodies has led to identification of antigens that are on the surface of endothelial cells and not on lymphocytes.

Major histocompatibility complex (MHC) class I-related chain A (MICA) molecules show homology with HLA molecules. MICA is a highly polymorphic molecule and is found to be located about 60 kb centromeric of HLA-B on chromosome 6 in humans. MICA antigens are different than classical MHC molecules as they do not combine with β2 microglobulin, do not bind peptides for antigen presentation to T cells, and are not expressed on lymphocytes. There is emerging evidence for a role for allosensitization to MICA in allograft rejection.[18,19] A correlation between presence of anti-MICA antibodies in kidney transplant recipients was shown to be associated with an increased frequency of graft loss.[20,21]

Lack of commercially available and well-validated assays is a limiting factor for the progress in this field of anti-non-HLA antigens and antibodies. More recently, results from a study by Breimer et al. using endothelial cell precursors isolated from donors used in a crossmatch type assay to detect antibodies to donor reactive antibodies to endothelial cell antigen look promising.[22] The data show that presence of antibodies to donor endothelial cells as detected in an endothelial crossmatch test in a subject results in a significantly higher rate of rejection than those subjects who did not have antibodies to endothelial antigens 3 months post-transplantation. Interestingly, IgG and IgM anti-endothelial antibodies were associated with graft rejections.[22]

References

1. Marsh SG, Albert ED, Bodmer WF, Bontrop RE, Dupont B, Erlich HA, Geraghty DE, Hansen JA, Hurley CK, Mach B, Mayr WR, Parham P, Petersdorf EW, Sasazuki T, Schreuder GM, Strominger JL, Svejgaard A, Terasaki PI, Trowsdale J. Nomenclature for factors of the HLA system, 2004. *Int J Immunogenet* 2005; 32:107–159.
2. Auchincloss H Jr, Sultan H. Antigen processing and presentation in transplantation. *Curr Opin Immunol* 1996; 8:681–687.
3. Morin-Papunen L, Tiilikainen A, Hartikainen-Sorri AL. Maternal HLA immunization during pregnancy: presence of anti HLA antibodies in half of multigravidous women. *Med Biol* 1984; 62:323–325.
4. Macleod AM, Hillis AN, Mather A, Bone JM, Catto GR. Effect of cyclosporin, previous third-party transfusion, and pregnancy on antibody development after donor-specific transfusion before renal transplantation. *Lancet* 1987; 1:416–418.
5. Doxiadis II, Claas FH. The short story of HLA and its methods. *Dev Ophthalmol* 2003; 36:5–11.
6. Fussell H, Thomas M, Street J, Darke C. HLA-A9 antibodies and epitopes. *Tissue Antigens* 1996; 47:307–312.
7. Patel R, Mickey MR, Terasaki PI. Serotyping for homotransplantation. XVI. Analysis of kidney transplants from unrelated donors. *N Engl J Med* 1968; 279:501–506.
8. Marrari M, Duquesnoy RJ. Progress report on the ASHI/CAP Proficiency Survey Program in Histocompatibility Testing. I. HLA-A,B,C typing, antibody screening, and lymphocytotoxicity crossmatching. American Society for Histocompatibility and Immunogenetics. College of American Pathologists. *Hum Immunol* 1994; 39:87–95.
9. Duquesnoy RJ, Marrari M. Progress report on the ASHI/CAP Proficiency Survey Program in Histocompatibility Testing. II. HLA-DR, DQ serologic typing, antibody identification, and B-cell crossmatching. American Society for Histocompatibility of Immunogenetics. College of American Pathologists. *Hum Immunol* 1994; 39:96–105.
10. Lightbody JJ, Rosenberg JC. Antibody-dependent cell-mediated cytotoxicity in prospective kidney transplant recipients. *J Immunol* 1974; 112:890–896.

11. Gailiunas P Jr., Suthanthiran M, Busch GJ, Carpenter CB, Garovoy MR. Role of humoral presenitization in human renal transplant rejection. *Kidney Int* 1980; 17:638–646.
12. Kerman RH, Kimball PM, Van Buren CT, Lewis RM, DeVera V, Baghdahsarian V, Heydari A, Kahan BD. AHG and DTE/AHG procedure identification of crossmatch-appropriate donor-recipient pairings that result in improved graft survival. *Transplantation* 1991; 51:316–320.
13. Okuno T, Kondelis N. Evaluation of dithiothreitol (DTT) for inactivation of IgM antibodies. *J Clin Pathol* 1978; 31:1152–1155.
14. Lavee J, Kormos RL, Duquesnoy RJ, Zerbe TR, Armitage JM, Vanek M, Hardesty RL, Griffith BP. Influence of panel-reactive antibody and lymphocytotoxic crossmatch on survival after heart transplantation. *J Heart Lung Transplant* 1991; 10:921–929; discussion 929–930.
15. Loh E, Bergin JD, Couper GS, Mudge GH Jr.. Role of panel-reactive antibody cross-reactivity in predicting survival after orthotopic heart transplantation. *J Heart Lung Transplant* 1994; 13:194–201.
16. Tait BD, Hudson F, Cantwell L, Brewin G, Holdsworth R, Bennett G, Jose M. Review article: Luminex technology for HLA antibody detection in organ transplantation. *Nephrology (Carlton)* 2009; 14:247–254.
17. Pei R, Lee J, Chen T, Rojo S, Terasaki PI. Flow cytometric detection of HLA antibodies using a spectrum of microbeads. *Hum Immunol* 1999; 60:1293–1302.
18. Dragun D. Humoral responses directed against non-human leukocyte antigens in solid-organ transplantation. *Transplantation* 2008; 86(8):1019–1025.
19. Stastny P, Zou Y, Fan Y, Qin Z, Lavingia B. The emerging issue of MICA antibodies: antibodies to MICA and other antigens of endothelial cells. *Contrib Nephrol* 2009; 162:99–106.
20. Terasaki PI, Ozawa M, Castro R. Four-year follow-up of a prospective trial of HLA and MICA antibodies on kidney graft survival. *Am J Transplant* 2007; 7:408–415.
21. Zou Y, Stastny P, Süsal C, Döhler B, Opelz G. Antibodies against MICA antigens and kidney-transplant rejection. *N Engl J Med* 2007; 357:1293–1300.
22. Breimer ME, Rydberg L, Jackson AM, Lucas DP, Zachary AA, Melancon JK, Von Visger J, Pelletier R, Saidman SL, Williams WW Jr, Holgersson J, Tyden G, Klintmalm GK, Coultrup S, Sumitran-Holgersson S, Grufman P. Multicenter evaluation of a novel endothelial cell crossmatch test in kidney transplantation. *Transplantation* 2009; 87(4):549–556.

Chapter 5
Kidney Allocation: Role of UNOS and OPOs

Patricia L. Adams, Walter K. Graham, and Susan Gunderson

Part 1: What Is UNOS and How Are Kidneys Allocated?
Patricia L. Adams and Walter K. Graham

The UNOS is a not-for-profit, private, voluntary membership organization incorporated in the Commonwealth of Virginia, which qualifies as a tax exempt charity under IRC section 501(c)(3). Since 1986, it has been the sole holder of a contract from the federal government to operate the national OPTN. Its story is one of the many remarkable successes in organ transplantation.

History. In June 1969, the Public Health Service awarded seven contracts to transplant centers in the United States to study "the feasibility of procuring kidneys in one place and preserving, matching, and transporting them in a viable condition to another place for transplantation." One of the recipients was Dr. David Hume of the Medical College of Virginia on behalf of the SEROPP, a group of eight transplant programs in four states and the District of Columbia.[1] SEROPP implemented a computerized online kidney matching system in December of the same year that was renamed the UNOS in 1977. UNOS (the computer sharing system) and SEOPF (formerly SEROPP) grew to encompass a large part of the United States – at one point SEOPF had 49 members in 21 states from New York to Arizona – and the 24 h operation known as the Kidney Center was created in 1982 to deal with more complex sharing; its name was changed in 1984 to the present day Organ Center.

The Structure of UNOS

UNOS won the initial contract from the federal government to operate the OPTN, and its structure became the structure of the national system. UNOS is governed as

P.L. Adams (✉)
Section on Nephrology, WFU School of Medicine, Wake Forest University Baptist Medical Center, Medical Center Boulevard, NC Baptist Hospital, Winston-Salem, NC, USA
e-mail: padams@wfubmc.edu

D.B. McKay, S.M. Steinberg (eds.), *Kidney Transplantation: A Guide to the Care of Kidney Transplant Recipients*, DOI 10.1007/978-1-4419-1690-7_5,
© Springer Science+Business Media, LLC 2010

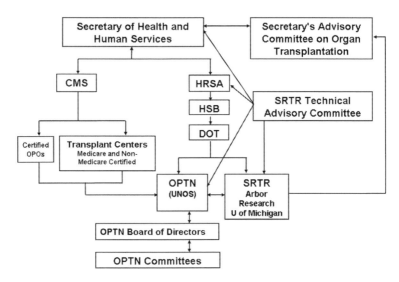

Fig. 5.1 Key players in the national solid organ transplant system

a representative democracy of its members – the transplant community. An administrative staff in Richmond, VA, led by an executive director carries out policy. In operating the OPTN, the board of directors and committees of UNOS act as the board and committees of the OPTN (Fig. 5.1).

Members. The members of UNOS include both institutional members and public members. The institutional members are transplant centers, OPOs, and histocompatibility laboratories. The public members include public not-for-profit organizations that promote organ donation, medical and scientific organizations that have members who are interested in organ transplantation, a limited number of individuals, and business members. The membership of UNOS and the membership of the OPTN are identical. All transplant centers and OPOs are required by federal law to belong to the OPTN, and they also all belong to UNOS.[2]

Regions. The nation is divided into 11 regions (Fig. 5.2). Each region elects a councillor, associate councillor, and a representative to each standing committee of UNOS every 2 years (Table 5.1). These individuals are responsible for representing their region at the national meetings, chairing their regional committee, and keeping the region informed about events in their area of responsibility. Each regional councillor sits on the UNOS board. The associate councillor represents the region on the all important MPSC.

The regional structure fosters regional cooperation and serves as a conduit for information and ideas from the UNOS leadership to the members. Unfortunately the current regional structure has some drawbacks. First, despite efforts to the contrary, the populations that each region contain vary in number and they vary in the number of member organizations. Comparing this with the US government, it would be as if each state had senators, but no representatives. Second, in regions with only a few

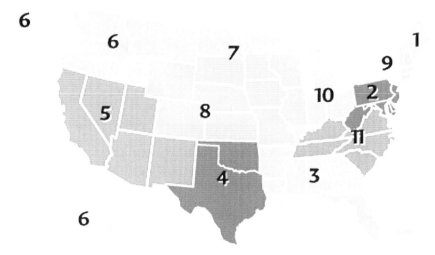

Fig. 5.2 The regions of UNOS

Table 5.1 UNOS (organ donation and transplantation) committees

Ad hoc disease transmission advisory
Ad hoc internal relations
Ethics
Executive
Finance
Histo compatibility
Kidney transplantation
Liver and intestinal organ transplantation
Living donor
MPSC
Minority affairs
Operations
OPO
Organ availability
Pancreas transplantation
Patient affairs
Pediatric transplantation
Policy oversight
Thoracic organ transplantation
Transplant administrators
Transplant coordinator

transplant centers, candidates waiting at other centers in the region have a better chance at an organ than when there are many transplant centers in the region. This inherent disequilibrium, compounded by varying organ procurement and transplant center acceptance rates, results in very different average wait times for candidates in different regions.

The Organ Center. The UNOS Organ Center is an electronic command post at UNOS headquarters in Richmond, Virginia, staffed 24/7 to facilitate organ sharing. It has been in continuous operation since 1982. Center personnel are available to assist with organ placement, organ transportation, donor information, and to answer all manner of questions from members, especially, it seems, during non-working hours when others are not available.

Government Oversight of Solid Organ Transplant

There have been several important pieces of legislation affecting the field of organ transplantation in the United States.

The first of these was NOTA, the *National Organ Transplant Act of 1984.*[3] This Act created the Task Force on Organ Transplantation, established the modern system of OPO, called for the creation of a SRTR, and outlawed the buying and selling of human organs and tissues. In 1987 the *Omnibus Budget Reconciliation Act* of that year added Section 1138 to the SSA requiring that OPOs and transplant hospitals belong to and abide by the rules and requirements of the OPTN in order to be eligible to receive any Medicare and Medicaid funds.[4] If these organizations did not join the OPTN and abide by its rules, the entire organization, not just the transplant programs, would be ineligible to be a Medicare/Medicaid provider.[5]

In 1989, the HCFA [now the CMS] announced that it would not enforce the new SSA provision until rules and requirements had been established for the OPTN. Contracts awarded to UNOS by HRSA for OPTN management between 1989 and 2000 called for a network in which policies were "voluntary guidance," not enforceable by the government. UNOS continued to operate by consensus and to be regulated by peer review. In 1995, HHS published "proposed federal regulations" for governance of the OPTN. This "proposed rule" underwent extensive public comment, public hearings, and discussions amongst transplant professionals and centers. It became a Final Rule in 1999.

The OPTN Final Rule of 1999 codified the regulations governing solid organ transplantation in the United States.[2] Together with NOTA, it established the nature, role, and legal authority of the OPTN. In 2006, HRSA announced a new interpretation of the Final Rule, giving the OPTN *oversight responsibility for living donation*, including the safety and well-being of donors.[6] Thus, transplant centers which heretofore were not subject to federal oversight if they did not use deceased donors or accept Medicare/Medicaid have become members of the OPTN and are subject to its rules, regulations, and safety policies.

In 2007, CMS published regulations defining *Medicare Conditions of Participation for transplant hospitals.*[7] Failure to comply with these conditions results in loss of Medicare monies to your transplant programs, not to your entire organization or center. The wording accompanying these regulations suggests that CMS now intends to assume the oversight function previously given to the OPTN, because "it does not have the statutory authority to delegate oversight responsibility to the OPTN. CMS is responsible for establishing minimum standards to protect patient health and safety and for implementing oversight mechanisms."[8] The OPTN's new primary responsibilities are to insure the effectiveness, efficiency, and equity of organ allocation; to increase the supply of organs; to collect and disburse data; and to designate transplant programs. This would appear to represent a paradigm shift from the previous practice of allowing medical professionals to establish patient safety standards. Also in 2007, legal impediments which prevented the OPTN from engaging in *paired donation* were removed, and UNOS is actively engaged in implementing a national policy and system to facilitate this process.

How Are Kidneys Allocated?

The allocation of deceased donor kidneys in the United States is extremely complex. For complete details, see the actual policy at www.Optn.org/policiesandbylaws/policies.asp. There are, however, several consensus principles which underlie the US system:

1. Former living donors have priority if they ever require a kidney transplant.
2. Pediatric candidates have priority due to the unique biological challenges children face with dialysis.
3. Allocation first to candidates in the area closest to the donor results in better outcomes.
4. Except in rare circumstances, blood type "O" kidneys are allocated to blood type "O" recipients and blood type "B" kidneys are allocated to blood type "B" recipients to promote parity in waiting times across blood types.
5. Some special groups require extra help to have equal access to organs (e.g., the sensitized candidate).

Presently in the United States, deceased donor kidneys are divided into two main types:

1. *ECD.* Since 2002, the allocation system has accommodated a new class of kidney organ from the ECD. The genesis for the ECD program came from the observation that viable kidneys were not allocated efficiently because of certain donor characteristics. Many transplant programs around the country refused organs that were subsequently transplanted at another program and the transplant succeeded.[9] A consensus conference was convened to develop guidelines for the use of these "expanded criteria kidneys."[10] An ECD kidney was defined as (1) from a donor age 60+ or (2) from a donor age 50+ with either a history of controlled hypertension, or a previous CVA, or both, with a Cr > 1.5 mg/dl (Fig. 5.3). These kidneys as a group have a RR of graft failure of greater than

Donor Condition	Donor Age Categories				
	<10	10-39	40-49	50-59	≥ 60
CVA + HTN + Creat > 1.5				X	X
CVA + HTN				X	X
CVA + Creat > 1.5				X	X
CVA or HTN alone					X
HTN + Creat> 1.5				X	X
Creatinine > 1.5					X
None of the above					X

CVA = CVA was cause of death
HTN = History of hypertension
Creat > 1.5 = Creatinine > 1.5 mg/dL

Fig. 5.3 The expanded criteria kidney donor

1.7 compared to standard criteria kidneys but they have been shown to provide a 3–10-year survival benefit over dialysis.[11]

2. *Kidneys from SCD do not meet the ECD criteria described above*

Either SCD or ECD may also meet the criteria for *DCD*. DCD donors are those whose families consent to controlled withdrawal of life support in the OR; donors who expire in the hospital but organ perfusion is maintained until consent can be given; or consented donors who experience CPR during organ recovery.

When candidates are listed on the UNOS/OPTN waitlist, they are asked if they would be willing to accept an ECD or a DCD kidney. These individuals are so noted in *DonorNet®* (the UNOS electronic organ offer system), and those who have consented participate in the allocation of ECD and SCD kidneys, including kidneys that are from DCD donors. All waitlisted individuals are automatically part of the SCD match.

Most kidney donations at the present time are facilitated by local OPO personnel. The OPO assigned to the DSA where the donor hospital resides is notified by hospital personnel of a potential donor. OPO personnel make the request for donation and, if necessary, manage the donor until surgery. Blood is sent for blood type and HLA determination on all consented donors well before any organs are removed. This histocompatability information, along with demographic information, clinical information related to the events of death and medical history are entered into *DonorNet®*.

Zero Antigen Mismatch Allocation Section

UNet® (the electronic matching system) then searches the waitlist for any blood type compatible potential recipients who are a zero MM with the donor (Fig. 5.4). If any such individual is found, then one kidney is allocated to that person. Preference is given to individuals who are blood type identical to the donor. If there are multiple potential zero mismatch individuals on the waitlist, the kidney goes first to any zero mismatch candidate in the local DSA with the highest point total, then to any regional zero MM candidate with the highest point total, and then to the zero mismatch individual anywhere in the United States with the highest point total. In the zero MM section of the match, candidates receive points as follows:

1. 1 point for each year waiting
2. 4 points for a CPRA of 80% or greater with defined unacceptable antigens
3. 4 points if age <11 years
4. 3 points if age 11–17 years
5. 4 points if previous donor of organ

	A	A	B	B	DR	DR	HLA LOCI
Recipient	1	2	7	8	1	3	
Donor 1	1	2	7	8	1	3	HLA IDENTICAL
Donor 2	1		7		1		0 - ABDR MM
Donor 3	2	1	7		1	3	0 - ABDR MM

Example of types of 0 - ABDR MM: When the recipient has all the alleles the donor has. If there is no allele number under the locus, it is presumed that the candidate has the same alleles at both loci.

Fig. 5.4 6-ABDR match vs. zero antigen mismatch

If only one kidney is allocated to a zero antigen mismatched candidate, then the second organ is allocated to a candidate who is not zero antigen mismatched unless there are two local zero MM candidates, and then both kidneys go to zero MM candidates. Offers of zero MM SCD kidneys must be made within 8 h of procurement. Offers of zero MM ECD kidneys must be made within 4 h of procurement.

The zero MM process has been retained in the allocation system for two reasons: (1) the survival of zero MM kidneys has historically been significantly better than any other match grade; (2) it gives recipients hope that a kidney may be available from the moment they are waitlisted. However, it is inherently unfair to minorities in the United States because the majority of donors are white and the HLA allele frequency differs in whites and minorities. Thus, whites have a greater chance of matching a white donor completely. For this reason, eliminating the zero

MM algorithm is evaluated each time changes are made to the allocation system. One such change began in January 2009. Now, zero MM shares will only be mandatory for adult candidates with CPRA > 20% and for all pediatric candidates.

The Main Allocation Section of the Match

The main allocation schema considers blood type *identity*, wait time, DR loci match, sensitization status as determined by %CPRA, former donor status, and pediatric age to determine a point total for each waitlisted individual. Kidneys from blood type "O" donors are allocated to "O" candidates. Kidneys from blood type "B" donors are allocated to "B" candidates. These policies help equalize waiting time across blood types. In certain circumstances, blood type "A" kidneys (which are typically allocated to blood type "A" or "AB" candidates), may be allocated to blood type "B" candidates. In the main allocation section of the match, candidates receive points as follows:
1. 0, 1, or 2 points for DR match (one point per locus match)
2. 4 points if prior living donor
3. 4 points if CPRA 80% or greater and defined unacceptable antigens
4. 1 point for each year waiting

Candidates 18 years of age or older may be listed as active on the waitlist at any time to be eligible for zero MM kidneys, but do not begin to accrue WT for all other kidneys until their GFR drops below 20 cc/min or they begin RRT. Candidates who are less than 18 years of age begin to accrue WT upon listing. In addition, SCD kidneys from donors less than 35 years of age are allocated first to candidates with CPRA of 80% or greater with the highest point total and then preferentially to candidates less than 18 years of age irrespective of point total.

The kidney is offered to the candidate first locally, then in the region, and finally, in the nation. If there are multiple individuals with the same eligibility, the kidney goes to the individual with the earliest list date. When equitable, the allocation system attempts to favor local donation because it has been shown that the adverse effect of the cold ischemia experienced by the organ during transport increases with the duration of the cold exposure.

The ECD Section of the Match

Candidates receive points and waiting time as in the standard section of the match. Only candidates who have agreed to accept ECD kidneys participate in the allocation of these kidneys.

The ECD program has been very successful. A review of 2 years of this program in 2004 showed the predictions of RR of graft failure to be accurate.[12] Both the recovery and the use of these kidneys have increased significantly.

OPO personnel also play an important role in the receipt of kidneys for transplantation. Each OPO maintains the local transplant waitlist for its designated geographic service area (DSA). An OPO may have only one member kidney transplant program – such as Life Share of the Carolinas in Charlotte, NC. In such a case, the DSA waitlist is the same as the Charlotte Memorial Hospital kidney program waitlist. Or, the DSA may contain several transplant programs – such as Carolina Donor Services in Raleigh, NC, where there are four kidney transplant programs. The waitlist at CDS is a combined waitlist of patients waiting at all four programs. The term "local donation" refers to the situation when the donor and the recipient reside within the same DSA.

At the present time, the rules of the OPTN allow candidates to be listed at multiple transplant centers. Such a practice should be considered for all candidates who are highly sensitized, i.e., have a high level of PRA in their blood resulting from previous blood transfusions, previous pregnancies, or previous transplants. High levels of PRA greatly reduce the number of organs available to a candidate. Listing such a candidate at a transplant center in a different DSA or a different region allows them exposure to *more* and *different* local and regional organs.

Kidney offers for a patient on the waitlist are made via *DonorNet*® to designated medical personnel at the kidney program, and the local OPO is notified because its personnel usually facilitate delivery of the organ. Physicians at the transplant program review all the information in *DonorNet*® about the donor and accept or refuse an organ offer for their patient. The final decision to accept a particular kidney remains the prerogative of the transplant surgeon or physician responsible for the care of the patient. Reasons for refusal might be that the patient is sick or cannot be found. A record of refusal codes is maintained by UNOS. If the organ is accepted, local transplant program protocols are begun to insure expeditious engraftment.

Recently, buoyed by the great success of the new lung allocation program which has essentially eliminated the waiting list for lung candidates, great effort has been devoted to the development of a new KAS. The goal has been to achieve equity and utility and to maximize "life years from transplant" (LYFT) and widespread input is being sought. Consensus has been difficult to achieve, and as of 2010, this project remains a work in progress.

UNOS, Data, and Research

Data collection has always been an integral part of UNOS and the OPTN. NOTA requires three foci for data:

- provide information to physicians and other health professionals regarding organ donation
- collect, analyze, and publish data concerning organ donation and transplants
- develop and maintain a scientific registry of the recipients of organ transplants

From 1987 until 2000, UNOS performed all this data collection and analysis. In 2000, HHS initiated a separate contract for operation of the scientific registry, and since then, the SRTR has been operated by Arbor Research/University of Michigan (Fig. 5.1).

Currently, the SRTR is responsible for publishing an annual report on the state of solid organ transplantation in the United States and for performing any additional studies requested by HHS. The expertise of the SRTR staff and the registry database may be utilized by UNOS committees when they are evaluating policy changes. A current example of this collaboration is the ongoing evaluation of the KAS.

UNOS retains responsibility for *all* data collection – both for the OPTN and the SRTR – and for analysis and process improvement of the operations of the OPTN. Additionally, individual investigator requested studies from the OPTN membership are handled by the scientific staff at UNOS. This is a wonderful opportunity for researchers in the field of transplantation to avail themselves of expert research and statistical assistance.

Part 2: What Is an OPO and How Does It Work?

Patricia L. Adams and Susan Gunderson

An OPO is a non-profit organization federally designated by CMS to operate within a DSA to procure solid organs for transplant. Usually, the OPO also serves as the procurement agent for tissues – skin, bone, heart valves, etc. – within the same DSA. The primary mission of the OPO is to maximize organ donation within the designated area and to facilitate placement of organs for transplant to centers both within the local region and across the country.

History. Some OPOs have been in existence for many decades. The NEOB, for instance, was founded in 1968.[13] Initially, organizations were formed by groups of transplant centers that banded together to facilitate organ sharing. As strange as it may seem today, most organ donation programs in the 1970s and 1980s were operated by transplant centers and procurement was the responsibility of transplant center personnel – surgical transplant fellows, transplant faculty, urology faculty, or fellows. At times, such as when multiple donors were available, it severely taxed surgical staff to complete all the donations and the subsequent transplants. Additionally, since the transplant centers were focused understandably on the recipients, promoting organ donation was a secondary focus. In the late 1980s, as more and more organs were transplanted, it became clear that the transplantation enterprise needed a group focused primarily on serving donors and donor families to ensure that organs are provided for all the waiting candidates.

Legislative Governance

While the donation process has evolved with several national and state legislative directives, the seminal legislation for OPO activity was the *Uniform Anatomical Gift Act of 1968* which provided a uniform environment for organ and tissue donation in the United States and created the legal right for individuals to donate organs and tissues.[14] This act was amended in 1987 and again in 2006. The most recent amendments focus on honoring the choice of an individual to be or not to be a donor and strengthening the language barring others from overriding a donor's decision to make an anatomical gift.

Other important legislative directives include *The NOTA of 1984*, which established the framework for the growth of OPOs as separate corporate entities from transplant centers.[3] The *OPO Certification Act of 2000* established regulations that governed the participation of OPOs in Medicare.[15] Between 1987 and 2008, the number of OPOs decreased to 58 in number: 50 independent organizations and 8 hospital-based programs (Fig. 5.5). The AOPO was formed and a national accreditation program was created. There are now 49 accredited OPOs within the United States.[16] Additionally, as mentioned above, more than 80% of OPOs currently recover tissue for medical use, but this function is certified by the AATB and regulated by the FDA, not CMS. A few OPOs are also involved in tissue processing and distribution. In 2006, *the Conditions of Participation for OPOs, Final Rule*, was published. This rule established process and outcome metrics to be met in the OPO certification process.[17]

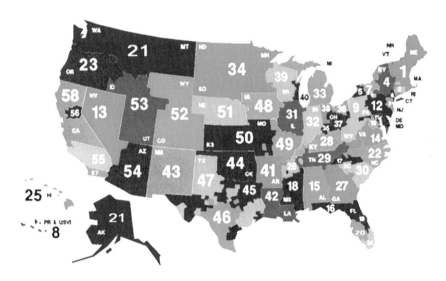

Fig. 5.5 Locations of currently active OPOs

OPO Organization

While all OPOs have a common mission of maximizing organ donation, size and service scope vary widely across the 58 entities, serving populations from 1 million to over 17 million and coordinating from fewer than 25 to over 400 organ donors annually. OPO oversight for independent OPOs is governed by a board of directors, typically comprised of community leaders, transplant center representatives, and individuals representing organ donors and transplant recipients.

Services provided by OPOs are usually organized around clinical, education/communication, tissue, and administrative functions. Clinical operations provide 24/7 service to respond to donor referrals; meet with families to seek donation authorization or validate the donor's decision; manage the donor to maximize organ function; direct organ placement with transplant centers; coordinate surgical retrieval and provide support to the donor family. OPO clinical staff work closely with UNOS and transplant centers to match donors and recipients.

Communications specialists are responsible for increasing public support for donation. Within the hospital setting, hospital services specialists are accountable for creating a highly functioning donor program. Tissue operations teams coordinate tissue recovery, typically within the donor hospital or medical examiner office.

The Organ Donor Breakthrough Collaboratives

The breakthrough collaboratives have been described as "the first innovative, universal partnership on a national level since the invention of required request."[18] In April 2003, HHS announced the first Organ Donation Breakthrough Collaborative. This was an initiative developed by the DOT of the HRSA branch of HHS, in concert with the IHI.[19] The intent was to reform organ donation in the United States by utilizing a "change package" derived from the best practices of the OPOs and large hospitals which had organ donation conversion rates (see glossary for definition) of 75% or better. The package initially had 4 strategies and about 30 key concepts. By the end of the first national collaborative meeting, it had morphed into a set of eight "First Things First Changes" necessary to achieve baseline donation rates at the national average and a set of six "High Leverage Changes" associated with getting to donation rates of 75% or greater.[19] These change packages were put into operation around the country. By the end of 2007, deceased organ donation had increased by a record 25% over the 2003 baseline. There have now been 4 national organ donation and transplantation breakthrough collaboratives and over 10 learning sessions. Deceased organ donation has continued to increase each year since 2004 (Figs. 5.6 and 5.7). DOT recognizes all donor hospitals, transplant centers, and OPOs which meet their performance goals at a yearly awards ceremony. However, DOT has announced that it will no longer be supporting future collaboratives financially, so other groups such as the Organ Donation and Transplantation Alliance are expanding their role to continue the focused national work of expanding organ donation.

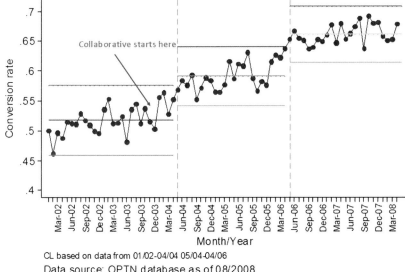

Fig. 5.6 Conversion rate by month, 1999–April 2008

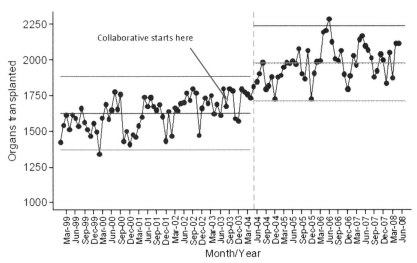

Fig. 5.7 Organs transplanted by month, 1999–May 2008

Role of the OPO in Organ Allocation

Although the P in OPO stands for procurement, OPO personnel are increasingly involved in organ allocation. To maximize each donated organ, OPO staff work to improve organ function through donor management, with the goal of ensuring that every transplantable organ can be utilized by a recipient. OPO personnel at the donor site enter information about the donor into *DonorNet*® and initiate the match run. Typically the OPO contracts with local surgical personnel for procurement of the donor organ, although some OPOs have their own staff for organ recovery. The OPO makes arrangements for surgical teams, both local and from other areas, which fly in to procure organs (often the case for liver, lung, or heart). OPO personnel are available to answer questions by phone from transplant centers and work closely with accepting transplant centers to maintain optimal organ function. They arrange transport for organs and on rare occasions even accompany the organ to its destination.

The OPO works closely with the transplant centers and programs within its service area, ranging from as few as 1 center to more than 12 within the DSA. Each OPO also maintains the combined "local" waitlist for all transplant centers within the DSA and receives organ offers for its centers from the Organ Center at UNOS or from other OPOs across the country. Some OPOs provide a very active service in receiving electronic organ offers from the Organ Center or screening calls from other OPOs with organ offers for candidates. Other OPOs are more passive in their participation, serving only as a relay service to the transplant center of the potential candidate. Ultimately, actual organ acceptance is always the prerogative of the transplant center. The OPO may also arrange local and distant transportation for the *incoming* organs. In short, OPO personnel are the ultimate facilitators: their role is to create a community and hospital culture supportive of donation, identify potential donors, honor designated donors decisions and seek authorization from family members when the donor's intent is unknown, and make sure that every precious donated organ makes it to its intended recipient. With no end in sight to the growing number of patients who can benefit from an organ transplant, the challenge to "ensure that every donation opportunity is fulfilled" will continue to be the mission of the OPO.

OPO Role in Living Donation

Historically, OPOs have not had much of a role in living donation. Living donors are typically identified and evaluated by the transplant center. However, in recent years, transplant centers have increasingly made use of "donor swaps" for their patients. In its simplest form, a donor swap occurs when there are two willing donors and two recipients, but each donor cannot give to his/her loved one, so the donors swap recipients. Common reasons for swaps are blood type incompatibility or a positive cross match between the original donor–recipient pairs. At the present time, some of these swaps involve five or more donor–recipient pairs, residing at multiple transplant centers across the nation. It seems inevitable that the OPO community, with its skill at organ transport and logistics, might eventually become involved in facilitating these swaps.

Glossary

AATB	American Association of Tissue Banks
AOPO	Association of Organ Procurement Organizations
CMS	Center for Medicare and Medicaid Services; one branch of HHS
CPRA	calculated panel reactive antibody; measures a recipient's preformed antibodies to donor antigens
Crossmatch	a histocompatibility test measuring the degree to which a recipient's immune system reacts against a donor
DCD	donation after cardiac death
DonorNet®	electronic donor information and organ offer system
Donor swaps	when two or more recipients exchange living donors because their original donors cannot donate to them because of incompatible blood type or positive crossmatch
DOT	Department of Transplantation
DSA	designated service area
ECD	expanded criteria donor
FDA	Federal Drug Administration
HCFA	Health Care Financing Administration; former name for CMS
HHS	Department of Health and Human Services
HRSA	Health Resources and Services Administration; one branch of HHS; home of the DOT
IHI	Institute for Healthcare Improvement
KAS	kidney allocation system
LYFT	life years from transplant
MPSC	Membership and Professional Standards Committee
NEOB	New England Organ Bank
NOTA	National Organ and Transplant Act of 1984
OPO	organ procurement organization
OPTN	Organ Procurement and Transplant Network
Organ donation conversion rate	number of actual donors as percent of eligible donors
RRT	renal replacement therapy
SCD	standard criteria donor
Sensitized candidate	has preformed anti-HLA antibodies (PRA) in the blood
SEROPP	South-Eastern Regional Organ Procurement Program
SEOPF	South-Eastern Organ Procurement Foundation
SRTR	Scientific Registry for Transplant Recipients

SSA   Social Security Act
Transplant center   usually a large hospital complex where multiple types of
                             transplants done
Transplant program   usually part of a transplant center; focused on one organ
Unet®   the electronic matching system
UNOS   United Network for Organ Sharing
0-ABDR MM   zero mismatch; this refers to the situation when the donor
                             has no allele which is different from the recipient even
                             though the donor does not have all the alleles of the
                             recipient

References

1. Pierce GA. UNOS history. In: Phillips MG (ed.), *Organ Procurement, Preservation and Distribution in Transplantation*. Richmond, VA, The William Byrd Press, Inc., 1991, pp. 1–3.
3. National Organ Transplant Act. 1984 Oct 19. Report No: Title 42, USC, Section 273.
2. Organ procurement and transplantation network. Health resources and services administration (HRSA). Final rule. *Fed Regist* 1999 Oct 20;64(202):56650–56661.
4. USC. Section 1138 of the Social Security Act 42. 2009. Report No: 1320.
5. Graham W. The 'Yin and Yang' of UNOS, A personal retrospective on UNOS' first two decades. UNOS Update 2008 Jun.
8. McDiarmid SV, Pruett TL, Graham WK. The oversight of solid organ transplantation in the United States. *Am J Transplant* 2008 April;8(4):739–744.
6. Health Resources and Services Administration (HRSA). Response to Solicitation on Organ Procurement and Transplantation Network (OPTN) Living Donor Guidelines. *Fed Regist* 2006 Jun 16;71:116.
7. Health Resources and Services Administration (HRSA). Medicare Program. Hospital conditions of participation: requirements for approval and re-approval of transplant center to perform organ transplants. Final rule. *Fed Regist* 2007 Mar 30;72:61.
9. Port FK, Bragg-Gresham JL, Metzger RA et al. Donor characteristics associated with reduced graft survival: an approach to expanding the pool of kidney donors. *Transplantation* 2002 Nov 15;74(9):1281–1286.
10. Rosengard BR, Feng S, Alfrey EJ et al. Report of the Crystal City meeting to maximize the use of organs recovered from the cadaver donor. *Am J Transplant* 2002 Sep;2(8):701–711.
11. Ojo AO, Hanson JA, Meier-Kriesche H et al. Survival in recipients of marginal cadaveric donor kidneys compared with other recipients and wait-listed transplant candidates. *J Am Soc Nephrol* 2001 Mar;12(3):589–597.
12. Sung RS, Guidinger MK, Lake CD et al. Impact of the expanded criteria donor allocation system on the use of expanded criteria donor kidneys. *Transplantation* 2005 May 15;79(9):1257–1261.
13. New England Organ Bank. 2007.
14. Uniform Anatomical Gift Act. 2006.
15. OPO Certification of 2000. Report No: Section 701 (c), 2000 Oct 13.
16. Association of Organ Procurement Organizations. 2004.
17. Health Resources and Services Administration (HRSA). Medicare and Medicaid Programs. Conditions for coverage for organ procurement organizations (OPO's). Final rule. *Fed Regist* 2006 May 31;71(104).
18. Mayes G. CMS proposes rules for organ procurement organizations aimed at increasing organ donation and improving performance. *Medscape Transplantation* 2005 May 20;6(1).
19. Organ Donation Breakthrough Collaborative. 2009 Oct 19.

Chapter 6
Live Donors: How to Optimally Protect the Donor

Robert Steiner

The purpose of this chapter is to offer evidence-based guidelines for donor selection practices – specific reasons to accept and specific reasons to refuse. This chapter also offers guidelines to assess the potential donor's understanding of the risks and benefits of donation.

What "Normal" Donors Face

There are no "normal" donors if "normal" means "safe." Young healthy donors are thought to be the least problematic, but in fact are at relatively high predonation "baseline" lifetime risk for ESRD. The prevalence of CKD stages 1–4 increased across the board from 10 to 13% in the United States in the past decade.[1] In 2006, there were 99,535 new ESRD patients.[2] In 2016, there are projected to be 136,166 new ESRD patients.[3] In 2002, for unselected young donors, the lifetime risk for dialysis was calculated to be 2–3% for whites and 6–7% for African Americans.[4] These disparate racial risk ratios persist for donors who need dialysis in later life.[5] Some apparently normal donors – particularly young donors – will inevitably fall prey to new onset glomerular disease, diabetic nephropathy, hypertensive-vascular nephropathy, or stone disease, although the risks in the general population are quite different for each of these entities.[6] Because ESRD is a disease of older patients, if all the ESRD a 25 year old donor were to experience in the next 20 years could be foreseen and these donors excluded, virtually all of their lifetime risk would remain. This risk is greater than the baseline risk of many middle aged nondiabetic otherwise normal hypertensive donors.[7] Many other middle aged donors with a variety of isolated medical abnormalities are probably at about the same or less baseline lifetime risk for ESRD as are young normal donors. Thus, it is futile for the nephrologist to try to identify safe donors, because all of them are at risk, e.g., for isolated medical abnormalities and the renal diseases with which they are associated.

R. Steiner (✉)
University of California at San Diego Medical Center, San Diego, CA, USA
e-mail: rsteiner@ucsd.edu

D.B. McKay, S.M. Steinberg (eds.), *Kidney Transplantation: A Guide to the Care of Kidney Transplant Recipients*, DOI 10.1007/978-1-4419-1690-7_6,
© Springer Science+Business Media, LLC 2010

As will be emphasized in this chapter, there is no firm dividing line between the counseling of "normal" donors and those with isolated medical abnormalities. Luckily, many important risks can be communicated clearly in a quantified fashion to all donors as they decide about the appropriateness of donation. Such "negative" information helps avoid donor inattention or romanticism. In our experience, this does not change the decision to donate but increases the comfort of the patients' physicians with donor selection, because donors know what they might expect in later life. Tools to help the practitioner assess the potential donor's motivation and understanding of the short and long-term risks are provided in this chapter (Testing Donors' Knowledge and Reasoning).

The Medical Evaluation and Operative Risk of Prospective Donors

A number of detailed protocols for the medical evaluation of potential donors have been proposed that are similar to the testing listed in Table 6.1.[8] The first tests ordered in the medical evaluation of the potential donor are the blood group typing (types A, B, AB, and O) and human leukocyte antigen (HLA) typing. If the blood groups are incompatible (e.g., potential donor is blood group A and potential recipient is blood group O), the donor evaluation stops, unless a donor "swap" is planned (see Chapter 8). If there are several potential donors, the HLA typing helps determine the closest genetic match (see Chapter 4). Closeness of match is often given great importance by donor families when there are several potential candidates and this might be a source of unjustified pressure for a partially matched donor.

Table 6.1 Tests to evaluate potential live kidney donors

Initial Tests:
    Blood Group Typing
    HLA Typing

History, physical and psychosocial examination
    Multiple blood pressure determinations
    Donor motivation and knowledge assessment

Urinalysis
    Dipstick for protein, blood and glucose
    Microscopy, culture
    Measurement of protein excretion if indicated

Renal Function
    24-hr urine for creatinine clearance (repeated if inaccurate collection)
    24-hr urine for calcium, urate or oxalate in stone formers

Blood screening

    Hematology

        CBC, coagulation screen, G6PD deficiency (if indicated)

    Chemistry Panel

        Creatinine, urea and electrolytes
        Liver function tests
        Urate
        Fasting plasma glucose
        Glucose tolerance test (if elevated FBG, family history of DM or obese)
        Lipid profile
        Thyroid function tests (if indicated)
        Pregnancy test (in all women of childbearing age)
        PSA

    Virology Screen

        Hepatitis B and C
        Toxoplasma
        Syphilis
        HIV
        HTLV 1 and 2
        Cytomegalovirus
        Epstein-Barr virus
        In persons from high risk regions also screen for: *malaria, babesiosis, west nile virus, schistosomiasis, coccidomycosis, HHV8, HSV, strongyloides, typhoid, brucellosis.*

Cardiopulmonary System

    Chest X-ray
    Electrocardiogram
    Exercise stress test
    Echocardiogram
    Angiography (when indicated)
    Pulmonary function tests (when indicated)

Assessment of renal anatomy

    Magnetic resonance angiography (MRA)
    Magnetic resonance imaging (MRI)

If the blood types are a match, the work-up proceeds with a medical and psychosocial evaluation of the potential donor. A thorough history and physical exam is conducted and blood pressures are assessed in the office and at intervals after the initial exam. A psychosocial evaluation is performed by a credentialed examiner. Extensive laboratory examinations are performed to determine glomerular filtration rate and to search for evidence of hereditary renal disease, nephrolithiasis, or evidence of urinary or renal vascular structural abnormalities. The medical evaluation also involves of testing for intrinsic cardiovascular or pulmonary diseases, evidence of malignancy, and evidence of either active or past infectious diseases as well as assessment of metabolic disorders.

The purpose of medically testing donors is to estimate operative risk, to detect transmissible disease, to ascertain kidney quality, and to help estimate the long-term baseline (2 kidney) renal risks of the donor. As no two donors will have exactly the same risks in most of these categories, medical testing is not necessarily performed to rule out donors at "increased risk," but to have information to counsel donors and their recipients about their risks. For example, the increasing number of donors with varying degrees of obesity that presents a spectrum of perioperative risks[9,10] and long-term risks for kidney disease are associated with the metabolic syndrome.

Any donor beginning a typically thorough donor examination must know that abnormalities may be discovered that will bear on his or her future ability to obtain insurance. Abnormalities may be discovered that warrant further evaluation for the sake of the potential donor's health. To minimize conflict of interest, we recommend that the involvement of the transplant center ceases at this point and that the donor candidate be evaluated by the donor's private physician according to the usual standard of practice. Donors must also know that the transplant center will not provide long-term care to them for any medical condition, even if it is present at the time of donation or otherwise related to donation.

Donors must also be aware that donation may impact their long-term insurability. If the donor develops renal disease after donation, he/she might not be insurable due to a "preexisting condition."

Surgical Risks

The surgical evaluation for donation includes review of the medical evaluation and review of the donor screening tests, including imaging exams (magnetic resonance angiography) to assess the vasculature of the donor kidney. The surgeon provides another opportunity for the donors to change their mind about donating; further assurance that the donation is voluntary. Counseling donors about the operative procedure itself is usually straightforward, as the risks are low and well characterized. Many donor nephrectomies are performed laparoscopically and the risks from 28 centers for complications of any type (atelectasis, infection, ileus, transfusion, etc.) are 10%, with major complications (vessel or other injury, acute renal failure, rhabdomyolysis, etc.) occurring in 4 out of 100 procedures. Perioperative death did not occur in over 3,000 procurements.[9,10] A discussion of laparoscopic donation can be found in Chapter 7.

Medical Testing of the Potential Donor

Donor Glomerular Filtration Rate (GFR)

GFRs can be measured most accurately by clearances of iothalamate or inulin, surrogates of GFR, which correlate imperfectly with creatinine clearances. The MDRD equation uses the serum creatinine to estimate a GFR normalized for body surface area, but it has only a 90% chance of being within 30% of the iothalamate GFR,[11] due to individual variations in creatinine production rates and possibly to degrees of obesity when body surface area (BSA) is calculated from height and weight. The MDRDE underestimates GFR at higher ranges, i.e., the range over which centers are concerned when evaluating their donors.[12] For these reasons GFRs estimated by the MDRD equation should not be used to profile renal function in potential donors. Although a measured 24 h creatinine clearance is not normalized for BSA and correlates imperfectly with the iothalamate GFR, most centers evaluate donors with creatinine clearances, which also supply information on creatinine production rates. Interestingly, when creatinine clearances are measured under controlled conditions, at the same time as inulin clearances, the correlation is extremely good.[13] A 24 h protein excretion rate can be determined at the same time, as can urine calcium, urate, and oxalate, if there is a question of risk of nephrolithiasis.

Whether GFR is normal or borderline reduced, the presence of actual renal disease (e.g., low clearance plus echodensity and/or abnormal urinalysis) in a donor candidate is another matter, as diseased kidneys do not hypertrophy well, either in the donor or in the recipient. As risk counseling cannot be performed, these donors are unacceptable, not necessarily because the risks are known to be high, but because the risks cannot be confidently or reasonably estimated.

Donors with borderline low GFR with no evidence of disease (no hematuria or dipstick proteinuria) are perhaps in a different category. There is biologic variation in GFR at any age, and GFR decreases with age. Therefore a borderline low GFR does not necessarily indicate intrinsic renal disease. In contrast, the degree of dipstick positive albuminuria is a predictor of subsequent deterioration in renal function.[14] When kidneys from older donors are transplanted, baseline GFR is lower, but hypertrophy and limitation of loss of GFR occur proportionally in the donor after donation.[15] Smaller donors will have lower GFRs but these may increase when normalized (i.e., standardized for donor size, usually measured as body surface area). The usual rule is to keep predonation clearance within two standard deviations of the normal clearance for the patient's age.[16] To predict long-term results, as discussed below, clearances fall by an average of about 5 cc/min/decade after an initial loss of about 20 cc/min at nephrectomy. Having said this, an older donor with a clearance of 80 cc/min, no matter how much above average that may be for the donor's age, will not provide as good a kidney as a younger donor with a clearance of 140 cc/min. As with most questions, it is easier to deal with paradigms than it is to agree on borderline cases, e.g., GFRs that will fall in the 70 cc/min range. In these borderline cases, GFR should be normalized for ideal body weight and a split function isotope scan should be performed to see how GFR is distributed between the two kidneys.

Risks of Donation for Those with Specific Medical Conditions

Diabetes Mellitus (DM)

Type II diabetes can be present for years, causing complications without clinical episodes that necessarily lead to detection of the state of glucose intolerance. The American Diabetes Association recommends screening by measurement of fasting blood sugar and provides a nomogram for calculating the risk of diabetes for various potential donors (www.diabetes.org). The presence of variable amounts of risk in a donor population does not automatically preclude donation, as various risks are universal, but calculating diabetic risk is the basis for effective donor counseling about future diabetes. Type I or type II diabetes is present for 20 years before proteinuria develops (in about 20% of patients), and about half of these patients develop ESRD in another 5 years.[17] Control of blood pressure seems to be far and away from the most effective preventative measure against nephropathy.[18]

The "obesity epidemic" in the United States has increased the number of potential donors who will be discovered as diabetic during the donor evaluation. Many potential donors with a positive glucose tolerance test develop diabetes and chronic renal failure in later life.[19] The presence of DM among adults in the United States was 6.9% in 1999, a 40% increase over the preceding 10 years.[20] The lifetime risk of DM for individuals born in the year 2000 is about one in three.[20] White males have about a one in four risk, and the risk in black males is about 50% greater. Hispanic males have another 10% increase in risk over blacks. The same lifetime risk ratios hold among white, black, and Hispanic females, but their risks at any age are 10–20% greater than for males.[20] There were over 48,000 new patients with ESRD due to DM in 2006, almost 45% of the total number of new patients.[2] Diabetic nephropathy therefore remains a major long-term risk for young donors after donation and therefore diabetic persons are not acceptable donor candidates.

A difficult situation occurs when evaluating a potential young donor with a strong family history of diabetes. The younger the donor the more difficult this dilemma becomes due to the risk of late onset diabetes, particularly in the setting of obesity. All young donors are at substantial risk, but in general those at highest risk for developing type 2 diabetes mellitus include persons with a family history of type 2 diabetes, a current BMI >30 kg/m^2, female gender, African American or Hispanic race, a history of gestational diabetes mellitus, and those with a history of excessive alcohol use.[8] If a potential donor has a personal history of diabetes, has a fasting blood glucose over 126 mg/dl (7.0 mmol/L) on at least two occasions or a 2 h oral glucose tolerance test blood level of over 200 mg/ml (11.1 mmmol/L), donation may be inadvisable on the basis of heroic or irrational risk as discussed below.[8]

Obesity

Obesity is defined as a body mass index (BMI) of >30 kg/m^2. Obese and morbidly obese (BMI>40 kg/m^2) potential donors are becoming more common due to the obesity epidemic in the United States. A BMI >35 kg/m^2 is considered a relative contraindication to donation at many transplant centers, particularly if there are associated comorbidities.[8] All obese donors should be screened for comorbidities such as diabetes mellitus, hypertension, cardiovascular disease, sleep apnea, liver disease, albuminuria, and dyslipidemia. Considering only long-term risk, apart from operative risk, as a large fraction of younger donors will become obese over time and develop comorbidities, centers may have to reconcile their policies of accepting young overweight, nonobese, healthy donors (particularly African American donors) while excluding middle-aged donors with minor obesity-related comorbidities who have no overt renal disease. This latter group may well be at lower overall lifetime risk for CKD (on the order of 1%) than many young "normal" candidates.

Obese donors should be encouraged to lose weight before donation and should be informed of short- and long-term risks associated with donation, such as hypertension, proteinuria, and renal disease.

Hypertension

Depending on how it is defined, hypertension is prevalent in about 25% of the US population of about 300 million people, so otherwise normal donor candidates who have blood pressures of 140/90 are not uncommon. Many centers reject potential donors with a blood pressure of 140/90 because they have a risk factor for ESRD.[21–23] The risk to donors with borderline elevation in blood pressure is very close to the risk for donors with high normal blood pressure. In fact, some donors who were considered normotensive and acceptable candidates in past decades are now considered hypertensive. Hypertension as a risk factor is discussed in more detail below.

Potential donors with mild, easily controlled hypertension can be considered to have an acceptable risk for donation if they meet defined criteria. These criteria are age >50 years, GFR >80 ml/min, and normal urinalysis. If these persons are accepted as donors, they should be counseled as to the presence of a risk factor as discussed below and know that they must have lifelong physician follow-up.[8] The method of blood pressure detection plays an important role in the evaluation of hypertension in donors. In patients that are older (>50 years) and those with high office blood pressures, the preferred method in difficult cases is ambulatory blood pressure monitoring.[8] Typical middle aged donor candidates with mild hypertension are probably at less risk than young normal donors[7].

Proteinuria

The presence of dipstick proteinuria is consistent with a long list of renal diseases, and the risk of ESRD is often strikingly proportional to the degree of proteinuria,[14,24] so a 20-year risk of ESRD cannot be estimated from proteinuria incidence and ESRD prevalence population statistics. However, cohort studies suggest that trace to 1+ proteinuria may have a less than 1 in 100 twenty-year risk of ESRD.[14,24] Proteinuria that is greater than or equal to 2+ (100 mg/dl) has five times the risk for ESRD than does an eGFR of <60 cc/min/1.73 m2.[14] Insofar as dipstick proteinuria often indicates significant parenchymal damage that may limit posttransplant hypertrophy as discussed above, the transplant may be inadvisable on those grounds alone.

Programs that accept or refuse donors with minimal degrees or proteinuria should have some basic data in mind to underlie selection and counseling of possibly acceptable donors. Microalbuminuria (MA) and nonalbumin (non-dipstick) proteinuria must be discussed separately. Microalbuminuria is present in about 5% of the "normal" general population[25] and is a risk for general cardiovascular disease, not renal disease. The risk of MA is greater, in fact, in the upper range of normal blood pressures.[26] Elevated nonalbumin proteinuria (e.g., when a 24 h collection shows 300 mg/day of such protein) is far more common than even low-grade dipstick proteinuria.[27] With this finding, the 20-year risk for ESRD would be well under one in 100, and the risk for values close to the upper range of normal is about the same as for those values in the upper range of normal.

Intrinsic Renal Disease

Kidneys with overt intrinsic disease should not be transplanted for two reasons: our functional expectations after transplantation for the recipient[28] and the donor[29] are probably based on the expectation of hypertrophy in the solitary kidney. This is most obvious in the adult recipient who receives transplanted pediatric kidneys. In the presence of mild donor disease one cannot be sure about posttransplant compensatory hypertrophy, in either the donor or the recipient. Even mild intrinsic renal disease at the time of donation increases the risk of eventual ESRD. Most centers consider this risk alone to be too heroic even for a willing and well-informed donor.

Recurrent and Familial Renal Disease

Recurrence of glomerular disease (GN) may be higher in normal kidneys transplanted from related donors, but such procedures are not contraindicated. Membranous GN, focal sclerosis, lupus nephritis, pauci-immune GN, IgA nephropathy, and membranoproliferative GN are relatively common diseases that recur. The overall damage from recurrent disease is somewhat unclear, as long-term graft survival is about the same when patients with these diseases are transplanted as it is for other ESRD diagnoses.[30] However, familial disease such as familial focal sclerosing glomerulonephritis may occur in sibling donors who do not have detectable disease at the time of donation. In general, the older the (normal) donor, the less the likelihood of missing significant familial disease. For example, "idiopathic" microscopic hematuria in an otherwise normal 55-year-old member of an Alport's kindred with a GFR of 100 cc/min might pose an acceptable donor risk to many centers. Polycystic kidney disease (PKD) is largely ruled out by the absence of cysts on ultrasound in a patient aged 30 or older.[16] CT scanning is more sensitive, and CT criteria have not been established. Two cysts in a candidate under 30 make the disease highly probable.[16] Genetic testing is expensive, complicated, and may not be entirely definitive but represents an advance over imaging alone for difficult cases. Just as in the general case, donor counseling here would include presenting the average loss of 20–25% of GFR at donation, with new onset CKD some time after donation proportionately abridging the time over which past donation disease progressed to dialysis by the same 20–25%. As discussed in the sections below, the same rate of progression has been documented in specific studies of two-kidney and one-kidney patients with either PCK or diabetic glomerular disease. What the donor seems to give up is the reduction in baseline function at which the progression of CKD would begin.

Nephrolithiasis

The donor candidate with a single small stone, past or present, meets with variable acceptance by transplant centers. Some are told they cannot donate because it is "too risky," but no risk estimate is offered or formulated. The high prevalence of stones in the general population and the low incidence of patients going on dialysis because of stones support a 20-year risk estimate for ESRD of one in several hundred for these donor candidates.[31]

The typical donor candidate who presents to most centers is among the lowest risk of the at-risk subgroup with stones. Studies of patients nephrectomized for recurrent stone disease are sometimes cited in discussing the risk of stone disease, but this severe form of stone disease is not representative of typical donor candidates. Furthermore, current imaging techniques may detect smaller stones,[32] and if such techniques were historically applied to the general population, they would increase the prevalence of stone disease, which lowers the risk estimate for ESRD from stones. A recent study from the Mayo Clinic suggests about a 50% increased risk of CKD and ESRD that is associated with diagnosed stone formers,[33] but causality is uncertain. Stones are widespread in the general population, but the number of new ESRD patients with ESRD specifically attributed to stone disease is not even 1% of the yearly total.[31]

Microhematuria

Many centers accept selected donors with isolated microscopic hematuria (IMH).[21–23,34] As discussed below, population risk factor prevalence and ESRD incidence data suggest that the 20-year risk for ESRD is less than 1 in 100 for these candidates.[6] A long-term study of a cohort with IMH suggests a similar risk.[35] If biopsy in these patients shows glomerular disease, it is IgA or other mesangial disease in about half the candidates.[36,37] By definition, these candidates have no proteinuria, and, as with many renal diseases, the absence of proteinuria for IgA nephropathy is correlated with the most stable and benign prognosis.[38] To counsel about what risks to expect if progressive IgA nephropathy develops, the counseling projections based on an initial loss of 20–25% of GFR with donor nephrectomy would apply. If a donor is biopsied and abnormalities of any sort are found, what is to be told to the donor? It is not usual practice to routinely biopsy "normal" donors, whom we know to do extremely well after nephrectomy. However, one study of 231 such unselected "normal" donors found more than half of all biopsies showed interstitial and/or vascular changes, and 12% showed mesangial expansion. Small differences within the normal range in serum creatinine and proteinuria between the two groups were noted.[39] This study probably tells us what lies "beneath the surface" in the many studies of donors who have maintained excellent renal function after donation.

Malignancy

All donors should be screened to exclude malignancy. A prior history of several malignancies excludes donation. These include melanoma, testicular cancer, renal cell carcinoma, choriocarcinoma, hematological malignancy, bronchial cancer, breast cancer, and monoclonal gammopathy.[8] In certain cases a prior history of malignancy is acceptable. These cases include cancers in which the primary malignancy is thought to be cured, assurance that renal impairment did not result from treatment of the cancer, and assurance that potential transmission of the cancer can be reasonably excluded (e.g., a lengthy time has elapsed since treatment). It is important though to be sure the donor and recipient understand that transmission of cancer cannot be assured completely.

Counseling Donors with Isolated Medical Abnormalities (IMAs)

Certain universal donor selection issues are hotly debated when discussing donors with common IMAs such as a past or present kidney stone, or intermittent microhematuria.[21–23,34] Very often the risk of these conditions varies with the severity of the single abnormality, and these severity/risk relationships are also present across the spectrum of the normal range.

In many cases, no agreement exists among centers about the acceptability of donors with isolated hematuria, mild hypertension, etc., but some centers do accept these donors with varying frequency. Various forums and consensus gatherings have proposed guidelines for accepting donors with IMAs, but the explicit ethical framework that should govern rules for donor selection and the risk estimations that are conceptually mandated by these guidelines are usually incompletely developed, if at all. Many typical donor candidates with IMAs face a slight risk of renal impairment. But, many will still have an expected incidence of ESRD over 20 years of less than 1%.[6,31] Young normal donors have major risks of developing IMAs over a long lifetime, so like it or not, centers always have to deal with a continuum of risk that does not permit easy decisions if one approaches this area honestly.[7] But such decisions are always easier when actual risk data are available to all parties who are involved in the decision. Even if a center accepted all of its donors with

IMAs, this would not greatly increase the overall transplant rates.[28] The purpose of risk estimation is rather to accept and reject donors defensibly, on the basis of a well thought out philosophy and the data to back it up.

Estimating Risks Associated with Donation and the Example of Hypertension in Donor Candidates

Donor risk should be estimated because such quantification is the basis for rational donor selection (i.e., acceptance as well as refusal). Risk must be expressed as the risk of something over some period of time. Populations with risk factors for ESRD (e.g., hypertension, hematuria) have been followed for development of ESRD. When the risk that is found in such studies is expressed as, e.g., 1 per 10,000 patient years, the 20-year risk of ESRD is 20/10,000, or 1 in 500. The US population has an estimated prevalence of hypertension of about 25% of 300 million people and a yearly incidence of hypertensive ESRD of 28,000 cases.[2] Otherwise normal donor candidates who have blood pressures of 140/90, for example, are not uncommon.

Many centers reject these candidates because they have a risk factor for ESRD.[21-23] Actual yearly risk – expressed as the expected incidence of ESRD per year per patient in this national cohort of hypertensive patients – can be estimated as 28,000 divided by 75,000,000, which equals about 1 in 3,000. The 20-year risk is 20 times this rate or 2 in 300 or 1 in 150. This figure overestimates risk for a typical donor candidate, i.e., it represents a "limiting value." Many hypertensive patients do not have ESRD from hypertension itself but suffer primarily from other factors causing parenchymal injury and secondary hypertension,[40,41,7] leading to an over-diagnosis of hypertensive ESRD and overestimation of the risks. The typical donor candidate will be in the "low risk" part of the cohort, but there is also a continuum of risk extending through the normal range of blood pressures,[42] which extends through marginally hypertensive donors.

The baseline risks for ESRD for some hypothetical donors may be estimated at less than 1 in 100 over 20 years. This is not intended to suggest that a risk of 1 in 100 is acceptable or unacceptable. Deciding on the acceptability of any risk is a separate process that must consider acceptable risk taking decisions in other areas of life and what risk the public – whose support is essential to the transplantation effort – would think acceptable in the donor's individual context, especially if harm eventually came to the donor.

The Effect of Nephrectomy on Long-Term Kidney Function

The effect of nephrectomy on long-term kidney function is probably the single most important issue for donors because it applies to the increase in "uremia" caused by loss of renal function from nephrectomy and the effect of uninephrectomy on the course of renal disease that might be acquired in the years after donation.[28,29] A reasonable approach to the potential donor query regarding the risk of donation might be "If you donate, renal-related problems that might happen after donation will be worse by about 20–25%." The actual figure from a meta-analysis of over 3,000 nephrectomies is an average loss of GFR of 17% and a further loss of about 6 cc/min/decade thereafter.[43] This rate of decline is significantly less than for the unselected, general population. In another meta-analysis of proteinuria and loss of GFR in kidney donors,[44] 6 years after donation, the average GFR was 86 and the decrement in GFR was 26 cc/min, or 23% from predonation. (This figure would have included a "normal" gradual loss of several cc/min over the 6 years after donation.) The same review also includes pooled data showing that GFR was only 10 cc/min lower in donors compared to (two kidney) controls, a figure that sounds too low for losing half of one's total renal mass.

In summary, whatever GFR a potential donor is fated to have with 2 kidneys at any point in his life, predicting on the average a donation-induced 20–25% worsening of uremia at that same time point seems reasonable. This would correspond to an increase in serum creatinine from 1 mg/dl without donation to 1.2 or 1.3 mg/dl after donation. If a hypothetical donor were fated to develop a "two kidney" creatinine of 5 mg/dl in 20 years, all else being equal, the creatinine would be 6.0–7.0 mg/dl if donation had occurred 20 years earlier. The precise health effects of this loss of GFR are not clear, but the poor prognosis associated with even mild decreases in GFR in the general population probably relate mainly to coexisting vascular disease and the metabolic syndrome, not the decrease in GFR itself.[45] A number of short-term studies attempting to separate risks associated with the metabolic syndrome from the risk associated with increased uremia after donation have found no increase in cardiovascular risk after donor nephrectomy.[45,46] Both in longevity and in preservation of GFR, living kidney donors seem to do better than the general two-kidney population [47] no doubt in part due to their good medical condition at the time of screening. Different well-informed practitioners might come to somewhat different opinions, but they should be debated within this general framework.

Nephrectomy itself causes hyperfiltration in the remaining kidney. A less-than-normal decline in renal function decade by decade in uninephrectomised patients supports the position that the effect of nephrectomy on the loss of GFR with ageing is small. After nephrectomy, hypertension eventually occurs in 30% of patients[48]; the loss of GFR decade by decade is still less than in the normal population.[43]

The increased glomerular capillary pressure associated with post-donation compensatory hypertrophy has been thought to accelerate "two-kidney" renal diseases.[49] However, such hyperfiltration probably occurs early in the course of most progressive renal disease as intact nephrons attempt to compensate for those with greater damage. Thus, hyperfiltration would not be unique to disease in the remaining kidney in a previous donor and, for this reason, may not be much of an additional factor in predicting deterioration in renal function. The best data on this question has come from a cohort of uninephrectomised polycystic patients, who lost renal function at the same rate as a two-kidney cohort.[50] Small cohorts of uninephrectomised patients with diabetic nephropathy who lost renal function slowly have been reported,[51] but data were limited. A recent study of uninephrectomised patients with diabetic nephropathy suggests that the rate of development of diabetic glomerular disease is about the same for patients with two kidneys and patients with one kidney.[52] Angiotensin II inhibitors classically lower glomerular pressure and preserve renal function in the renoprival state, and these agents may also slow progression of disease after nephrectomy.

Testing Donors' Knowledge and Reasoning

Donor testing is appropriately performed by transplant center social workers or donor advocates. But it can be done informally in the office when the donor medical evaluation is reviewed. Although these techniques have been recommended to transplant centers,[53] they can be adapted by the general nephrologist in his or her role as donor counselor. As with teaching of important information in other areas of life, it is not enough just to present information to donors – they must be tested. In our hands, such testing has not been difficult. When testing reveals donor candidates who are poorly informed or not thinking through the issues that justify donation, they are more likely to be thinking irrationally, uncommitted to donation, coerced, or even perhaps surreptitiously paid. In all these cases the donor needs to be protected from proceeding with donation until these questions can be resolved.

Donor testing is simple and the application is straightforward. These tests can be written or they can be read to the donor so that he or she may answer. A donor does not have to get every question right the first time, but letting the donor perform in a structured setting roots out misconceptions, inattentiveness (when donation is because of pressure or payment), and irrational thinking. Testing the donor makes him or her an active participant and reinforces the idea that he or she is making a decision that should be based on risk and benefit, not romanticizing.

There is no downside to teaching and testing even the most legitimately motivated donor (e.g., parent to young child) this way. It has been argued that "emotionally motivated" donors – like the distraught parent – do not need counseling. However, distraught parents still basically feel that their donating is benefiting the child, and therefore teaching the nature of that benefit – and confirming the donor's understanding of what he or she is risking – is essential to a defensible donation. Testing donors assures that corners are not being cut and self-interest not indulged. Potential donors should be made to understand that they will not be allowed to donate until they retain and process the essential facts that are contained in defensible donor education.

In general, a donor must be provided with all relevant information about the donation. As can be seen from the examples provided in this chapter that includes a significant amount of "negative" information that might dissuade a donor. To insure donor protection, if the initial impulse is not to provide information because it might deter donation, that is a good reason to provide it in the teaching materials.

True–false testing (Fig. 6.2). Questions presented as part of a testing instrument can be used by transplant centers, but the same thing can be done conversationally in the office of a general nephrologist. Fifteen true–false questions that cover many essential facts are shown in Table 6.2. The purpose of true–false testing is to probe the donor's knowledge of specific facts about the risks of donation.

Table 6.2 True–false questions for donor candidates

"The lifetime risk of dialysis varies from almost 3% to over 7% in the general population." (True. Over a 75 year lifetime, the risk for whites approaches 3%, and for blacks 7%.)

"Passing the donor medical exam reduces my lifetime risk of dialysis to zero." (False. The lifetime risk for most acceptable donors is probably less than 1 in 100 depending on personal risk factors. But medical conditions may arise in later life that will lead to kidney failure. If this happens, having donated will bring about the need for dialysis at an earlier time than if donation did not occur.)

"On average, donating a kidney will cause immediate loss of about 25% of my total kidney function." (True. This figure is an average from a large number of patients and will vary from maybe 15 to 25%.)

"How closely a donor and recipient are matched should not be the deciding factor in selecting a donor." (True. Donors and recipients need to be compatible, which is common, but so-called perfect matches are rare. Only a perfect match gives significant additional benefit.)

"Kidneys from deceased donors usually only work 2 or 3 years." (False. Half of these kidneys will be working at 9 years.)

"About half the people who begin dialysis in the US are over 60." (True. Many kidney diseases begin in middle age or later and worsen slowly.)

"Kidney transplantation is life-saving." (False. While transplantation appears to lengthen the life span of a dialysis patient, most good candidates can live on dialysis for years while waiting for a deceased donor kidney.)

"Very few transplant candidates will live long enough on dialysis to receive a deceased donor kidney." (False. Especially with good compliance, many people live on dialysis and are active for years.)

"A living donor kidney transplant can be expected to last 20 years." (False. One out of two living donor kidney recipients will be back on dialysis in about 15 years.)

"Less than 1 out of 100 living donor transplants are lost in the first year." (False. National experience predicts that almost 1 of 20 will be back on dialysis by 1 year.)

"Donating a kidney will cause me to develop kidney disease." (False. Donation will decrease the overall kidney function you would have when you developed a kidney disease. Donation would be responsible for someone having to begin dialysis only if the remaining kidney developed cancer or a very severe blockage, or was severely damaged by an accident, a stabbing, etc.)

"The need for transplantation is so urgent that time should not be wasted on learning about donating." (False. Kidney transplantation is not lifesaving because patients can be supported by dialysis. The only really good decision for anyone is based on knowing the risks, benefits, and alternatives.)

"I will earn the gratitude of the center by donating." (False. you will earn the gratitude of the center by being honest about misgivings and fully recognizing your RIGHT not to have to donate to anyone.)

"If I develop kidney disease or risk factors in later life, the center will provide me free medical care." (False. Only the testing for donation, the donor operation, and specific, immediate follow up of that operation is covered by donor insurance. Besides this, the center cannot provide free checkups, medications, or other care to its donors, for any medical problem.)

"Once I decide to donate I cannot change my mind." (False. You can change your mind even up to the day the operation is scheduled.)

Questions that are missed should prompt special attention. Donors who are ultimately acceptable need not get everything right the first time, although many will do so. Most ultimately acceptable donors will get most answers right at an early point after their donor teaching is completed. When questions are incorrectly answered, sometimes the problem is only linguistic or the misconceptions are minor. But in any case, the correct answers must be taught and re-tested, either at the same sitting or at another time.

The donor belief profile (DBP): a test for rational thought (Table 6.3). This instrument is a bit different than the true–false questions and is intended to test for rational thought, i.e., how well does the decision to donate fit with the donor's other goals, needs, and beliefs? To varying degrees, all centers assess donors for rational thought by spending time with them and forming an impression of the way they are processing information to decide on donation. Without a correct donor opinion on the DBP questions, which cover a number of issues that are highly relevant to donation, the rationality of donation is dubious. The donor must have *an* opinion on these issues and also have the *correct* opinion. For example, an acceptable donor must believe that "living donation has sufficient advantages over deceased kidney donation" and "dialysis is a less acceptable alternative than transplantation." The DBP again reminds the donor that he or she must process important information that would support reasonable donation. A donor who thinks dialysis is better than transplantation or has no opinion on the acceptability of dialysis for the recipient is not thinking clearly, because one goal of donation precisely is to avoid dialysis.

Table 6.3 Donor belief profiling

The following issues must be correctly decided by donor candidates who are making a rational decision to donate. Wishing to donate but not having decided these issues correctly could be a sign of a distracted donor, a pressured donor, a donor who is driven by guilt, a paid donor, etc. In any case, the only defensible decision for the donor is one that is grounded in the following:

- Transplantation is sufficiently better than dialysis for the recipient.
- Living donor transplantation is sufficiently better than deceased donor transplantation.
- My transplanted kidney will probably work for the recipient for a reasonable period of time.
- I understand the facts and issues (risks, benefits, and alternatives) well enough to make a reasoned decision to donate.
- My life situation will permit donation at this time.
- I am not deciding to donate because of pressure from someone else.
- I choose to take risks of donation to try to achieve benefit for my recipient.

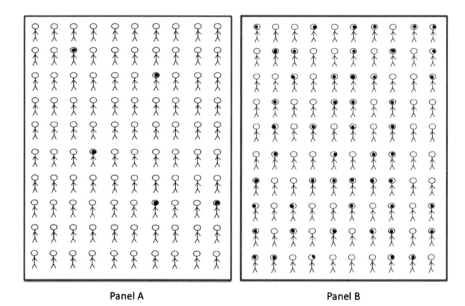

	Panel A			Panel B	

Fig. 6.1 Panels **A** and **B**. Quantitative teaching of risk and benefit. The *first panel* displays a 5 out of 100 incidences, e.g., the 5% graft failure rate of living donor kidneys at 1 year. The *second panel* displays a 50% incidence, e.g., the 50% rate of graft loss at 14–15 years

Teaching risk quantitatively with stick figure diagrams (Figs. 6.1a, b). Simply calling donation "high risk" or "low risk" does not convey much actual information. Often, transplant physicians call donation "high risk" because they cannot estimate risk at all, not because they know the risk to be high. As has been discussed, "risk" has to mean "risk of something" (e.g., ESRD) over an "interval of time" (e.g., 20 years). The task of a donor counselor is to put risk data in this teachable and understandable form. Risk then becomes relatively easy to teach using stick figure diagrams. These fields of 100 or 1,000 stick figures present percentage data less pejoratively than saying "high risk, low risk" and convey actual data as well. The stick figure diagram also illustrates to donors the "all or nothing" nature of some bad outcomes. That is, a 20% chance of dialysis for ESRD shows 20 of 100 stick figures on dialysis, not 100 stick figures each of whom is 20% worse off.[54]

Assuring Confidentiality

Donor testing reinforces to the donor that he/she is making an important decision that is supported by donor values and the facts of donor risk and recipient benefit. Donors and their families should be told from the outset that counseling will be one on one, and donor information will not be directly shared with the recipient or other interested parties. We ask that donors come to their appointments without the recipient or anyone else that might conceivably be a source of pressure to donate. Even if that person is sitting in the waiting room while donation is discussed, clear contemplation of the option not to donate may be difficult. Larger sessions with family and recipient together can be scheduled separately.

Ethical Issues

Perfectly safe donation would be a boon to transplant professionals, as donors would not need to be counseled about the baseline two-kidney risks of ESRD in later life or the effect of nephrectomy on the progression of later life chronic kidney disease (CKD). But "first of all do no harm" does not, in a straightforward sense, apply to living kidney donation, as donors always take risk and are always harmed by the donor nephrectomy. The same ethical criteria govern the selection of all donors: donors must be informed, uncoerced, and deciding rationally, and their acceptance must not unavoidably threaten the public trust in the transplantation effort.[28] Certain situations may invite special scrutiny in any of these areas, e.g., when donors are met over the Internet[29] or when they seem to be willing to take heroic risk.[28] The real mission of the transplant team is a systematic approach that protects the donor by informing him/her of the spectrum of risks and probabilities of good and bad outcomes, tests him/her for the rationality of his choice, assesses for coercion, and at times denies an ethically valid, legitimate "heroic" donation to limit public distrust that might be generated by bad outcomes.

Some conscientious transplant physicians, concerned with their responsibilities and sensitive to the negative effects of potential criticism, deal with uncertainty by denying donors out of hand when any problems arise. The ethics of this response can be questioned, as transplant professionals hold themselves out to be responsible decision makers who should make defensible decisions to say no as well as to say yes. Denying a donor may indeed be appropriate if there is enough uncertainty and that uncertainty is unavoidable. However, the step that most donor counselors have not taken is to try to develop a body of knowledge about donor risk that can be used to formulate selection policy and to teach to donors. Some will feel that attempting to calculate donor risk is a step backward that will promote a cavalier approach. But because there is no safe transplantation, we have no choice. The donor counselor must not necessarily deny donation out of hand but must "know what he or she is talking about" when asked to address isolated medical abnormalities such as hypertension or a renal stone that is discovered in the donor evaluation. The transplant community has appropriately focused on preventing unethical selection of kidney donors, but donors who are refused for insubstantial reasons, when the donor counselor is not well informed about risk, are also not well served. It does not somehow make one more ethical to deny transplantation as "too risky" simply because of unfamiliarity with the body of medical fact that relates to donor risk.

Protecting the potential living kidney donor requires knowledge and teaching of the facts surrounding living kidney donation. It also involves the ability to test the donor's knowledge of both short- and long-term risk and the spectrum of outcomes that are possible for the recipient. Protecting the donor requires that he or she decides be deciding to donate in a structured and rational manner. These are the characteristics of a decision to donate that is defensible to the public, whose support is vital to the transplant effort. They do not preclude emotion and compassion but they should underlie the decisions of even the most compassionate donors.

We cannot completely protect donors from harm and risk, but even the lowest risk donors have the right to say no and should be refused if they are not appropriately deciding to proceed. We must accept the reality of donor harm and risk and see that the correct processes are undertaken and that the correct criteria are met. This is the best way we can protect our donor candidates and the larger transplant effort by ensuring good, defensible donor decisions.

References

1. Coresh J, Selvin E, Stevens LA, Manzi J, Kusek JW, Eggers P, Van Lente F, Levey AS. Prevalence of chronic kidney disease in the United States. *J Am Med Assoc* 2007; 298: 2038–2047.
2. Collins AJ, Foley RN, Herzog C, Chavers B, Gilbertson D, Ishani A, Kasiske B, Liu J, Mau LW, McBean M, Murray A, St Peter W, Guo H, Li Q, Li S, Li S, Peng Y, Qiu Y, Roberts T, Skeans M, Snyder J, Solid C, Wang C, Weinhandl E, Zaun D, Arko C, Chen SC, Dalleska F, Daniels F, Dunning S, Ebben J, Frazier E, Hanzlik C, Johnson R, Sheets D, Wang X, Forrest B, Constantini E, Everson S, Eggers P, Agodoa L. United States Renal Data System 2008 annual data report abstract. *Am J Kidney Dis* 2009; 53:vi–vii, S8–S374.
3. Gilbertson DT, Liu J, Xue JL, Louis TA, Solid CA, Ebben JP, Collins AJ. Projecting the number of patients with end-stage renal disease in the United States to the year 2015. *J Am Soc Nephrol* 2005; 16:3736–3741.
4. Kiberd BA, Clase CM. Cumulative risk for developing end-stage renal disease in the US population. *J Am Soc Nephrol* 2002; 13:1635–1644.
5. Gibney EM, King AL, Maluf DG, Garg AX, Parikh CR. Living kidney donors requiring transplantation: focus on African Americans. *Transplantation* 2007; 84:647–649.
6. Steiner RW, Danovitch G. The medical evaluation and risk estimation of end-stage renal disease for living kidney donors. In: RW Steiner (ed.), *Educating, Evaluating, and Selecting Living Kidney Donors*. Kluwer Academic Publishers, Dordrecht, The Netherlands, 2004, pp. 51–79.
7. Steiner, RW. 'Normal for Now' or 'At Future Risk': A double standard for selecting young and older living kidney donors. *Am J Transplant* 2010. (In Press)
8. Delmonico F. A report of the Amsterdam forum on the care of the live kidney donor: data and medical guidelines. *Transplantation* 2005; 79:S53–S66.
9. Kavoussi LR. Laparoscopic donor nephrectomy. *Kidney Int* 2000; 57:2175–2186.
10. Patel S, Cassuto J, Orloff M, Tsoulfas G, Zand M, Kashyap R, Jain A, Bozorgzadeh A, Abt P. Minimizing morbidity of organ donation: analysis of factors for perioperative complications after living-donor nephrectomy in the United States. *Transplantation* 2008; 85: 561–565.
11. Levey AS, Bosch JP, Lewis JB, Greene T, Rogers N, Roth D. A more accurate method to estimate glomerular filtration rate from serum creatinine: a new prediction equation. Modification of Diet in Renal Disease Study Group. *Ann Intern Med* 1999; 130: 461–470.

12. Issa N, Meyer KH, Arrigain S, Choure G, Fatica RA, Nurko S, Stephany BR, Poggio ED. Evaluation of creatinine-based estimates of glomerular filtration rate in a large cohort of living kidney donors. *Transplantation* 2008; 86:223–230.
13. Lemann J, Bidani AK, Bain RP, Lewis EJ, Rohde RD. Use of the serum creatinine to estimate glomerular filtration rate in health and early diabetic nephropathy. Collaborative Study Group of Angiotensin Converting Enzyme Inhibition in Diabetic Nephropathy. *Am J Kidney Dis* 1990; 16:236–243.
14. Ishani A, Grandits GA, Grimm RH, Svendsen KH, Collins AJ, Prineas RJ, Neaton JD. Association of single measurements of dipstick proteinuria, estimated glomerular filtration rate, and hematocrit with 25-year incidence of end-stage renal disease in the multiple risk factor intervention trial. *J Am Soc Nephrol* 2006; 17:1444–1452.
15. Rook M, Bosma RJ, van Son WJ, Hofker HS, van der Heide JJ, ter Wee PM, Ploeg RJ, Navis GJ. Nephrectomy elicits impact of age and BMI on renal hemodynamics: lower post-donation reserve capacity in older or overweight kidney donors. *Am J Transplant* 2008; 8:2077–2085.
16. Marson LP, Lumsdaine JA, Forsythe JLR, Hartmann A. Selection and evaluation of potential living kidney donors. In: RS Gaston, J Wadstom (eds.), *Living Donor Kidney Transplantation*. Taylor and Francis, Abingdon, Oxon, 2005, pp. 33–54.
17. Ritz E, Orth SR. Nephropathy in patients with type 2 diabetes mellitus. *N Engl J Med* 1999; 341:1127–1133.
18. Havas S. The ACCORD Trial and control of blood glucose level in type 2 diabetes mellitus: time to challenge conventional wisdom. *Arch Intern Med* 2009; 169:150–154.
19. Ritz E. Metabolic syndrome: an emerging threat to renal function. *Clin J Am Soc Nephrol* 2007; 2:869–871.
20. Narayan KM, Boyle JP, Thompson TJ, Sorensen SW, Williamson DF. Lifetime risk for diabetes mellitus in the United States. *J Am Med Assoc* 2003; 290:1884–1890.
21. Mandelbrot DA, Pavlakis M, Danovitch GM, Johnson SR, Karp SJ, Khwaja K, Hanto DW, Rodrigue JR. The medical evaluation of living kidney donors: a survey of US transplant centers. *Am J Transplant* 2007; 7:2333–2343.
22. Kasiske BL, Bia MJ. The evaluation and selection of living kidney donors. *Am J Kidney Dis* 1995; 26:387–398.
23. Reese PP, Feldman HI, McBride MA, Anderson K, Asch DA, Bloom RD. Substantial variation in the acceptance of medically complex live kidney donors across US renal transplant centers. *Am J Transplant* 2008; 8:2062–2070.
24. Iseki K, Ikemiya Y, Iseki C, Takishita S. Proteinuria and the risk of developing end-stage renal disease. *Kidney Int* 2003; 63:1468–1474.
25. Jones CA, Francis ME, Eberhardt MS, Chavers B, Coresh J, Engelgau M, Kusek JW, Byrd-Holt D, Narayan KM, Herman WH, Jones CP, Salive M, Agodoa LY. Microalbuminuria in the US population: third National Health and Nutrition Examination Survey. *Am J Kidney Dis* 2002; 39:445–459.
26. Knight EL, Kramer HM, Curhan GC. High-normal blood pressure and microalbuminuria. *Am J Kidney Dis* 2003; 41:588–595.
27. Kannel WB, Stampfer MJ, Castelli WP, Verter J. The prognostic significance of proteinuria: the Framingham study. *Am Heart J* 1984; 108:1347–1352.
28. Steiner RW, Gert B. Ethical selection of living kidney donors. *Am J Kidney Dis* 2000; 36: 677–686.
29. Friedman AL, Lopez-Soler RI, Cuffy MC, Cronin DC 2nd. Patient access to transplantation with an Internet-identified live kidney donor: a survey of U.S. centers. *Transplantation* 2008; 85:794–798.
30. Choy BY, Chan TM, Lai KN. Recurrent glomerulonephritis after kidney transplantation. *Am J Transplant* 2006; 6:2535–2542.
31. Steiner RW. Risk appreciation for living kidney donors: another new subspecialty? *Am J Transplant* 2004; 4:694–697.

32. Winchester P, Kapur S, Prince MR. Noninvasive imaging of living kidney donors. *Transplantation* 2008; 86:1168–1169.
33. Rule A, Bergstralh E, Melton LJ, Li X, Weeaver A, Lieske J 2008. Kidney stones are associated with and increased risk of developing chronic kidney disease. In *American Society of Nephrology Annual Meeting 2008*. [F-FC202], Mayo Clinic; Health Sciences Research.
34. Thiel GT, Nolte C, Tsinalis D. Living kidney donors with isolated medical abnormalities: the SOL-DHR experience. In: RS Gaston, J Wadstom (eds.), *Living Donor Kidney Transplantation*. Taylor and Francis, Abingdon, Oxon, 2005, pp. 55–73.
35. Yamagata K, Takahashi H, Tomida C, Yamagata Y, Koyama A. Prognosis of asymptomatic hematuria and/or proteinuria in men. High prevalence of IgA nephropathy among proteinuric patients found in mass screening. *Nephron* 2002; 91:34–42.
36. Topham PS, Harper SJ, Furness PN, Harris KP, Walls J, Feehally J. Glomerular disease as a cause of isolated microscopic haematuria. *Q J Med* 1994; 87:329–335.
37. McGregor DO, Lynn KL, Bailey RR, Robson RA, Gardner J. Clinical audit of the use of renal biopsy in the management of isolated microscopic hematuria. *Clin Nephrol* 1998; 49:345–348.
38. Ibels LS, Gyory AZ, Caterson RJ, Pollock CA, Mahony JF, Waugh DA, Roger SD, Coulshed S. Primary IgA nephropathy: natural history and factors of importance in the progression of renal impairment. *Kidney Int Suppl* 1997; 61:S67–S70.
39. Mancilla E, Avila-Casado C, Uribe-Uribe N, Morales-Buenrostro LE, Rodriguez F, Vilatoba M, Gabilondo B, Aburto S, Rodriguez RM, Magana S, Magana F, Alberu J. Time-zero renal biopsy in living kidney transplantation: a valuable opportunity to correlate predonation clinical data with histological abnormalities. *Transplantation* 2008; 86: 1684–1688.
40. Kincaid-Smith P. Hypothesis: obesity and the insulin resistance syndrome play a major role in end-stage renal failure attributed to hypertension and labelled 'hypertensive nephrosclerosis'. *J Hypertens* 2004; 22:1051–1055.
41. Roland AS, Hildreth EA, Sellers AM. Occult primary renal disease in the hypertensive patient. *Arch Int Med* 1964; 113:101–110.
42. Vasan RS, Larson MG, Leip EP, Evans JC, O'Donnell CJ, Kannel WB, Levy D. Impact of high-normal blood pressure on the risk of cardiovascular disease. *N Engl J Med* 2001; 345:1291–1297.
43. Kasiske BL, Ma JZ, Louis TA, Swan SK. Long-term effects of reduced renal mass in humans. *Kidney Int* 1995; 48:814–819.
44. Garg AX, Muirhead N, Knoll G, Yang RC, Prasad GV, Thiessen-Philbrook H, Rosas-Arellano MP, Housawi A, Boudville N. Proteinuria and reduced kidney function in living kidney donors: A systematic review, meta-analysis, and meta-regression. *Kidney Int* 2006; 70:1801–1810.
45. Prasad GV, Lipszyc D, Huang M, Nash MM, Rapi L. A prospective observational study of changes in renal function and cardiovascular risk following living kidney donation. *Transplantation* 2008; 86:1315–1318.
46. Garg AX, Prasad GV, Thiessen-Philbrook HR, Ping L, Melo M, Gibney EM, Knoll G, Karpinski M, Parikh CR, Gill J, Storsley L, Vlasschaert M, Mamdani M. Cardiovascular disease and hypertension risk in living kidney donors: an analysis of health administrative data in Ontario, Canada. *Transplantation* 2008; 86:399–406.
47. Fehrman-Ekholm I, Elinder CG, Stenbeck M, Tyden G, Groth CG. Kidney donors live longer. *Transplantation* 1997; 64:976–978.
48. Mullaney SR, Zeigler MG. The risk of end stage renal disease for hypertensive kidney donors. In: RW Steiner (ed.), *Educating, Evaluating, and Selecting Living Kidney Donors*. Kluwer Academic Publishers, Dordrecht, The Netherlands, 2004, pp. 81–97.
49. Weir MR. The renoprotective effects of RAS inhibition: focus on prevention and treatment of chronic kidney disease. *Postgrad Med* 2009; 121:96–103.

50. Zeier M, Geberth S, Gonzalo A, Chauveau D, Grunfeld JP, Ritz E. The effect of uninephrectomy on progression of renal failure in autosomal dominant polycystic kidney disease. *J Am Soc Nephrol* 1992; 3:1119–1123.

51. Sampson MJ, Drury PL. Development of nephropathy in diabetic patients with a single kidney. *Diabet Med* 1990; 7:258–260.

52. Chang S, Caramori ML, Moriya R, Mauer M. Having one kidney does not accelerate the rate of development of diabetic nephropathy lesions in type 1 diabetic patients. *Diabetes* 2008; 57:1707–1711.

53. Steiner RW, Frederici CA. The education and counseling process for potential donors and donor attitudes after living kidney donation. In: RW Steiner (ed.), *Educating, Evaluating, and Selecting Living Kidney Donors*. Kluwer Academic Publishers, Dordrecht, The Netherlands, 2004, pp. 51–79.

54. Steiner RW, Gert B. A technique for presenting risk and outcome data to potential living renal transplant donors. *Transplantation* 2001; 71:1056–1057.

Chapter 7
Laparoscopic Donor Nephrectomy: Essentials for the Nephrologist

Arturo Martinez

History of Live donation

As of December 31, 2006, the United States Renal Data System (USRDS) reported that there were 506,256 patients with end-stage renal disease (ESRD)[1] and 83,559 died as a result of their ESRD.[2] As of November 21, 2008, there were 82,797 patients on the kidney transplant waiting list and 11,838 had undergone a transplantation with an expected >95% graft and patient success rate. Unfortunately, 2,742 died and 1,062 removed from the list because they were too sick for transplantation.[3] The success of transplantation has made it more common and available to a greater number of patients who previously would not have been candidates for transplantation. This success has also led to the explosion of the number of people waiting for a transplant and therefore the desire to expand the potential live and deceased donor pools. Prior to the development of laparoscopic surgery, the only viable means of extracting a kidney was to make a large flank or abdominal incision. Although all involved appreciated the inherent morbidity associated with the technique, it required the donor to sustain a protracted recovery with the potential for long-term discomfort. Laparoscopic surgery is a minimally invasive technique that seeks to accomplish the same goals of open surgery (i.e., remove or repair the target organ), but diminishing the morbidity and making it available to a wider group of patients.

A great deal has transpired since the first live donor transplant. In the last 20 years, 90,619 live donor nephrectomies have been performed since 1988.[4] The open technique was the only available technique for approximately 40 years. The procedure most commonly was performed via a flank approach in which an oblique incision, starting posteriorly from the 11th or 12th rib and extending to the lateral

A. Martinez (✉)
Department of Urology, The Permanente Medical Group, San Francisco, CA, USA
e-mail: havmar@sbcglobal.net

D.B. McKay, S.M. Steinberg (eds.), *Kidney Transplantation: A Guide to the Care of Kidney Transplant Recipients*, DOI 10.1007/978-1-4419-1690-7_7,
© Springer Science+Business Media, LLC 2010

edge of the rectus muscle, was made to gain access to the retroperitoneum. It was common to remove all or part of the rib during the procedure. The goal was to remove the kidney in the least traumatic fashion possible in order to preserve the kidney function, prevent post-transplant complications, and insure that the donor would be minimally affected. The outcome of the open approach was excellent. Open donor nephrectomy patients were found to have a normal or extended life expectancy[5] and an overall improved health compared to age-matched controls.[6] Although they were found to have a slight elevation in systolic blood pressure and mild proteinuria, the incidence of CKD was less than or equal to the general population.[7,8] Morbidity associated with the flank incision included the development of a pseudo hernia from the denervation of the flank muscles, pain associated from removing a rib, and a prolonged recovery from such a large incision.

First Laparoscopic Nephrectomy

The first laparoscopic nephrectomy was performed in 1990 by Dr. Ralph Clayman at the University of Washington, St Louis.[9] The case was notable for taking approximately 8 h. The rationale for this first case, of course, was to prove its feasibility and see if there could be improved results with regard to patient recovery. Since then innumerable laparoscopic nephrectomies have been performed for malignant and benign disease. In addition, laparoscopic partial nephrectomies, pyeloplasties, renal explorations, and ureteral reconstructions are now commonplace and represent only a small example of the urologic procedures that can be done via a minimally invasive approach. Numerous studies have demonstrated a lower morbidity of the laparoscopic nephrectomy and it has now become the standard of care in the majority of circumstances. With this experience in hand, extending the technique to live kidney donors was obvious in order to provide them the same benefit of smaller incisions, quicker recovery, a safe approach, reduced blood loss, and improved visualization.

First Laparoscopic Donor Nephrectomy (LDN)

The first LDN was performed by Ratner and associates in 1995.[10] Despite initial concerns about feasibility, trauma to the kidney, increased rates of transplant rejection, primary non-function, venous thrombosis, and questions as to whether the right kidney could be removed safely, studies demonstrate equal transplant outcomes with the technique.[11]

Current Number of Donors

Live donor kidneys account for 45% of all kidney transplants in the last 20 years in the United States.[12] An estimated 6,000 will be performed in 2008. These donors represent a very special group of people who are making the ultimate gift of life – a piece of themselves so that another human can have a better life.

Selection Criteria

Any new procedure should offer some advantage over the standard technique without compromising quality, outcome, or safety. Guidelines are published by the American Society of Transplant Physicians.[13] There should be strict adherence to safety and emotional stability of the potential donor.

Expanding Donors

The goal of all transplant centers is to find the best available kidney for their recipient in a timely manner. With the ever increasing waiting list and wait times, everyone involved is looking for ways to expand the potential donor pool. Laparoscopic donation has expanded the potential pool of donors by making it more palatable for patients and transplant professionals. The selection criteria for potential laparoscopic donors will not only be the same group of patients who would have normally donated but because of the reduced morbidity, it also encompasses a wider group of potential donors. Donors who would not normally have donated because of morbidity associated with a large operation, large scar, cosmetic issues, body image issues, logistical issues (prolonged time off work or school), and financial constraints are now more willing to donate. In addition, because of the smaller incisions associated with laparoscopic donor nephrectomies, patients who would have been excluded from donation are now more freely considered such as patients who are obese or who may have minor medical problems such as kidney stone disease and essential hypertension.[14]

Contraindications to Laparoscopic Donor Nephrectomy

At present the only contraindication to laparoscopic donation, in an otherwise viable donor, is available access to the kidney and experience of the surgical team with different approaches. Any kidney that can be removed open should be able to be removed via a minimally invasive technique if a working space can be developed. Prior abdominal procedures with significant abdominal adhesions might preclude a transabdominal approach. In this situation, if the surgical team is experienced in the retroperitoneal approach, the kidney can be extracted safely. Other anatomical considerations include renal fusion anomalies such as horseshoe kidneys, ectopic kidneys, multiple arteries, multiple veins, and duplicated collecting systems.

Approaches

There are three options for laparoscopic donor nephrectomy: transabdominal, retroperitoneal, and hand-assisted transabdominal. All approaches are very successful in experienced surgeons. They all require a 6–8 cm incision to extract the organ. The transabdominal approaches are the most common because the anatomy presents itself in a more conventional manner. The retroperitoneal approach has a steeper learning curve and requires readjusting one's perspective while keeping the anatomic landmarks clear. Most centers tend to use the pure laparoscopic transabdominal approach. It requires an incision and an extraction bag in order to remove the kidney after it has been devascularized. Injuries to the vessels and collecting system have occurred with this technique. The hand-assisted transabdominal approach has the advantage of using the required incision site to allow the surgeon to insert his/her hand during the dissection process. This approach has a shorter learning curve, has the potential of using fewer ports, and obviates the need for an extraction device that might cause injury to the kidney since the hand is used to remove the kidney once it has been devascularized.

How I Do It

I prefer the hand-assisted laparoscopic technique. I vary the operation based on which kidney is to be removed, gender, body habitus, prior incisions, and body image expectation of the donor. For younger patients, or for those who do not want to have an upper abdominal incision, the hand port incision for a left nephrectomy is a Pfannenstiel incision that can easily be concealed with underwear or bikini bottoms (Fig. 7.1). On the right side, a low oblique inguinal incision is also an option (Figs. 7.2 and 7.3). For all other patients whose left kidney is to be removed, the hand port is placed in the upper midline position (Fig. 7.4). The ergonomics for the

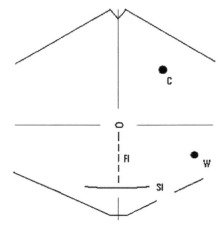

Fig. 7.1 Left nephrectomy via Pfannenstiel incision. SI, skin incision (7 cm); FI, fascial incision (8–10 cm); C, camera port; W, working port

Fig. 7.2 Right nephrectomy
via Pfannenstiel incision. SI,
skin incision (7 cm); FI,
fascial incision (8–10 cm); C,
camera port; W, working port

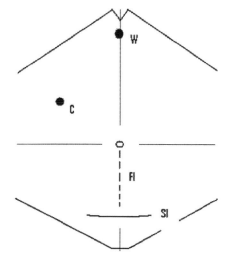

Fig. 7.3 Right nephrectomy
via oblique right lower
quadrant incision. SI, skin
incision (7 cm); FI, fascial
incision (8–10 cm); C,
camera port; W, working port

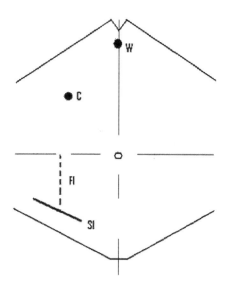

surgeon, in this position, are much better. Two additional working ports are used in
all situations: one for the camera and a working port for instruments.

A single incision technique is currently being developed which will obviate the
need of the two additional port sites. All instruments are introduced through the
single incision with the use of specialized articulating instruments or a robot.[15]

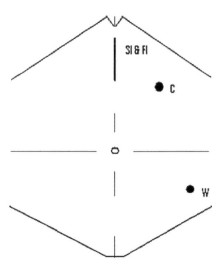

Fig. 7.4 Left nephrectomy via upper midline incision. SI, skin incision (7 cm); FI, fascial incision (8–10 cm); C, camera port; W, working port

Surgical Complications of Laparoscopic Donor Nephrectomies

The true complication rate is unknown for the procedure. There is currently no central donor registry to track all the live donor nephrectomy outcomes. Potential and known complications of the procedure include

  Wound infection
  Bowel injury
  Spleen, adrenal, and liver injury
  Neuropraxias from positioning
  Vascular injury during the extraction process
  Internal herniation
  Hemorrhage from malfunction of a vascular occlusive device
  Incisional hernias
  Injury to the kidney

Note: bowel injury and internal herniation can be avoided with the retroperitoneal approach.

Delayed Graft Function (DGF) and Acute Tubular Necrosis (ATN) with Laparoscopic Donor Nephrectomies

There is still controversy with regard to whether LDN causes an unacceptable rate of ATN and DGF in experienced centers today. According to Duchene and Winfield: "A critical analysis of DGF after LDN revealed that female donor kidneys into male

Table 7.1 Open vs. laproscopic donor nephrectomy

	Open nephrectomy[18]	Laparoscopic nephrectomy[16]
Surgical time	164 min [92–298] $n=50$	213 min [130–329] $n=1,872$
Blood loss	240 ml [20–1,800] $n=50$	160 cc [30–1,024] $n=1,772$
ATN/DGF rates	<1%	3.9% [2.6–11%] $n=1,472$
Patient recovery: LOS	3–5 days	1.1 days
Return to work	15 weeks	4–6 weeks

recipients and highly mismatched donors were significant factors in DGF, but no variable related to the LDN procedure itself (prolonged carbon dioxide pneumoperitoneum, warm ischemia time, renal artery length, use of right kidney) affected the functional outcome of the allograft".[16,17] Table 7.1 summarizes data from several large series of both open and LDN.

In my own experience, I decreased the ATN/DGF rate by making some simple but important technical changes to the procedure. The donor is aggressively hydrated with lactated ringer or normal saline at a rate of 1 l/h along with 12.5 g of Mannitol/l starting as soon as the IV is placed in the pre-op area and continued throughout the operation until the donor artery is clipped. Typically donors will receive 2–3 l of fluid during the entire procedure. Intraoperatively, the peritoneal pressure is maintained at 12 mmHg or less, care is taken to not stretch the artery unduly to avoid vascular spasm and the kidney is not removed unless there is a brisk diuresis. Furosemide 10 mg IV is sometimes used. With a hand-assisted approach, warm ischemia is minimized.

In conclusion, laparoscopic donor nephrectomy encompasses a number of approaches that have achieved the desired goal of producing a viable allograft and minimizing donor morbidity compared to the historical standard open approach.

References

1. http://www.usrds.org/2008/ref/B_Prevalence_08.pdf
2. http://www.usrds.org/2008/ref/H_Mortality_&_Causes_of_Death_08.pdf
3. OPTN: Organ Procurement and Transplantation Network 2008 report: Removal Reason, Kidney, http://www.optn.org/latestData/rptData.asp
4. http://www.optn.org/latestData/rptData.asp
5. Fehrman-Ekholm I et al. Kidney Donors Live Longer 1. *Transplantation* 1997 Oct 15; 64(7):976–978.
6. Anderson CF, Velosa JA, Frohnert PP et al. The risks of unilateral nephrectomy: status of kidney donors 10 to 20 years postoperatively. *Mayo Clin Proc* 1985; 60:367–374.
7. Provoost AP, Brenner BM. Long-term follow-up of humans with single kidneys: the need for longitudinal studies to assess true changes in renal function. *Curr Opin Nephrol Hypertens* 1993; 2:521–526.
8. Ohishi A, Suzuki H, Nakamoto H, Katsumata H, Hayashi K, Ryuzaki M et al. Status of patients who underwent uninephrectomy in adulthood more than twenty years ago. *Am J Kidney Dis* 1995; 26:889–897.

9. Clayman RV, Kavoussi LR, Soper NJ et al. Laparoscopic nephrectomy: initial case report. *J Urol* 1991; 146(2):278–282.
10. Ratner LE, Ciseck LJ, Moore RG et al. Laparoscopic live donor nephrectomy. *Transplantation* 1995; 60(9):1047–1049.
11. Derweesh IH, Goldfarb DA, Abreu SC, Goel M, Flechner SM, Modlin C, Zhou L, Streem SB, Novick AC, Gill IS. Laparoscopic live donor nephrectomy has equivalent early and late renal function outcomes compared with open donor nephrectomy. *Urology* 2005 May; 65(5): 862–866.
12. http://www.optn.org/latestData/rptData.asp
13. Delmonico FL, Dew MA. Living donor kidney transplantation in a global environment. *Kidney Int* 2007; 71:608–614. DOI:10.1038/sj.ki.5002125; published online 7 February 2007.
14. Schweitzer EJ, Wilson J, Jacobs S et al. Increased rates of donation with laparoscopic donor nephrectomy. *Ann Surg* 2000; 232(3):392–400.
15. Gill IS, Canes D, Aron M, Haber GP, Goldfarb DA, Flechner S, Desai MR, Kaouk JH, Desai MM. Single port transumbilical (E-NOTES) donor nephrectomy. *J Urol* 2008 Aug; 180(2):637–641; discussion 641. Epub 2008 Jun 12.
16. Duchene DA, Winfield HN. Laparoscopic donor nephrectomy. *Urol Clin North Am* 2008; 35:415–424.
17. Abreu SC, Goldfarb DA, Derweesh I et al. Factors related to delayed graft function after laparoscopic live donor nephrectomy. *J Urol* 2004; 171(1):52–57.
18. Kok NFM et al. Comparison of laparoscopic and mini incision open donor nephrectomy: single blind, randomised controlled clinical trial. *Br Med J* 2006 Jul 29; 333(7561):221.

Chapter 8
New Sources in Living Kidney Donation

Ruthanne L. Hanto, Alvin E. Roth, M. Utku Ünver, and Francis L. Delmonico

History

The first successful living kidney transplantation occurred in 1954 when Ronald Herrick donated a kidney to his identical twin brother, Richard, at the Peter Bent Brigham Hospital in Boston, Massachusetts. There was no possibility of a rejection of the kidney because the brothers were genetically identical twins. Since then, however, the field of kidney transplantation has evolved so that genetic identity or matching is no longer a necessary criterion for success. Advances in immunosuppressive drugs (and changes in attitudes toward non-directed living donation) currently allow successful kidney transplantation between donors and recipients even with a complete human leukocyte antigen (HLA) mismatch. Despite these advances, the risk of hyperacute rejection has prohibited kidney donation and transplantation between ABO blood type incompatible donors and renal transplant candidates. Transplantation of a kidney to a candidate who has developed antibody reactive to donor-specific HLA (alloantibodies) incurs an even greater risk. Candidates develop antibodies when exposed to foreign HLA antigens as the result of pregnancy, blood transfusion, previous organ transplant, and occasionally autoimmune disorders. To avoid kidney rejection in candidates who are sensitized (have developed preformed alloantibodies), a crossmatch of donor and candidate blood is performed prior to transplant. A positive crossmatch predicts rejection of the transplanted kidney and the donation would not occur.

Approximately one-third of potential living donors are unable to donate to their intended candidates due to either ABO incompatibility or antigen incompatibility indicated by a positive crossmatch.[1] Previously either of these incompatibilities prevented donation and transplantation. Transplantation across the ABO barrier has a reasonable success rate if one utilizes protocols that remove natural isoagglutinin antibodies and recipients are closely monitored after transplantation.

R.L. Hanto (✉)
New England Organ Bank, New England Program for Kidney Exchange, Organ Procurement Organization, Newton, MA, USA
e-mail: rhanto@neob.org

D.B. McKay, S.M. Steinberg (eds.), *Kidney Transplantation: A Guide to the Care of Kidney Transplant Recipients*, DOI 10.1007/978-1-4419-1690-7_8,
© Springer Science+Business Media, LLC 2010

Desensitization protocols that remove donor preformed HLA alloantibodies reactive to the donor antigens are increasing in utilization; however, these protocols are technically demanding and expensive with long-term outcomes unknown at this time. Kidney paired donation (KPD) and kidney list donation (KLD) are alternative options for candidates with an incompatible living donor.

The concept of KPD was initially conceived by Rapport in 1986,[2] but it was not implemented until 1991 when the first KPD transplants were performed in South Korea.[3] The United States performed its first KPD transplant in 2000 at Rhode Island Hospital when two adult children who were incompatible with their mothers each donated a kidney to the other's mother.[4] The first KLD in New England occurred in 2001.

New England Implementation

In February 2001, Region 1 of the United Network for Organ Sharing (UNOS) initiated a system of kidney transplantation that would enable renal transplant candidates to participate in either KPD or KLD among the 14 transplant centers and 2 organ procurement organizations (OPO) in New England.[5] This laid the groundwork for the establishment of the New England Program for Kidney Exchange (NEPKE)[6] in 2004.

Kidney List Donation

Kidney list donation, also known as living donor/deceased donor list exchange, occurs when the donor in an incompatible pair donates to someone on the UNOS deceased donor waitlist. In exchange for donating a kidney to a candidate on the waitlist, their incompatible candidate is allocated a kidney from the deceased donor pool (Fig. 8.1). Regions must apply for a variance from UNOS in the allocation of kidneys from deceased donors to participate in kidney list donation.

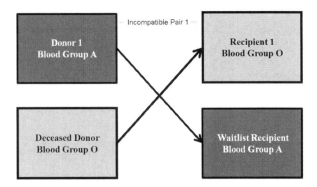

Fig. 8.1 Kidney list donation

Kidney Paired Donation

The NEPKE system identifies various types of KPDs, also known as kidney exchange. These include both cyclical exchanges and chains. Cyclical exchanges involve either two or three donor/recipient (D/R) pairs. Chains begin with an unpaired donor and/or end with a recipient on the UNOS deceased donor waitlist. The initial proposal for a computerized KPD system called for the consideration of large cycles and chains.[7] However, for logistical reasons, early exchanges were limited to two pairs, with the computer system adapted to find the optimal set of two-way matches.[8] Today two and three-pair exchanges as well as non-directed donor (NDD) chains are common.

Two-Pair Exchange: Two-pair exchanges begin when the donors in two D/R pairs are incompatible with their intended recipients. If the donors are both compatible with the recipient in the opposite pair, an exchange of kidneys can occur [8,9] (Fig. 8.2).

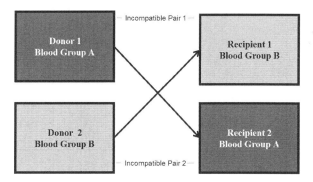

Fig. 8.2   Kidney paired donation: two-pair exchange

Three-Pair Exchange: As the name three-way exchange indicates, a third incompatible pair is added to the match. As shown in Fig. 8.3, pairs 1 and 2 are incompatible due to ABO, while pair 3 is incompatible due to positive crossmatch. In this exchange, paired donor 1 donates to recipient 2, while donor 2 donates to recipient 3 and donor 3 donates to recipient 1.[10]

Non-directed Donor Chain: A NDD, commonly referred to as a Good Samaritan or altruistic donor, does not know someone who needs a kidney transplant, he/she would like to donate to anyone in need. When a NDD enters a KPD program, they allow pairs to match who otherwise would not. As a result, two or three recipients undergo kidney transplantation following the gift of one NDD. Figure 8.4 illustrates how a NDD entering a KPD system donates to a recipient of an incompatible donor, that first donor donates to a recipient of a second incompatible pair and that pair's donor donates to someone on the UNOS waitlist. Traditionally, the NDD would donate directly to the waitlist, with only one person benefiting from transplantation. As incentive for transplant programs to enter NDDs into the NEPKE system, the

Fig. 8.3 Kidney paired
donation: three-pair exchange

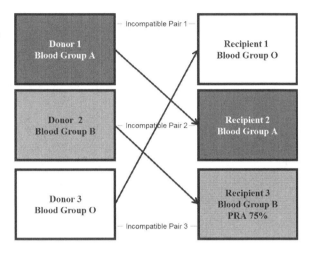

Fig. 8.4 Kidney paired
donation: NDD chain

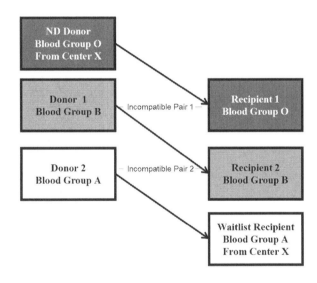

evaluating center receives the kidney at the end of the chain to transplant a candidate on their center's waitlist. In some KPD programs, rather than the third donor donating to the waitlist, they return to the KPD pool and become the next NDD to begin a new chain.[11]

List Exchange Chain: A list exchange chain combines KPD and KLD. A pair who meets criteria for a standard KLD enters the KPD system. This pair is matched with another pair, a recipient on the UNOS waitlist and a deceased donor. The initial KLD eligible donor provides a kidney to the recipient in another incompatible pair, the second donor donates to someone on the UNOS waitlist, and the initial KLD candidate is allocated a kidney from the deceased donor pool[11] (Fig. 8.5).

Fig. 8.5 Kidney paired donation: list exchange chain

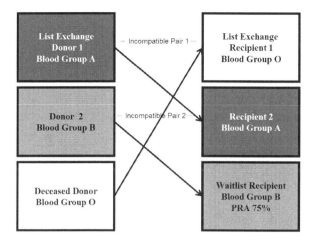

Benefits of KPD

The recipient of a paired donation receives all the benefits of a living donor kidney transplant. Transplants from living kidney transplants, both related and unrelated, have greater graft survival than deceased donor transplants, benefiting the individual recipient. Graft survival for living unrelated is similar to living related kidney transplant, providing the recipients of paired donation the same benefits of directed living donation.[12,13] In addition to individual benefits, KPD and KLD increase the number of kidneys available for transplant, removing the intending recipient from the deceased donor list or pre-empting the need for placement on the list, benefiting all kidney transplant candidates.

Computer Optimization

Prior to computer optimization programs, exchanges involved matching of ABO incompatible pairs and two-way exchanges only. The development of a mechanism based on computer optimization algorithms, specifically designed for kidney matching, revolutionized KPD.[6] Initially algorithms were adapted to handle only two-pair exchanges in New England[6] and later elsewhere.[9] As logistical ability has improved, flexible integer programming formulations were developed that allow optimization to specify the maximum size cycles and chains that will be considered,[14] these too have been adopted elsewhere. Compatibility is based on ABO blood type, HLA typing, and predicted crossmatch results (based on candidate alloantibody screening). The first task of the computer is to generate a compatibility matrix, which searches for recipients who are ABO compatible with all registered donors. If a recipient has an identified unacceptable antigen to a donor's HLA, the computer eliminates the unacceptable match from further consideration. Optimization techniques identify incompatible recipients who would potentially receive a transplant through KPD. Integer programming then determines maximal two- and three-way exchanges, NDD chains, and list exchange chains based on a set of priorities listed in Table 8.1.

Table 8.1 NEPKE matching priority

1. Candidate is a prior living donor
2. PRA $\geq$ 80% (Class I or II)
3. Maximum number of kidneys transplants
4. Candidate < 18 years old
5. PRA 50–79%
6. Collective wait time of matched pairs

For example, suppose there are eight patient–donor pairs registered to the database through the participating transplant centers. Further, suppose that all pairs have the same priority. Thus, we would like to find a set of exchanges that serves the largest number of pairs.[14] The computer defines the compatibility matrix as demonstrated in Table 8.2. The rows denote the recipients and columns denote the donors. D1 is the paired donor of recipient R1; D2 is the paired donor of recipient R2; and so on. NEPKE software finds the compatible and incompatible donors for each recipient and the reasons for incompatibility.

Table 8.2 Compatibility matrix for kidney paired donation

	D1	D2	D3	D4	D5	D6	D7	D8
R1	ABO	OK	OK	ABO	HLA	ABO	HLA	OK
R2	OK	HLA	ABO	OK	ABO	OK	HLA	ABO
R3	OK	HLA	ABO	HLA	ABO	OK	ABO	ABO
R4	ABO	OK	ABO	ABO	ABO	ABO	ABO	ABO
R5	ABO	OK	ABO	ABO	ABO	ABO	ABO	ABO
R6	ABO	HLA	HLA	ABO	OK	ABO	HLA	HLA
R7	ABO	HLA	HLA	ABO	HLA	ABO	HLA	OK
R8	ABO	HLA	ABO	ABO	ABO	ABO	ABO	ABO

The second task for the computer is to identify optimal exchanges using the information generated from the compatibility matrix. In this example, there are four possible exchanges (Fig. 8.6). Without using optimization, one can choose Exchange 1, but none of the other exchanges will be feasible due to the same pair involved in multiple matches. In this case, pair 1 and pair 2 donate and receive transplants. However, by using optimization the computer identifies a maximal two- and three-way match choosing Exchanges 3 and 4. Using optimization pairs 1, 2, 3, 5, and 6, all benefit from kidney exchange with an additional three transplants performed.[15] In this step the computer uses integer programming techniques to maximize the number of pairs matched under the given possible exchange cycles. Other objectives (as summarized in Table 8.1) are also utilized by these techniques.

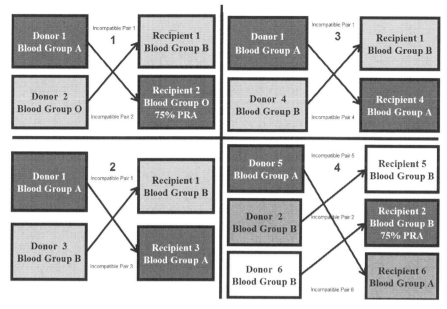

Fig. 8.6 Four possible exchanges generated. Using optimization, the computer software identifies matches 2 and 4 as providing the greatest number of transplants

Types of KPD Programs

There are several models of KPD programs currently in use in the United States. In a center-specific program, all pairs are registered at the same transplant center. The major advantage of a center-specific program is that the logistics of coordinating an exchange are less complicated and no travel is necessary for the donor or the kidney. In a multicenter regional program exchanges are determined between pairs registered at two or more transplant centers in same region. Advantages are short travel time for either the donor who will travel to their match center for surgery or reduced cold ischemic time if the kidney shipped to the match center after recovery. A cross-regional program involves the exchange between pairs at two or more transplant centers in different UNOS regions. The advantage of this type of program is an increase in the number of pairs entered in the system, which increases the number of potential matches and transplants. Finally, a national program would involve the exchange between pairs entered in a centralized national database in which any UNOS-affiliated transplant program has the ability to enter pairs.

Multiregional Application

The benefits of expanding the pool of D/R pairs in KPD programs are well established.[16,17] In an effort to increase the chance that NEPKE pairs would fine a match, NEPKE works with individual transplant centers and other paired donation programs outside Region 1. In 2006 the Mid-Atlantic Paired Exchange Program (MAPEP), organized through the New Jersey Sharing Network, and their five affiliated transplant centers began entering incompatible D/R pairs into the NEPKE system. Combining NEPKE and MAPEP increases the number of pairs in both systems thereby increasing the number of potential matches and actual transplants. Although the matching process remains the same, MAPEP developed their own consent forms and policies on issues such as donor evaluation and antibody screening. These policies are consistent with NEPKE policies and have not posed an impediment to programs working together.

Candidacy for Kidney List Donation

Candidates for list donation must be eligible for a kidney transplant and have a medically suitable living donor who is incompatible by blood type. The candidate wishing to enter the KLD program must meet specific criteria prior to acceptance. Criteria include first deceased donor kidney transplant; currently treated with dialysis; unsensitized, defined as a PRA less than 10%; on the list of New England candidates awaiting a kidney transplant (with an established care relationship with a UNOS Region 1 center); and has waited 45 days to find a KPD match prior to moving to KLD[5] (Table 8.3).

Table 8.3 Region 1 candidate requirements for kidney list donation

- First deceased donor transplant
- Currently on dialysis
- Unsensitized (<10%)
- Has established care relationship with UNOS Region 1 center
- On New England Region 1 waiting list
- Has waited at least 45 days for a Kidney Paired Donation

Kidney List Donation Allocation

The UNOS Kidney Committee has sponsored an alternative allocation system for the original intended candidates of living donors. In this system for standard donors less than 35 years of age, the original intended candidate of a living donor comes after zero ABDR mismatches, local prior living organ donors, local highest scoring high PRA candidates, local pediatric candidates, and payback debts and credits. The local original intended candidates come right before the local candidates on the match run. For standard donors over 35 years of age, the original intended candidate of a living donor comes after zero ABDR mismatches, local prior living organ donors, and payback debts and credits but before local kidney alone candidates (this

Table 8.4 Region 1 allocation priority for standard criteria donors

1. Kidney + lifesaving extra-renal
2. Region 1 emergency kidney
3. Region 1 zero antigen MM K/P w/ PRA > 80%
4. National zero antigen MM K/P w/ PRA > 80%
5. Region 1 standard K/P top 12 unsensitized
6. Zero antigen MM (region and national)
7. Prior living donors
8. Region 1 KLD recipients
9. Region 1 highest scoring high-PRA recipients (category on donors ≤35)
10. Pediatric priority recipients (category on donors ≤35)
11. UNOS paybacks
12. Region 1 list

allocation does not have separate classifications for local highest scoring high PRA candidates and local pediatric candidates). Four regions have adopted the UNOS Kidney Committee allocation while Region 1 and others have adopted a slightly different allocation policy (Table 8.4).[18]

Candidacy for Kidney Paired Donation

As with KLD, the candidate for KPD must also be eligible to receive a kidney transplant; however, they may participate in KPD pre-emptive of the initiation of dialysis. The candidate may be incompatible to their intended donor by blood type and/or positive crossmatch. In addition, there is no limit to the number of previous kidney transplants from either living or deceased donors.

Donor Candidacy for KPD and KLD

Donors entered into NEPKE must meet one of the following criteria: the living donor must be willing but unable to donate a kidney to their intended candidate due to an incompatible blood type, positive crossmatch, and/or some other incompatibility or be a NDD. Donor medical and psychosocial suitability is determined by individual transplant center criteria with a recommendation of the following: the UNOS Guidance for the Development of Program-Specific Living Kidney Donor Medical Evaluation Protocols[19] and Guidelines for the psychosocial evaluation of living unrelated kidney donors in the United States.[20] To decrease the number of potential matches in which a donor is later found to be medically or psychosocially unsuitable for donation, a standard minimum donor evaluation for all NEPKE donors is required prior to entering the program.

Alloantibody Screening

Prior to registration in NEPKE antibody screening is required for all candidates with a PRA greater than 10%. Class I and II antibody screening can be performed by FlowPRA, Luminex, or ELISA. If screen is positive, solid phase specific/panel assay for Class I and/or II is performed. Report must include all HLA alloantibody specificities. If PRA is high and/or antibody specificities cannot be determined, single antigen solid phase assay is performed. Any additional routine screening by the transplant center is performed using the center's standardized tests. Additional testing does not need to be reported to NEPKE. The candidate, however, may benefit from additional solid phase screening if there is a significant decrease in PRA.

Consent for Participation

Once suitability for KPD is determined, donors and candidates are given the opportunity to make an informed decision regarding program participation. A transplant center representative reviews the components of NEPKE with each recipient and their donor(s) separately providing accurate and complete information regarding participation in the NEPKE. After review, each individual participant is asked to sign a separate consent form if he/she agrees to participate in KPD. The consent form outlines what KPD and NEPKE are; the KPD procedure; information that will be entered into the database and how it will be used; how confidentiality will be maintained; and the risks, benefits, and alternatives to participating in the program.

The transplant team provides a preliminary review of the general risks for kidney transplant and donor nephrectomy surgeries, including risk that surgery may not occur due to unforeseen events in the operating room such as hypotension, myocardial infarction, unexpected findings. The surgical team responsible for the operative procedure of each specific patient in the exchange reviews the risks and benefits of surgery and obtains informed consent.

Exchange Process

Once a potential match has been accepted by all involved centers, more detailed donor information is exchanged between centers and if this is acceptable, preliminary crossmatches are conducted between the candidate and their matched donor. Flow crossmatch is strongly recommended when appropriate. For candidates with high levels of alloantibodies ($\geq 80\%$), detailed analyses including autocrossmatch testing and testing of several historical serum samples are encouraged. Donor blood is generally sent to the histocompatibility laboratory of their matched candidate for crossmatch, that is, the crossmatch is performed at the potential recipient's histocompatibility laboratory. Transplant centers update donor medical and psychosocial evaluation as needed. The center that will actually perform the donor's surgery meets that donor, reviews their medical history, obtains any new testing that is warranted, and obtains the legal surgical consent signature. Candidates are re-evaluated by their transplant center to determine current suitability for transplant. Transplant centers consider psychosocial issues specific to KPD and discuss with both the donor and recipient. Transplant centers and participants agree to date and time of simultaneous donor nephrectomies immediately followed by candidate kidney transplant. Final crossmatches between the candidate and their matched donors are conducted prior to surgery according to transplant center guidelines; flow crossmatch are recommended when appropriate.

A conference call is scheduled with involved transplant centers several days prior to the surgery date to discuss logistics of the donation and transplant, donor follow-up, and D/R correspondence/meeting. Donor surgeons speak to each other in the operating room prior to incision. If any donor nephrectomy is delayed, all donor nephrectomies are rescheduled to occur simultaneously.

Ethical and Legal Issues in Kidney Paired Donation and Kidney List Donation

Legal and ethical issues have arisen involving the practice of KPD and KLD in the United States. Ambiguity in the National Organ Transplant Act (NOTA) delayed the universal acceptance of these exchanges as standard practice. NOTA prohibits the buying and selling of human organs by making it unlawful to exchange "valuable consideration" for human organs for use in transplantation.[21]

Legal concerns raised under NOTA caused many transplant centers and the UNOS to hesitate implementation of KPD and KLD programs. The solution to legal ambiguities and threat of possible lawsuits required legislative clarification of valuable consideration as it relates to KPD and KLD.

In March 2007, Department of Justice, C. Kevin Marshall Deputy Assistant Attorney General in a memo to the Department of Health and Human Services concluded "that valuable consideration term as used in section 301 does not apply to KLD or KPD, because neither involves the buying or selling of a kidney or otherwise commercializes the transfer of kidneys."[22] It is important to note that in NOTA "The term 'valuable consideration does not include the reasonable payments associated with their removal, transportation, implantation, processing, preservation, quality control, and storage of a human organ or the expenses of travel, housing, and lost wages incurred by the donor of a human organ in connection with the donation of the organ.'[21] These exclusions address types of 'payments' and 'expenses' that may otherwise fall within the term 'valuable consideration' on the theory that they involve monetary benefits or at least a monetary transfer. Any benefits received in the KPD/KLD exchanges, on the other hand, are not monetary. The lack of comparable exclusion for non-monetary benefits may suggest that non-monetary KPD and KLD exchanges do not involve valuable consideration."[22]

The Charlie W. Norwood Living Organ Donation Act, signed into law in 2007, amends NOTA to clarify that valuable consideration and associated criminal penalties do not apply to KPD. Section 301 274e states that "it shall be unlawful for any person to knowingly acquire, receive, or otherwise transfer any human organ for valuable consideration for use in human transplantation if the transfer affects interstate commerce." The Charlie W. Norwood Act added, "The preceding sentence does not apply with respect to human organ paired donation."[21] Although earlier versions of the bills addressed KLD, the final version does not.

National Pilot Program

The Charlie W. Norwood Living Organ Donation Act allows UNOS to move forward with a National Pilot KPD program. A national system will (1) allow centers not large enough to participate at the single center level access to KPD, (2) provide greater opportunity for difficult to match pairs to find an exchange, and (3) increase the total number of kidney donors, benefiting all candidates waiting.

In order for a national KPD program to be successful, it will require participation of a large number of transplant centers. In order to engage transplant centers, the national program will need to be flexible enough to satisfy the diverse needs of different transplant programs. Current optimization programs permit this flexibility, allowing a menu of clinical and logistical options that accommodate the varying needs of different transplant centers and their patients.[23] In June 2008, the OPTN/UNOS Board of Directors approved a proposal for a national KPD pilot program administered by the OPTN.[24] This proposal will accommodate the various needs of individual transplant programs and patients, providing the flexibility needed for participation.

Proposed Operational Guidelines

Optimization and Prioritization

The national optimization protocol will look at every possible matching from the list of potential D/R pairs (compatibility matrix similar to NEPKE).[25] The computer program will compare the possible matches using predetermined weights based on objectives established for the program. The program then selects the matches with the greatest number of points. Priority points assigned are listed in Table 8.5.

Options for Individual Patients and Transplant Programs

In the current plan for the national pilot program, transplant programs will be able to choose to participate in either two-way alone or two- and three-way matches.

Table 8.5   Priority points for national KPD pilot program

1. Zero antigen mismatch between donor and candidate
2. Highly sensitized candidate (PRA ≥ 80%)
3. Prior living donor status of the candidate
4. Pediatric candidate (age < 18 years)
5. Waiting time accumulated within the KPD program
6. Geographic proximity (transplant center, local, or regional)

Table 8.6   Transplant program choices in KPD

Donor	Candidate
Distance willing to travel	Distance willing to travel
Nephrectomy type (open/laparoscopy/either)	Acceptable donor age
Nephrectomy side	Acceptable donor BMI
Willing to participate in an open NDD chain	Donor blood pressure limits
Willing to participate in a close NDD chain	Donor CMV status
	Donor EBV status
	Donor history of cancer
	Willing to participate in an open NDD chain
	Willing to participate in a close NDD chain

This allows centers who are new to KPD to start with logistically easier matches if desired. Transplant programs as well as patients will have the opportunity to choose between lists of options regarding logistics and medical criteria (Table 8.6).

Crossmatching

As the number of pairs in a system increases, the accuracy of virtual crossmatching will become increasingly important. In the national pilot program donors and candidates will be typed for HLA – A, B, Bw4, Bw6, Cw, DQ, DR, Dr51, DR52, DR53, and DP. Centers will have the option to enter unacceptable antigens at levels of high and low stringency for each candidate in the program. High stringency is defined as all HLA antigens to which the candidate has antibodies and low stringency as only unacceptable antigen that are highly likely to cause a positive crossmatch. These options provide flexibility for each transplant program based on their individual center protocols and the individual needs of each candidate. Crossmatches usually take place at the histocompatibility laboratory affiliated with the matched candidate; however, some programs recommend that using a centralized tissue typing laboratory to perform preliminary crossmatches may be more efficient than exchanging blood among participating transplant centers. Until such a laboratory can be established, a national KPD program will need to utilize currently available resources.

Living Donor Evaluation

The potential living donor will need to undergo a medical evaluation similar to the NEPKE requirements with professional consultations by a nephrologist and local transplant or donor nephrectomy surgeon, as well as a psychosocial evaluation by a social worker or psychologist. The medical evaluation should adhere to the guidelines set forth in the Amsterdam Forum On the Care of the Live Kidney Donor[26] and consist of at least a history and physical examination; blood and urine testing; creatinine clearance; tissue typing, ABO blood typing; a duplex ultrasound of both native kidneys documenting size, presence of cysts, and/or other abnormalities; and age-appropriate cancer screening. Transplant programs will be required to use consent process outlined in "The Resource Document for Informed Consent for Living Donors"[27] developed by the UNOS Living Donor committee and approved by the Executive Committee. As the UNOS Board of Directors approves other resource documents, such as recommendation for the medical and psychosocial evaluation of living kidney donors, the Kidney Committee will work to incorporate these resource documents into the national KPD pilot program.

Program Evaluation

Monitoring participation of transplant programs in a national KPD program is vital to its success. The UNOS Kidney Committee will evaluate the national KPD program every 6 months for the first 3 years, recommending adjustments to the system as needed. Additional enhancements to the program will be considered on a regular basis, such as NDD chains involving altruistic living donors. Making enhancements and maintaining flexibility will enable a national KPD program to accommodate the diverse needs of individual transplant programs and their candidates, increasing the transplant opportunity for all participants.

Acknowledgments We thank Dr. Kenneth Andreoni, Chair of the OPTN/UNOS Kidney Paired Donation Work Group Committee, and Elizabeth F. Sleeman MHA, UNOS Policy Analyst, for their valuable assistance and insightful comments.

References

1. Montgomery RA, Zachary AA, Ratner LE et al. Clinical results from transplanting incompatible live kidney/donor recipient pairs using kidney paired donation. *JAMA* 2005;294: 1655–1663.
2. Rapaport FT. The case for a living emotionally related international kidney donor exchange registry. *Transplant Proc* 1986;18:5–9.
3. Park K, Moon JI, Kim SI, Kim YS. Exchange donor program in kidney transplantation. *Transplantation* 1998;67(2):336.
4. Living donor transplants by donor relation. U.S. OPTN Network and the SRTR. Available at: http://www.optn.org/latestData/rptData.asp. Accessed Oct 8, 2008.
5. Delmonico FL, Morrissey PE, Lipkowitz GS et al. Donor kidney exchanges. *Am J Transplant* 2004;4:1628–1634.

6. Roth AE, Sönmez T, Ünver UM. A kidney exchange clearinghouse in New England. *Am Econ Rev Papers Proc* May 2005;95(2):376–380.
7. Roth AE, Sönmez T, Ünver UM. Kidney exchange. *Q J Econ* 2004;119(2):457–488.
8. Roth AE, Sönmez T, Ünver UM. Pairwise kidney exchange. *J Econ Theory* 2005 Dec;125(2):151–188.
9. Gentry SE, Segev DL, Montgomery RA. A comparison of populations served by kidney paired donation and list paired donation. *Am J Transplant* 2005;5:1914–1921.
10. Saidman S, Roth AE, Sönmez T, Ünver UM, Delmonico FL. Increasing the opportunity of live kidney donation by matching for two and three way exchanges. *Transplantation* 2006;81(5):773–782.
11. Roth AE, Sönmez T, Ünver UM, Delmonico FL, Saidman SL. Utilizing list exchange and nondirected donation through "chain" paired kidney donations. *Am J Transplant* 2006;6:1–12.
12. Davis C, Delmonico FL. Living-donor kidney transplantation: a review of the current practices for the live donor. *Clin J Am Soc Nephrol* 2005;16:2098–2110.
13. Abecassis M, Barlett St, Collins AJ et al. Kidney transplantation as primary therapy for end-stage renal disease: a national kidney foundation/kidney disease outcomes quality initiative (NKF/KDOQITM) conference. *Clin J Am Soc Nephrol* 2008 Mar;3(2):471–480.
14. Roth AE, Sönmez T, Ünver UM. Efficient kidney exchange: coincidence of wants in markets with compatibility-based preferences. *Am Econ Rev* 2007 Jun;97(3):828–851.
15. How does the computer do the matching? New England Program for Kidney Exchange. Available at: http://www.nepke.org/math.htm. Accessed Feb 17, 2009.
16. Kaplan I, Houp JA, Leffell MS, Hart JM, Zachary AA. A computer match program for paired and unconventional kidney exchanges. *Am J Transplant* 2005;5:2306–2308.
17. Simpkins CE, Montgomery RS, Hawxby AM et al. Cold ischemia time and allograft outcomes in live donor renal transplantation: is live donor organ transport feasible? *Am J Transplant* 2007 Jan;7(1):99–107.
18. Board of Director meeting minutes. UNOS. Richmond, VA, Jun 24–25, 1999:21; Jun 15–16:14, 2000; Nov 16–17, 2000:1; Jun 27–28, 2002:27; Nov 20–21, 2003:8.
19. Policies: Living Donation. UNOS. Available at: http://www.unos.org/living_donation. Accessed Jul 8, 2008.
20. Dew MA, Jacobs CL, Jowsey SG, Hanto R, Miller C, Delmonico FL. Guidelines for the psychosocial evaluation of living unrelated kidney donors in the United States. *Am J Transplant* 2007;7:1047–1054.
21. Shared Content Documents, National Organ Transplantation Act. UNOS. Available at: http://www.unos.org/SharedContentDocuments/NOTA_as_amended Jan_2008.pdf. Accessed Oct 8, 2008.
22. Legality of alternative organ donation practices under 42 U.S.C. 274e. United States Department of Justice, Office of Legal Counsel. Available at: http://www.usdoj.gov/olc/2007/organtransplant.pdf. Accessed Oct 9, 2008.
23. Rees MA, Roth AE, Unver U et al. Designing a National Kidney Exchange Program. *Unpublished.*
24. United Network for Organ Sharing. Committee Reports. UNOS. Available at: http://www.unos.org/CommitteeREports/board_main_Kidney Transplantation Committee December 18, 2006. pdf. Accessed Feb 17, 2009.
25. Andreoni K, Sleeman E, Hanto R et al. Development of a National Kidney paired Donation Pilot Program. *ATC 09. Poster Presentation.* Boston, MA. May 30, 2009–Jun 3, 2009.
26. Delmonico F. Council of the Transplantation Society. A report of the Amsterdam forum on the care of the live kidney donor: data and medical guidelines. *Transplantation* 2005 Mar 27;79(6 Suppl.):S53–S66.
27. Resource document for informed consent for living donors. UNOS. Available at: http://www.unos.org/SharedContentDocuments/Informed_Consent_Living_Donors.pdf. Accessed Feb 20, 2009.

Chapter 9
What Are Immunosuppressive Medications? How Do They Work? What Are Their Side Effects?

Peter Chung-Wen Chang and Donald E. Hricik

Introduction

Effective suppression of the transplant recipient's immune system has improved short-term outcomes in renal transplantation. The immunologic basis for graft rejection is described in Chapter 3. Although there are infrequent reports of patients requiring little or no immunosuppressive medications, most patients require life-long immunosuppression.

Most transplant centers employ multidrug regimens that minimize the toxicity of any single agent and inhibit the recipient's immune system via separate or synergistic mechanisms. Each of the immunosuppressive agents has side effects that variably contribute to cardiovascular disease, infection, and malignancy – the main causes of mortality in transplant recipients. A concern for long-term side effects has fueled the development of "minimization strategies" designed to reduce exposure to toxic immunosuppressants in long-term survivors of kidney transplants (see Chapter 10). A dilemma of minimization is that poor kidney function also contributes to comorbidites (such as cardiovascular disease), and therefore maintenance of kidney function is paramount.

Many new immunosuppressant drugs, including a variety of biologic agents, are currently being tested in clinical or pre-clinical trials. Several of these new agents will likely be available in the future. This chapter focuses on medications currently used for induction therapy, for maintenance immunosuppression, and for treatment of acute rejection.

Antibodies Used for Induction Therapy

Induction therapy is defined as immunosuppressive medication given before, or at the time of, transplantation. Practically, induction therapy is administered through intravenous delivery of antibodies that are directed to cells of the recipient immune

P.C.-W. Chang (✉)
Division of Nephrology and Hypertension, Department of Medicine, University Hospitals Case Medical Center, Cleveland, OH, USA
e-mail: pcwchang@hotmail.com

D.B. McKay, S.M. Steinberg (eds.), *Kidney Transplantation: A Guide to the Care of Kidney Transplant Recipients*, DOI 10.1007/978-1-4419-1690-7_9,
© Springer Science+Business Media, LLC 2010

system. The use of induction antibody therapy varies around the world but has become increasingly popular in the United States over the past 15 years; more than 70% of patients currently receive one of the agents described below.

The idea of induction therapy is to dampen the immune system of the recipient before it has a chance to "recognize" the grafted organ. Patients that benefit most from this therapy are those with preformed anti-HLA antibodies (e.g., patients with a history of blood transfusions or prior transplantation) and patients in selected high-risk groups (African American, Hispanic). The benefits of using induction therapy to reduce acute rejection must be weighed against the cost of the induction medications (at least $8,000 for a minimal course of induction therapy) and the risks of over-immunosuppression (including serious infections and malignancy).

The medications used for induction therapy include antibodies directed against the recipient immune cells. The antibody solution is usually administered intra-venously to the patient in the operating suite, sometimes even before the transplant procedure, and continues to be given for some time after transplantation; the time course depends on the type of induction antibody.

There are two general types of induction antibodies: lymphocyte depleting or non-depleting antibodies. Lymphocyte depleting antibodies target antigens on the surface of recipient immune cells that lead to their removal (depletion) whereas non-depleting antibodies block receptors on the surface of immune cells, thereby inactivating the cells.

Within each category of induction antibodies, there are both monoclonal agents directed against specific antigenic targets of lymphocytes and polyclonal agents containing a pool of antibodies directed against multiple antigens. Each category will be discussed below, focused on the antibodies most commonly used.

In recent years, some centers have developed "desensitization" protocols that are administered prior to transplantation in kidney transplant candidates with high titers of antibodies against HLA antigens[1-4] or ABO incompatibility.[5,6] These protocols involve some combination of plasmapheresis and/or administration of intravenous immune globulin (IVIG) and antibodies directed against the CD20 molecule on B cells (anti-CD20 antibodies), but are beyond the scope of this chapter.

Lymphocyte Depleting Antibodies

Polyclonal Depleting Antibodies

Polyclonal antibodies are produced by immunization of a live animal, resulting in a mixture of immunoglobulin molecules recognizing different epitopes (part of the molecule to which the antibody binds) of the immunizing antigen. The most common polyclonal agent currently used in the United States for induction therapy is rabbit anti-thymocyte globulin (rabbit ATG; Thymoglobulin®). A horse-derived polyclonal antibody (ATGAM®) is available in the United States, but now rarely used. Although Thymoglobulin is the most frequently prescribed induction agent in the United States, rabbit ATG is approved by the FDA only for treatment of rejection and is technically used off-label as an induction therapy. However, when compared to no induction antibody therapy, ATG and other polyclonal agents have been shown to reduce the incidence of acute rejection and to prolong graft survival.[7,8] A randomized trial suggested that rabbit ATG is superior to basiliximab, a non-depleting antibody, in preventing acute rejection in patients deemed to be at high risk for immune graft injury.[9]

Lymphocytes are cleared from the circulation during active administration of ATG; the anti-thymocyte globulin is slowly infused daily for 3–10 days posttransplant. The starting dose is 1.5 mg/kg/day and the first dose is often administered intraoperatively. Thrombocytopenia and leukopenia are common side effects, often resulting in the need for dose modification. Fever, chills, and myalgias are observed commonly with the initial infusion, but can be mollified by concomitant administration of corticosteroids. Anaphylactic reactions to ATG are rare.

Monoclonal Depleting Antibodies

Monoclonal antibodies are produced from a single cell line and the resulting immunoglobulins are homogenous. Upon binding to a specific antigenic epitope, the depleting antibody leads to the destruction (deletion) of the cell.

Alemtuzumab (Campath 1H) is a humanized monoclonal antibody that binds to a receptor (CD52) that is present on all T and B lymphocytes, as well as the majority of macrophages, monocytes, and natural killer cells.[10] Alemtuzumab was originally approved in the 1980s as an agent for the treatment of B-cell chronic lymphocytic leukemia and is currently used off-label in transplantation. This monoclonal antibody produces significant and prolonged (>12 months) leukopenia. The drug is easily administered peripherally, given in a single (30 mg) or double dose in the perioperative period.

Alemtuzumab has been used primarily to facilitate "minimization" of maintenance immunosuppression immediately following the transplant surgery.[11–13] The toxicity profile is still under investigation, but myelosuppression can occasionally be severe. Some transplant centers have reported a relatively high incidence of humoral (antibody-mediated) acute rejection in patients treated with alemtuzumab,[13,14] and repeated courses of therapy have been associated with the emergence of autoantibodies and autoimmune disorders.

Another depleting monoclonal antibody, OKT3 (Orthoclone Muromonab-CD3®), targets a receptor present on all T cells (the CD3 complex of the T-cell receptor – see Chapter 3), and binding to T cells causes profound impairment of both T-cell activation and proliferation. Although this drug proved to be useful as an induction agent in the 1980s,[15] it is rarely employed for induction in the United States in the modern era, mostly because of its cost and toxicities (see below).

Non-depleting Antibodies

The major type of non-depleting monoclonal antibody in current use is directed against the alpha chain of the interleukin 2 (IL-2) receptor. The IL-2 receptor is a trimeric receptor (consisting of alpha, beta, and gamma chains) that becomes expressed on the surface of activated T cells. Binding to the alpha chain of the IL-2R receptor (also called the CD25 molecule) blocks the proliferative signals normally mediated by IL-2 without causing profound depletion of lymphocytes. Basiliximab (Simulect®) is a chimeric anti-CD25 antibody (30% murine, 70% human). Daclizumab (Zenapax®) is a humanized anti-CD25 antibody (10% murine, 90% human). Together, these two anti-CD25 antibodies are the second most frequently prescribed induction antibodies in the United States, next to rabbit ATG.

When compared to placebo, treatment with either basiliximab[16] or daclizumab[17] is associated with lower rates of early acute rejection. Basiliximab is typically administered at a dose of 20 mg IV on day 0 (usually administered intraoperatively) and again on postoperative day 4. Although daclizumab was originally intended to be delivered at a standard dose of 1 mg/kg IV on transplant day 0 and again at 2, 4, 6, and 8 weeks post-transplant for a total of five doses, some centers have reported successful outcomes with one[18] or two dose[19] regimens. Both of these antibodies have long half-lives and are well tolerated with few, if any, side effects. Anaphylactic/hypersensitivity reactions are exceedingly rare.

Maintenance Immunosuppressants

The recipient immune system must be effectively suppressed after transplantation to prevent rejection of the donor graft. To accomplish effective immunosuppression, patients are prescribed a combination of medications that target different limbs of the immune system. The medications most commonly used are corticosteroids, calcineurin inhibitors, and antiproliferative agents. Each maintenance immunosuppressive agent will be discussed below, highlighting mechanism of action, dosing, and side effects. There are differences between drug use and dosing at different transplant centers and so only general guidelines for their use will be provided.

Corticosteroids

Mechanisms of Action

Corticosteroids exert two principal effects on the recipient immune system. First, within 4–8 h of administration, they alter the circulation of lymphocytes causing them to be sequestered in the reticuloendothelial system. Second, corticosteroids inhibit the function of lymphocytes by interfering with soluble signals that are important for the recruitment of several types of immune cells to the rejection process (i.e., lymphokines and cytokines). The action of commonly prescribed glucocorticoids is not limited to immune cells though, as the molecule easily diffuses into all cells and binds to cytoplasmic receptors that are present in almost all cells of the body.[20] The widespread bioavailability accounts for additional pharmacologic effects commonly associated with glucocorticoids, such as anti-insulin activity, protein catabolism, lipolysis, stimulation of fat synthesis. Therefore, it is understandable why transplant physicians try to use as low a dose as possible of glucocorticoids.

Dosing

The synthetic corticosteroids commonly used to prevent and treat rejection are prednisone, prednisolone, and methylprednisolone. These agents have been employed to prevent and treat acute allograft rejection for more than 40 years. Prednisone is the oral steroid preparation most commonly prescribed for maintenance therapy in the United States; its activity depends on the conversion to prednisolone by the liver enzyme 11-β-hydroxydehydrogenase. Prednisolone is usually prescribed to patients with hepatic insufficiency. Methylprednisolone is a modified form of prednisolone that has greater potency than either prednisolone or prednisone and is usually used intravenously to treat acute rejection.

Corticosteroids are prescribed according to fixed and empiric dose-tapering schedules. General guidelines for the dosing of corticosteroids are shown in Table 9.1. While many transplant physicians use doses of prednisone as low as 5 mg daily beyond the several months after transplantation, the well-known side effects of steroids have led to steroid-sparing regimens. While controversial, complete withdrawal of corticosteroids in low-risk patients has become common in many transplant centers.[21] Further discussion about the risks and benefits of steroid avoidance or withdrawal can be found in Chapter 10.

Table 9.1 Guidelines for maintenance immunosuppressive drug dosing[a]

Medication	0–3 months	3–12 months	>1 year
Prednisone	10–20 mg/d	5–10 mg/d	5–10 mg/d
Azathioprine	1–2 mg/kg	1–2 mg/kg[b]	1–2 mg/kg[b]
CellCept®	1,000–1,500 mg BID	1,000–1,500 mg BID	1,000–1,500 mg BID
Myfortic®	720 mg BID	720 mg BID	720 mg BID
Ideal Blood levels[c]			
Cyclosporine (ng/ml)	200–400	100–200	100–200
Tacrolimus (ng/ml)	8–15	5–15	5–15

[a]These are guidelines only, drug dosing may vary by transplant center.
[b]Dosage may need to be lowered for leukopenia.
[c]CNI dosing is generally based on blood level, and doses are lower when simultaneously prescribed a TOR inhibitor.

Side Effects

The side effects of corticosteroids are well recognized by most physicians. In addition to increasing the risk of infection, the major side effects include weight gain, Cushingoid appearance, hypertension, fluid retention, osteopenia and osteonecrosis, acneform rash or ecchymoses, and psychiatric disturbances. Metabolic side effects include glucose intolerance and hyperlipidemia.

Calcineurin Inhibitors

Mechanisms of Action

Calcineurin inhibitors (CNIs) have formed the cornerstone of solid-organ transplant immunosuppressive regimens since the introduction of cyclosporine (CsA) in the early 1980s. CsA is a small cyclic polypeptide of fungal origin. The other available CNI is tacrolimus, a macrolide antibiotic compound available in the United States since the mid-1990s. Tacrolimus is the most commonly used CNI in the United States. As described below, CsA and tacrolimus have different side effects. Whether the two agents are comparably efficacious in preventing rejection or prolonging graft survival remains a subject of great debate.[22]

Both CsA and tacrolimus inhibit the function of a cytoplasmic molecule found in most cells called calcineurin. Calcineurin is an intracellular phosphatase that functions to dephosphorylate certain nuclear regulatory proteins, allowing them to pass through the nuclear membrane and activate cytokine genes (i.e., interleukins 2 and 4, interferon alpha, and tumor necrosis factor alpha), that are essential to T-cell activation.

Dosing

The original oral formulation of CsA was Sandimmune®, which exhibits relatively poor bioavailability with great intra- and inter-patient pharmacokinetic variability. A newer microemulsion formulation, Neoral®, was later developed to improve absorption and minimize variation in bioavailability.[23] Several generic forms of CsA are now available. Tacrolimus is currently available as Prograf®, but generic forms of tacrolimus will be available soon. Because of variations in absorption and genetic differences in the expression and function of the cytochrome P450-3A4 system responsible for metabolism of CNIs (see below), drug level monitoring is still considered necessary for optimal management of all of the available CNIs.[24,25]

Due to subtle variations in pharmacokinetics between different formulations, it is best to avoid switching from brand name compounds to generics. However, if conversion is necessary, close monitoring of drug levels and renal function is suggested in the short term. Both CNIs (CsA and tacrolimus) are excreted in the bile with minimal renal excretion; therefore, there is no need for dose adjustment in the presence of renal impairment.[23,24] CsA can be administered intravenously, generally using

30% of the oral dose as a constant infusion over 24 h. Intravenous tacrolimus is extremely toxic and should be used with caution.

The typical starting dose of CsA is 8–12 mg/kg per day with maintenance dose of 3–5 mg/kg per day divided into twice daily doses. For tacrolimus, the typical starting dose is 0.15–0.3 mg/kg per day divided into twice daily doses. There is a reasonably good correlation between trough blood levels of tacrolimus and overall drug exposure. This correlation is less reliable with CsA. Nonetheless, due to convenience and cost, trough drug levels are most commonly used in monitoring all CNIs.[23,26]

There are two general methods for measuring whole blood concentration of CNIs. High-performance liquid chromatography (HPLC) is the most specific method, but is also more expensive and labor intensive. Whole blood immunoassays are cheaper and more readily available for use in automated analyzers. The typical target levels for CNIs measured by immunoassays are shown in Table 9.1. Lower starting doses of CNIs and lower trough target levels are used when these agents are prescribed with a TOR inhibitor, as the combination of agents increases the risk of nephrotoxicity.[27]

Drug Interactions

CNIs are metabolized by cytochrome P450 3A4 enzyme system located in the liver and gastrointestinal tract. Because many drugs can upregulate or downregulate the P450 enzyme system, vigilance is needed to avoid potential drug interactions between CNIs and commonly prescribed medications (Table 9.2).

Drugs that reliably decrease CNI concentration by inducing the P450 enzyme system include rifampin and anticonvulsants such as barbiturates and phenytoin. If these drugs are required, the dose of CNI often needs to be increased to maintain therapeutic levels. Other drugs that decrease CNI levels less predictably include nafcillin, trimethoprim, imipenem, cephalosporins, and ciprofloxacin. St John's wort, an herbal mood enhancer, also can induce the P450 enzyme system. Whenever any of these medications are used, CNI trough levels should be monitored closely. Lastly, corticosteroids are also inducers of the P450 enzyme system. When steroids are tapered, CNI levels should be monitored closely to determine need for CNI dose reduction.[23,24,27]

Drugs that increase CNI concentration by inhibiting P450 activity include nondihydropyridine calcium channel blockers, such as diltiazem and verapamil; the azole antifungal agents, such as ketoconazole, itraconazole, voriconazole, and fluconazole; and erythromycin and its analogs (except for azithromycin). Drugs such as diltiazem or ketoconazole are occasionally prescribed in conjunction with CNIs in an effort to lower the CNI dose and reduce cost. Other medications that inhibit P450 activity less predictably include isoniazide, oral contraceptives, amiodarone, and carvediol. With the advent of highly active antiretroviral therapy (HAART), some centers are now providing organ transplants to HIV-positive patients. Therefore, it is worth noting that protease inhibitors – particularly Ritonavir – are potent inhibitors of P450 enzyme. Lastly, a special dietary concern for all patients on

Table 9.2 Common calcineurin inhibitor drug interactions[a] (This is a partial list; many other medications have potential interactions with CNIs)

Increase CNI levels[b]	Decrease CNI levels[c]
Erythomycin	Rifampin
Diltiazem	Barbituates
Verapamil	Phenytoin
Ketoconazole	Nafcillin
Itraconzazole	Trimethoprim
Voriconazole	Imipenem
Fluconazole	Cephalosporins
Isoniazide	Ciprofloxacin
Oral contraceptives	St. John's wort
Amiodarone	Corticosteroids
Carvediol	
Ritonavir	
Grapefruit juice	

[a]In all cases check CNI blood level before making any dose adjustments.
[b]May need to decrease CNI drug dose to compensate for an increase in CNI blood level.
[c]May need to increase CNI drug dose to compensate for a decrease in CNI blood level.

a CNI is grapefruit juice that can result in higher drug levels from increased absorption.[23,24,27] Non-P450 enzyme-related drug interactions can occur with cholestyramine and GoLYTELY® which may interfere with absorption of CNIs. Concomitant use of CNIs and HMG-CoA reductase inhibitors alter the pharmacokinetics of the "statin," resulting in a longer half-life and a greater risk for rhabdomyolysis.[23,28]

Side Effects

The CNIs have several noteworthy side effects (see Table 9.3), including nephrotoxicity. In the short term, CNIs cause a dose-related, reversible renal vasoconstriction resulting in decreased renal blood flow. Concomitant use of other nephrotoxic agents, such as aminoglycosides and NSAIDs, should therefore be avoided.[23,27] CsA has a greater vasoconstrictive effect than tacrolimus, which could explain its tendency for sodium retention and hypertension.[30] In the long term, CNI use may lead to interstitial fibrosis, although it remains unclear whether this is more likely with CsA than with tacrolimus.[29] Glomerular capillary thrombosis, progressing to graft failure and sometimes associated with full-blown hemolytic uremic syndrome also has been reported with CNIs.[23]

Table 9.3 Side effects of maintenance immunosuppressive medications

Common side effects of calcineurin inhibitors		
Side effects	Cyclosporine	Tacrolimus
Nephrotoxicity	+++	+++
Hypertension	++	+
Hyperlipidemia	++	+
Glucose intolerance	++	+++
Neurologic (tremors/dysesthesias)	+	++
Electrolyte abnormalities (low Mg/high K)	++	++
Gout	+	
Hirsutism	+++	
Hair loss		++
Gingival hyperplasia	+++	

Common side effects of azathioprine	
Hematologic	Leukopenia, thrombocytopenia, anemia
Gastrointestinal	Hepatitis, cholestasis, nausea, pancreatitis,
Cosmetic	Alopecia
Malignancy	Especially non-melanoma skin cancers and non-Hodgkin's lymphoma

Common side effects of mycophenolate mofetil derivatives	
Gastrointestinal Gastritis, ulcer, hemorrhage, diarrhea, bloating, abdominal pain, nausea/vomiting	Diarrhea, colitis
Hematologic	Anemia, leukopenia, thrombocytopenia

Common side effects of mTOR inhibitors	
Impaired wound healing	Lymphoceles; wound dehiscence
Renal	Potentiate nephrotoxicity of CNI; prolong delayed graft function; proteinuria
Electrolyte	Hypokalemia; hypomagnesemia
Endocrine	Potentiate new onset of post-transplant diabetes
Metabolic	Hypercholesterolemia and hypertriglyceridemia
Pulmonary	Noninfectious interstitial pneumonia
Hematologic	Pancytopenia – especially thrombocytopenia
Other	Oligospermia; low libido; aphthous ulcers; edema; myopathy; progressive multifocal leukoencephalopathy (PML); birth defects
Malignancy	May be protective

Besides sodium retention, CNIs can also induce hyperkalemia as a result of impaired aldosterone production and response. Avoidance or cautious use of potassium-sparing diuretics is therefore prudent. CNIs can also downregulate tubular transport proteins causing magnesuria and calciuria. Although both CNIs are associated with hyperuricemia, CsA is more commonly associated with gout.[23,24,27]

Of the two drugs, tacrolimus is reported to pose less net cardiovascular risk. Besides its association with hypertension, CsA use also has been shown to cause higher serum cholesterol, triglycerides, and low-density lipoprotein levels.[30,31] CsA is also reported to accelerate atherosclerosis via endothelial cell damage and smooth muscle proliferation.[28] On the other hand, tacrolimus is more commonly associated with post-transplant hyperglycemia and new-onset diabetes mellitus (NODM).[22,29] This is a dose-related effect primarily resulting from decreased insulin secretion, although there is also evidence for insulin resistance.[32,33] Other potential cardiac effects with tacrolimus include prolonged QT interval and cardiomyopathy.[24,28]

Tacrolimus also has greater neurotoxicity, with tremor, dysesthesias, headache, and insomnia being common dose-related findings.[22,33] More severe effects such as seizures, confusion, psychosis, and coma are uncommon. Some cosmetic effects that may interfere with medication compliance include hirsutism, gingival hyperplasia, and coarsening of facial features among CsA users, while tacrolimus users may develop hair loss to frank alopecia.[26,33]

Antiproliferative Agents

Antiproliferative agents are integral to immunosuppressive regimens in transplantation because they block the proliferation of recipient lymphocytes that recognize the foreign donor antigens. There are three available antiproliferative agents: azathioprine (AZA), mycophenolic acid derivatives, and the TOR inhibitors.

Azathioprine

Mechanisms of Action

The oldest of the antiproliferative agents is azathioprine (AZA), first introduced in the 1960s. AZA is a metabolite of 6-mercaptopurine, which is processed intracellularly into purine analogues that inhibit purine synthesis from both the direct and salvage pathways.[34] In so doing, the drug suppresses gene replication and cell proliferation via inhibition of RNA and DNA synthesis. Although it is more selective for T lymphocytes, it can also suppress promyelocytes in the bone marrow resulting in leukopenia, thrombocytopenia, and/or anemia[36,38]

Dosing

AZA is available in both oral and IV formulations as Imuran® or in generic formulation. However, only half of the orally administered AZA is absorbed; therefore, equivalent IV dose is half that of the oral dose. The starting oral dose of AZA is 1–2 mg/kg administered once daily. There is no need for blood level monitoring, as the effectiveness of AZA does not correlate with its blood level. It is also not excreted by the kidney, so there is no need for dose reduction during episodes of acute renal insufficiency.[36] Dose adjustments are based on toxicity (see side effects below).

Drug Interactions

Unlike CNIs, AZA has only a few drug interactions. Since AZA is metabolized by xanthine oxidase it interacts with allopurinol and febuxostat (Uloric®), which also inhibit xanthine oxidase. Therefore, when allopurinol is combined with AZA, there can be prolonged AZA activity resulting in significant pancytopenia. To prevent pancytopenia, the AZA dose should be reduced by 75–80% if used in combination with allopurinol and the white blood cell counts should be followed closely.

Side Effects

The most important side effects of AZA are hematologic (see Table 9.3). Leukopenia is a common finding but thrombocytopenia and anemia also can occur. Patients treated with AZA should have a complete blood cell count measured at least weekly during the first month of therapy and less frequently thereafter, as long as the drug dose remains stable. If significant myelosuppression is observed, the dose should be reduced.[35,36]

Other reported side effects of AZA include hepatitis and cholestasis, which present as reversible elevations in transaminases and bilirubin levels. Pancreatitis has also been reported, although it is rare. AZA's antiproliferative effects can also suppress other rapidly dividing cells resulting in alopecia and GI toxicities, such as anorexia, nausea, and vomiting.[27,36]

Mycophenolic Acid Derivatives

Mechanisms of Action

Mycophenolate mofetil (MMF or CellCept®) is a prodrug of mycophenolic acid. It was approved for use in 1995 and has essentially replaced AZA as the antiproliferative agent of choice given its relatively few side effects and superior effects in preventing acute rejection.[37] More recently, an enteric-coated form of mycophenolate sodium (ECMPS or Myfortic®) became available in 2004.

MMF is a reversible inhibitor of inosine monophosphate dehydrogenase (IMPDH), which is a critical rate-limiting enzyme in de novo purine synthesis. MMF achieves its antiproliferative effect by blocking nucleic acid synthesis. However, its effect is relatively selective for lymphocytes because not only do lymphocytes have a more susceptible isoform of IMPDH but they also rely more heavily on de novo purine synthesis, while other cell types have an alternative salvage pathway.[33,38,39]

Dosing

MMF is available as capsules in either 250 or 500 mg dosages. The standard dose when used in conjunction with CsA is 1 g administered twice daily; African Americans may need a higher dose of 1.5 g twice daily to achieve adequate suppression when used with CsA.[27] ECMPS is available in 180 and 360 mg capsules and the standard dose is 720 mg administered twice daily, which is equivalent to 1 g twice daily of MMF.[40] Only MMF is available as an intravenous formulation and intravenous dosing that is identical to the oral dose.

MMF is hydrolyzed to mycophenolic acid in the liver, producing an initial peak drug concentration in 1–2 h followed by a second peak in 5–6 h through enterohepatic cycling.[34,40] The gastrointestinal side effects of MMF stem from this cycling. Not surprisingly, ECMPS has also been reported to have similar gastrointestinal side effects as MMF,[40] despite earlier reports that suggested ECMPS had less GI toxicity than MMF. To minimize side effects, daily doses can be split into three to four administrations a day. Like AZA, therapeutic drug monitoring is not mandatory although some centers measure trough levels of mycophenolic acid in an effort to individualize dosing and assure adequate drug administration.

Drug Interactions

There are few significant drug interactions with MMF. However, concomitant administration of other antiproliferative agents, such as AZA or TOR inhibitors, should be done with caution to avoid excessive myelosuppression. Drugs that decrease intestinal absorption of MMF include antacids, cholestyramine, and oral ferrous sulfate. CsA can also decrease MMF concentrations by interfering with the enterohepatic cycling, an effect not seen with tacrolimus[27] This explains the higher dose of MMF sometimes needed when used in conjunction with CsA compared to tacrolimus and sirolimus.

Side Effects

The most important side effects for MMF are gastrointestinal in nature (see Table 9.3). Patients often complain of diarrhea and less commonly of nausea, bloating, dyspepsia, or emesis. Esophagitis, pancreatitis, and gastritis with occasional gastrointestinal hemorrhage also have been reported. These gastrointestinal side effects are dose dependent and usually respond to dose reduction.[27,35] Although MMF is more selective for lymphocytes than AZA, bone marrow suppression can still occur. Although all immunosuppressants increase the risk of infection, CMV infections have been reported to be more common with MMF.[35] Dose reduction, or discontinuation, has been associated with increased acute rejection, even in a previously stable patient. Therefore, the drug should be reintroduced as soon as possible, as dictated by the clinical course.[27,39] MMF and ECMPS are contraindicated in pregnancy (see Chapter 20).

mTOR Inhibitors

Mechanisms of Action

The newest antiproliferative agents are the mTOR inhibitors. mTOR stands for "mammalian target of rapamycin", which is a regulatory molecule that is needed for entry into the cell cycle. There are two medications in this class. Sirolimus (Rapamune®), also known as rapamycin, is a macrolide antibiotic compound structurally related to tacrolimus. Everolimus (Certican®) is a chemical variant of sirolimus, but is not used as frequently as sirolimus. Sirolimus is the only mTOR inhibitor approved by the FDA at this time. Initially, there was great enthusiasm for using sirolimus as an alternative to CNIs. However, as the side-effect profile of mTOR inhibitors emerged, enthusiasm for de novo uses of this mTOR inhibitor has waned.[41-43]

Because sirolimus is structurally similar to tacrolimus, it also binds the same intracellular binding protein used by tacrolimus (FKBP). However, the sirolimus–FKBP ligand does not block calcineurin, but instead blocks the effects of mTOR. As mentioned, mTOR is a key regulatory molecule in cell division; hence its blockade leads to the inhibition of cellular proliferation. The mTOR pathway also has an angiogenic effect, so unlike other antiproliferative agents, sirolimus has been reported to have unique antiangiogenic properties.[44]

Dosing

Sirolimus was initially formulated as an oral solution, but has been replaced by a more convenient oral form that comes in 1 and 5 mg capsules. Its usual dose is 2–5 mg daily. Sometimes an initial loading dose (up to 15 mg daily for 3 days) is used to more rapidly reach a steady state.[27,43] Like the CNIs, sirolimus is metabolized by the P450 enzyme and so has the same variations in inter- and intra-patient bioavailability as the CNIs. Therefore, blood level monitoring is required. The target level ranges from 10 to 20 ng/ml, with a lower target of 8–12 ng/ml in stable patients.[34] Because sirolimus has a long half-life, averaging 62 h, drug levels do not need to be checked until several days after dose adjustments. Since it is minimally excreted in the urine, there is no dose adjustment needed with renal impairment.[27]

Drug Interactions

Given that both CNIs and sirolimus are metabolized by P450, there is potential for interaction when these two classes of medication are administered together. It has been shown that when sirolimus is administered with CsA, there can be a significant increase in sirolimus levels. However, this effect can be decreased if the sirolimus is administered 4 h after CsA.[27] Tacrolimus does not appear to increase sirolimus levels. And like CNIs, sirolimus has similar drug interactions with increased drug levels from concomitant use of nondihydropyridine calcium channel blockers, azole antifungal agents, erythromycin, and grape fruit juice while decreased drug levels are observed with anticonvulsants such as phenytoin and carbamazepine.[45]

Side Effects

Sirolimus has many potential side effects (see Table 9.3), the most important of which are hyperlipidemia and myelosuppression. Poor wound healing stems from its antiproliferative and antiangiogenic properties.[45,46] Taken together with reports that the agent increases the risk of lymphoceles and delayed graft function,[43,45,46] use of sirolimus as a de novo maintenance immunosuppressant has fallen into disfavor.

In addition to myelosuppression, other rapidly dividing cells can also be affected resulting in oligospermia and apthous mouth ulcers. Unlike the CNIs, sirolimus is not thought to be nephrotoxic, but when administered with a CNI, there is a potentiation of CNI nephrotoxicity.[43,47] To avoid nephrotoxicity, the dose of CNI should be reduced when used in combination with sirolimus. A note of caution is that sirolimus has been reported to directly affect podocytes and to cause proteinuria, leading to nephrotic syndrome.[27,45] Recent reports also suggest that sirolimus may be diabetogenic, especially when used in combination with CNIs.[48] It can also cause myopathy, cholestasis, low testosterone levels with associated decreased libido, and edema that is resistant to diuretic therapy. One idiosyncratic reaction with sirolimus is noninfectious interstitial pneumonia. The diagnosis is one of exclusion and it usually resolves after 2–3 weeks of drug discontinuation. Sirolimus has shown antineoplastic effects in patients with renal cell carcinoma and Kaposi's sarcoma.[45,49]

Maintenance Drug Combinations

The number of available maintenance immunosuppressants for transplant recipients has greatly increased the number of potential drug combinations that can be used to prevent allograft rejection. The most popular combination of drugs currently used in the United States consists of tacrolimus and a mycophenolic acid derivative with or without prednisone. CsA-based regimens have declined in popularity. As mentioned above, de novo use of sirolimus is no longer common, although some centers convert patients from a CNI to sirolimus several months after transplantation. AZA is most often reserved for patients who are intolerant of the side effects or costs of the other antiproliferative agents.

Treatment of Acute Rejection

Treatment of acute rejection is best handled at the patient's transplant center. Some transplant centers obtain a percutaneous renal transplant biopsy to facilitate treatment decisions in patients with suspected rejection and others employ empiric treatment. Cases of acute cellular rejection that are deemed to be clinically or histologically mild are often treated initially with large "pulse" doses of corticosteroids (typically methylprednisolone in doses ranging from 250 to 1,000 mg intravenously daily for 3–5 days or oral prednisone 200 mg per day for 3–5 days). Patients who do not respond to pulse steroid therapy and those with clinically or histologically severe rejection are treated with anti-lymphoctye preparations including rabbit anti-thymocyte globulin or OKT3. The use of OKT3 for treatment of acute rejection has decreased greatly in the past decade, largely owing to its cost and significant first-dose side effects including a "cytokine storm" syndrome consisting of fever, headache, flu-like symptoms, and, more rarely, acute respiratory failure. Traditional anti-lymphocyte antibodies are often employed to treat antibody-mediated rejection, based on the concern for simultaneous cellular rejection. However, treatment with plasmapheresis, anti-CD20 antibodies (e.g., rituximab), and/or intravenous immune globulin (IVIg) is now commonly used as either primary or adjunctive therapy for humoral rejection.

References

1. Jordan SC, Tyan D, Stablein D et al. Evaluation of intravenous immunoglobulin as an agent to lower allosensitization and improve transplantation in highly sensitized adult patients with end-stage renal disease: report of the NIH IG02 trial. *J Am Soc Nephrol* 2004;15:3256–3262.
2. Stegall MD, Gloor J, Winters JL et al. A comparison of plasmapheresis versus high-dose IVIg desensitization in renal allograft recipients with high levels of donor specific alloantibody. *Am J Transplant* 2006;6:346–351.
3. Gloor JM, DeGoey SR, Pineda AA et al. Overcoming a positive crossmatch in living-donor kidney transplantation. *Am J Transplant* 2003;3:1017–1022.
4. Montgomery RA, Zachary AA. Transplanting patients with a positive donor-specific cross-match: a single center's perspective. *Pediatr Transplant* 2004;8:535–542.
5. Tyden G, Kumlein G, Genberg H et al. ABO incompatible kidney transplantations without splenectomy using antigen specific immunoadsorption and rituximab. *Am J Transplant* 2005;5:145–148.
6. Schwartz J, Stegall MD, Kremers WK et al. Complications, resource utilization and cost of ABO-incompatible living donor kidney transplantation. *Transplantation* 2006;82:155–163.
7. Szczech LA, Berlin JA, Aradhye S et al. Effect of antilymphocyte induction on renal allograft survival: a meta-analysis. *J Am Soc Nephrol* 1997;8:1771–1777.
8. Belitsky P, MacDonald AS, Lawen J et al. Use of rabbit anti-thymocyte globulin for induction immunosuppression in high-risk kidney transplant recipients. *Transplant Proc* 1997;29(Suppl 7A):16.
9. Brennan DC, Daller JA, Lake KD et al. Rabbit antithymocyte globulin versus basiliximab in renal transplantation. *N Eng J Med* 2006;355:1967–1977.
10. Bloom DD, Hu H, Fechner JH et al. T-lymphocyte alloresponses of campath 1-H treated kidney transplant patients. *Transplantation* 2006;81:81–87.
11. Shapiro R, Basu A, Tan H et al. Kidney transplantation under minimal immunosuppression after pretransplant lymphoid depletion either thymoglobulin or campath. *J Am Coll Surg* 2005;200:505–515.
12. Watson CJ, Bradley JA, Friend PJ et al. Alemtuzumab (CAMPATH 1H) induction therapy in cadaveric kidney transplantation – efficacy and safety at five years. *Am J Transplant* 2005;5:1347–1353.
13. Barth RN, Janus CA, Lilesand CA et al. Outcomes at 3 years of a prospective pilot study of campath-1H and sirolimus immunosuppression for renal transplantation. *Transpl Int* 2006;19:885–892.
14. Flechner SM, Friend PJ, Brockmann J et al. Alemtuzumab induction and sirolimus plus mycophenolate mofetil maintenance for CNI and steroid-free kidney transplant immunosuppression. *Am J Transplant* 2005;5:3009–3014.

15. Norman DJ, Kahana L, Stuart FP et al. A randomized clinical trial of induction therapy with OKT3 in kidney transplantation. *Transplantation* 1993;55:44–50.

16. Nashan B, Moore R, Amlot P et al. Randomized trial of basiliximab versus placebo for control of acute cellular rejection in renal allograft recipients. *Lancet* 1997;1:1193.

17. Vincenti F, Kirkman R, Light S et al. Interleukin-2 receptor blockade with daclizumab to prevent acute rejection in renal transplantation. *N Engl J Med* 1998;338:161–165.

18. Ahsan N, Holman MJ, Jarowenko MV et al. Limited dose monoclonal IL-2R antibody induction protocol after primary kidney transplantation. *Am J Transplant* 2002;2:568–573.

19. Ter Meulen CG. Two doses of Daclizumab are sufficient for prolonged interleukin-2R chain blockade. *Transplantation* 2001;72:1709–1710.

20. Hollenberg SM, Evans RM. Multiple and cooperative trans-activation domains of the human glucocorticoid receptor. *Cell* 1988;55:899–906.

21. Augustine JJ, Hricik DE. Steroid sparing in kidney transplantation: changing paradigms, improving outcomes, and remaining questions. *Clin J Am Soc Nephrol* 2006;1:1080–1089.

22. First MR. Improving long-term renal transplant outcomes with tacrolimus: speculation vs evidence. *Nephrol Dial Transplant* 2004;19(Suppl 6):17–22.

23. Dunn CJ, Wagstaff AJ, Perry CM et al. Cyclosporin: an updated review of the pharmacokinetic properties, clinical Efficacy and tolerability of a microemulsion-based formulation (neoral) in organ transplantation. *Drugs* 2001;61:1957–2016.

24. Scott LJ, McKeage K, Keam SJ et al. Tacrolimus: a further update of its use in the management of organ transplantation. *Drugs* 2003;63:1247–1297.

25. Waiser J, Slowinski T, Brinker-Paschke A et al. Impact of the variability of cyclosporin A trough levels on long-term allograft function. *Nephrol Dial Transplant* 2002;17:1310–1317.

26. Fung JJ. Tacrolimus and transplantation: a decade in review. *Transplantation* 2004;77 (9 Suppl):S41–S43.

27. Danovitch GM. Immunosuppressive medications and protocols for kidney transplantation. In: Danovitch GM, (ed.), Handbook of Kidney Transplantation. Philadelphia, PA, Lippincott Williams & Wilkins, 2005, pp. 72–134.

28. Miller LW. Cardiovascular toxicities of immunosuppressive agents. *Am J Transplant* 2002;2:807–818.

29. Jurewicz WA. Tacrolimus versus ciclosporin immunosuppression: long-term outcome in renal transplantation. *Nephrol Dial Transplant* 2003;18(Suppl 1):7–11.

30. Claesson K, Mayer AD, Squifflet JP et al. Lipoprotein patterns in renal transplant patients: a comparison between FK506 and cyclosporine A patients. *Transplant Proc* 1998;30: 1292–1294.

31. Jensik SC. Tacrolimus (FK506) in kidney transplantation: three-year survival results of the US multicenter, randomized, comparative trial. FK 506 Kidney Transplant Study Group. *Transplant Proc* 1998;30:1216–1218.

32. Heisel O, Heisel R, Balshaw R et al. New onset diabetes mellitus in patients receiving calcineurin inhibitors: a systematic review and meta-analysis. *Am J Transplant* 2004;4: 583–595.

33. Tanabe K. Calcineurin inhibitors in renal transplantation. *Drugs* 2003;63:1535–1548.

34. Siegel CT. Maintenance immunosuppression. In: Hricik DE, (ed.), Kidney Transplantation. Chicago, IL, Remedica, 2007, pp. 55–75.

35. Braun WE. Renal transplantation: basic concepts and evolution of therapy. *J Clin Apher* 2003;18:141–152.

36. Chan GLC, Canafax DM, Johnson CA. The therapeutic use of azathioprine in renal transplantation. *Parmacotherapy* 1987;7:165–177.

37. Meier-Kriesche HU, Steffen BJ, Hochberg AM et al. Mycophenolate mofetil versus azathioprine therapy is associated with a significant protection against long-term renal allograft function deterioration. *Transplantation* 2003;75:1341–1346.

38. Allison AC, Eugui EM. Mechanism of action of mycophenolate mofetil in preventing acute and chronic allograft rejection. *Transplantation* 2005;80(2 Suppl):S181–S190.

39. Pelletier RP, Akin B, Henry ML et al. The impact of mycophenolate mofetil dosing patterns on clinical outcome after renal transplantation. *Clin Transplant* 2003;17:200–205.
40. Sollinger H. Enteric-coated mycophenolate sodium: therapeutic equivalence to mycophenolate mofetil in de novo renal transplant patients. *Transplant Proc* 2004;36(Suppl):S517–S520.
41. Flechner SM, Kobashigawa J, Klintmalm G. Calcineurin inhibitor-sparing regimens in solid organ transplantation: focus on improving renal function and nephrotoxicity. *Clin Transplant* 2008;22:1–15.
42. Johnson RW. How should sirolimus be used in clinical practice? *Transplant Proc* 2003;35(3 Suppl):S79–S83.
43. Kuypers DR. Benefit-risk assessment of sirolimus in renal transplantation. *Drug Saf* 2005;28:153–181.
44. Chueh SC, Kahan BD. Clinical application of sirolimus in renal transplantation: an update. *Transpl Int* 2005;18:261–277.
45. Augustine JJ, Bodziak KA, Hricik DE. Use of sirolimus in solid organ transplantation. *Drugs* 2007;67:369–391.
46. Valente JF, Hricik D, Weigel K et al. Comparison of sirolimus vs mycophenolate mofetil on surgical complications and wound healing in adult kidney transplantation. *Am J Transplant* 2003;3:1128–1134.
47. Webster AC, Lee VW, Chapman JR et al. Target of rapamycin inhibitors (sirolimus and everolimus) for primary immunosuppression of kidney transplant recipients: a systematic review and meta-analysis of randomized trials. *Transplantation* 2006;81:1234–1248.
48. Romagnoli J, Citterio F, Nanni G et al. Incidence of posttransplant diabetes mellitus in kidney transplant recipients immunosuppressed with sirolimus in combination with cyclosporine. *Transplant Proc* 2006;38:1034–1036.
49. Kauffman HM, Cherikh WS, Cheng Y et al. Maintenance immunosuppression with target-of-rapamycin inhibitors is associated with a reduced incidence of de novo malignancies. *Transplantation* 2005;80:883–889.

Chapter 10
Optimizing Immunosuppression

Alexander C. Wiseman and James E. Cooper

Rationale for Optimizing Current Immunosuppressant Strategies

While short-term outcomes in kidney transplantation have improved significantly over the last decades, questions remain regarding long-term improvements in graft survival. Whereas long-term graft survival was reported to improve significantly from the mid-1980s to the mid-1990s,[1] a more recent analysis has shown an equivalent relative risk of graft failure for those transplanted in 1995 through 2000 despite a reduction in acute rejection rates of nearly 50% during that time.[2] Thus, attention has shifted to medication regimens that not only prevent early acute rejection but also take into consideration drug side-effect profiles, ease of use, and effect on long-term graft function.

One potentially modifiable factor in improving long-term graft function is the avoidance of nephrotoxicity caused by calcineurin inhibitors (CNIs). CNI nephrotoxicity may be present in 33% of protocol biopsies at 1 year and nearly 100% of all biopsies at 10 years.[3] Recipients of non-kidney solid organ transplants are not exempt from CNI nephrotoxicity, as over 90% of liver, heart, and lung transplant patients remain on CNI at 1 year,[4] with rates of chronic kidney disease (GFR < 30 ml/min) of 10–20% over the long term.[5] In addition to their nephrotoxic effects, CNIs are associated with post-transplant diabetes, hypertension, hyperlipidemia, hirsutism, neurotoxicity, and alopecia. With the development of newer agents, considerable effort has been devoted to safely reducing exposure of kidney transplant recipients to CNIs over the last decade.

While steroids have not been implicated in chronic graft loss, they are associated with numerous complications that have significant effects on patient morbidity and dissatisfaction. As with CNIs, steroid use causes hypertension and hyperlipidemia, but can also result in obesity, glucose intolerance, osteonecrosis, avascular

A.C. Wiseman (✉)
Kidney and Pancreas Transplant Program, Department of Nephrology, University of Colorado, Aurora, CO, USA
e-mail: alexander.wiseman@ucdenver.edu

D.B. McKay, S.M. Steinberg (eds.), *Kidney Transplantation: A Guide to the Care of Kidney Transplant Recipients*, DOI 10.1007/978-1-4419-1690-7_10, © Springer Science+Business Media, LLC 2010

necrosis, glaucoma, cataracts, myopathy, cushingoid features, and neuropsychiatric complications. An economic analysis of chronic steroid therapy in kidney transplant recipients estimated a $5,300 cost per patient year in 1996,[6] concluding that elimination of steroids from immunosuppressive regimens would be cost equivalent even if associated with an 11% increase in acute rejection rates. Importantly, patients perceive steroids to be less desirable than CNIs and if given an option to discontinue one medication, 65% would prefer steroid elimination vs. 19% that would prefer CNI elimination.[7] The metabolic, cardiovascular, and cosmetic side effects associated with chronic corticosteroid use have inspired numerous trials to limit their use. Figure 10.2 illustrates common side effects encountered with chronic steroid and CNI use.

Current State of Transplant Immunosuppression

Despite the diversity of agents available for the clinician caring for kidney transplant patients, combination therapy with a CNI, an antiproliferative agent, and prednisone remains the primary strategy at present. Figure 10.1 illustrates the trend of immunosuppressive regimens at time of discharge over recent years. Calcineurin inhibition remains the foundation of immunosuppression, with 94% of patients discharged on a CNI after transplant (Table 10.1, 2007 OPTN/SRTR annual report, table 5.6e). Over the last decade tacrolimus has largely replaced cyclosporine (CsA) as the preferred CNI after reports of improved graft outcomes with use of the former.[8-10] A similar trend can be seen in the antiproliferative category, with MMF used in 87% of discharge regimens vs. <1% receiving azathioprine (OPTN/SRTR 2007 annual report, table 5.6e). Sirolimus (SRL) was prescribed to 8% of transplant recipients

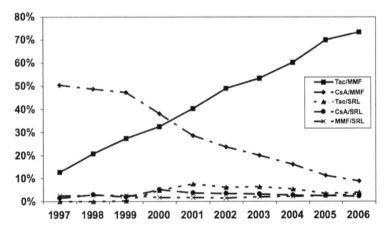

Fig. 10.1 Trends in immunosuppression regimens at the time of hospital discharge 1997–2006. CsA, cyclosporine; MMF, mycophenolate mofetil; Tac, tacrolimus; SRL, sirolimus (Source: OPTN/SRTR annual report, table 5.6e)

Table 10.1 Acute allograft rejection and 1-year allograft survival by era and associated developments in immunosuppression agents

Era	Immunosuppression developments[a]	Acute rejection (%)	1-Year graft survival (%)
1960s–1970s	Azathiaprine/prednisone/polyclonal antibodies	Near 100	30–50
1980s	Cyclosporine and OKT3 introduced	50	80
1990s	Mycophenolate, tacrolimus, thymoglobulin introduced	25	90
2000s	IL-2 receptor antibodies, sirolimus introduced	10–15	95

[a]The development of newer agents has markedly decreased acute rejection rates and improved short-term graft survival

at discharge in 2007 and has seen a steady decline in use since its peak of 17% in 2001. Similar trends are apparent in immunosuppressant maintenance regimens at 1 year post-transplant, with 64% of patients on a combination of tacrolimus + MMF, followed by 10% on CSA + MMF. Tacrolimus + SRL and CsA + SRL regimens comprise smaller percentages of maintenance regimens at 4 and 2%, respectively (OPTN/SRTR 2007 annual report, table 5.6d) (Fig. 10.1). Acute allograft rejection and 1-year allograft survival by era is shown in Table 10.1 and drug side-effect profiles is shown in Fig. 10.2.

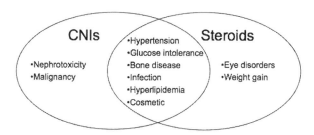

Fig. 10.2 Common side effects associated with chronic steroid and CNI use

Corticosteroid Minimization

Given the side-effect profile and patient dissatisfaction with chronic steroid use, a number of immunosuppression strategies have been studied to test the necessity of chronic prednisone use in kidney transplantation. These methods can generally be categorized into those that discontinue steroids later (3 months) after transplant, those that discontinue steroids early (days to weeks) after transplant, and those that avoid exposure altogether (Table 10.2).

Table 10.2 Summary of selected corticosteroid minimization studies

Author/year	N	Protocol	Induction	Results
Vanrenterghem (2000)[a] *Late withdrawal*	300	Steroids w/d at 3 months vs. standard taper, CsA + MMF maintenance	~33% each group (Atgam or OKT3)	• AR in 25% of w/d group vs. 15% of controls at 6 months follow-up • Lower blood pressure and cholesterol in w/d group
Ahsan (1999)[a] *Late withdrawal*	266	Steroids w/d at 3 months vs. standard taper, CsA + MMF maintenance	~30% each group	• Study terminated early due to 22% AR in w/d group vs. 5% in controls
Matas (2005) *Early withdrawal*	589	Steroids w/d at 6 days vs. standard taper, CNI + MMF or SRL maintenance	Thymoglobulin	• 5-year actuarial graft survival 84% with 1 AR rates 11% • Compared to historical controls, w/d group with less PTDM, AVN, CMV
Kaufman (2005) *Early withdrawal*	278	Steroids w/d at 3 days and Tac + MMF maintenance in all patients	Campath (123) or basiliximab (155)	• Retrospective analysis comparing two induction regimens demonstrating excellent AR rates (15%) with either agent
Kumar (2006)[a] *Early withdrawal*	300	Steroid w/d at 2 days vs. standard taper, CNI + MMF or SRL maintenance	Basiliximab	• Similar 1-year AR and 3-year actuarial graft survival between groups • Protocol biopsies with similar subacute and chronic rejection in each group • Less PTDM and weight gain in w/d group
Woodle (2008) (*Astellas*)[a] *Early withdrawal*	397	Steroid w/d at 7 days vs. standard taper, Tac + MMF maintenance	Basiliximab, dacluzimab, or thymoglobulin	• No difference in primary composite endpoint (see text) at 5-year follow-up • Probability of AR higher in w/d group • No difference in cholesterol, blood pressure, or PTDM
Vincenti (2008) (*FREEDOM*)[a] *Avoidance and early withdrawal*	538	Complete steroid avoidance vs. steroid w/d at 7 days vs. standard taper, CsA + MMF maintenance	Basiliximab	• GFR at 12 months similar between arms • AR rates higher in avoidance (31%) and w/d (26%) arms vs. control (14%) • Lower BMI, lipid-lowering, and anti-hyperglycemic medication use in w/d or avoidance arms, no difference in bone density or blood pressure

[a]Prospective, randomized controlled studies.

CsA cyclosporine; *MMF* mycophenolate mofetil; *Tac* tacrolimus; *SRL* sirolimus; *AR* acute rejection; *w/d* withdrawal,

Late Steroid Withdrawal

With the development of new immunosuppressive agents, attempts have been made to eliminate prednisone from chronic immunosuppression. The introduction of CsA in the 1980s led to a number of steroid withdrawal trials that reported a wide range of acute rejection rates as high as 81% in the withdrawal groups. Steroid withdrawal in these early trials occurred from 6 days to 6 years post-transplant and generally utilized CsA in combination with azathioprine and steroids, while the use of polyclonal antibody induction therapy was not common.[11] A meta-analysis of trials performed during the CsA/azathioprine era reported a 48% acute rejection rate in steroid withdrawal arms compared to 30% in control arms.[12] Importantly, longer term follow-up suggested a detrimental effect on graft survival.[13,14] Discouraging as these results may have been, studies consistently reported favorable metabolic effects such as reduced hypercholesterolemia and less anti-hypertensive medication requirement.

The introduction of MMF in the mid-1990s led to two pivotal multicenter trials examining steroid withdrawal 3 months after transplant. A large double-blind placebo-controlled European study randomized 500 transplant recipients of low immunological risk to either steroid withdrawal or continuation at 3 months in addition to maintenance therapy with CsA and MMF. Induction therapy was optional and occurred in approximately 30% of each cohort. Acute rejection was more common in the steroid withdrawal group vs. the control group (23% vs. 14%),[15] while serum creatinine at 1 year was similar between the two groups. In this study, patients that had experienced acute rejection in the first 3 months post-transplant prior to randomization were not excluded, and interestingly this was the time period during which most rejection episodes occurred. When analyzing data from only those who had received induction therapy there was no significant difference in acute rejection rates between the two groups, raising the question of applicability of this and other similar induction-free or induction-optional studies to current practice in which a large majority of patients receive antibody induction.

A multicenter American trial was conducted with similar design. Patients were maintained on CsA, MMF, and steroids post-transplant until 3 months when steroids were either withdrawn or continued. The study population was slightly higher risk and included a proportion of African Americans. As in the European study, induction therapy was optional and occurred in approximately 30% of patients in each cohort. In contrast to its European counterpart, however, patients were excluded if any acute rejection episode occurred within the first 3 months. Enrollment into this study was halted by the data safety monitoring board after 266 of 500 patients were enrolled due to a fourfold to fivefold increase in acute rejection episodes in the steroid withdrawal group (22% vs. 5% in control).[16] This discrepancy was more pronounced in African Americans, 60% of whom in the steroid withdrawal group experienced acute rejection. As opposed to the European study, prior treatment with induction therapy had no impact on acute rejection rates.

Whereas the majority of late steroid withdrawal investigation has been undertaken in the setting of CsA maintenance, several smaller studies have addressed the issue while utilizing more recent maintenance therapeutic options. Results of late steroid withdrawal in transplant recipients maintained on tacrolimus and MMF have been reported in two unblinded European trials with low-risk populations. In both studies steroids were withdrawn after 3 months, and in both studies there was no significant difference in acute rejection episodes between groups.[17,18] Information on induction therapy is not available. Late steroid withdrawal with a background SRL-based maintenance immunosuppression has been reported in several small non-randomized studies. Hricik et al. observed the effects of steroid withdrawal at 3 months in a population of African American transplant recipients maintained on SRL and tacrolimus. With an average of 4 years follow-up, acute rejection was reported at 41%, with only 41% of patients still free of steroids.[19]

These data have created the general perception that late steroid withdrawal is associated with a higher risk of acute rejection, confirmed in a meta-analysis of six trials utilizing MMF and CNIs, in which the pooled relative risk of acute rejection was 2.28 for those who underwent late steroid withdrawal.[20] Though difficult to objectively measure, it is important to weigh the cost of an increased risk of acute rejection against the beneficial effects of reduced steroid exposure on metabolic side effects and subsequent potential impact on longer term cardiovascular outcomes. Indeed, the majority of late steroid withdrawal studies (mostly non-randomized) report improvements in parameters such as total cholesterol, mean arterial pressure, requirement for anti-hypertensive agents, and blood glucose in groups assigned to steroid removal. Thus, studies that show more acute rejection during a 6- or 12-month follow-up in those who underwent late steroid removal may have different conclusions if patient and graft survival was assessed at longer follow-up.

Early Steroid Withdrawal and Steroid Avoidance

The uninspiring experience with later steroid withdrawal has guided more recent steroid minimization efforts to concentrate on early steroid withdrawal within the first week after transplant, as well as complete steroid avoidance. While it may seem counterintuitive that these strategies could lead to better outcomes than late steroid withdrawal, it is possible that initial steroid use and later withdrawal may be detrimental. Corticosteroids decrease cytokine release but may upregulate cytokine receptors on T cells.[21] Following late steroid withdrawal, a subsequent increase in cytokine release with binding to upregulated receptors may then promote an enhanced T-cell response and lead to acute rejection. Clinically, the burden of steroid-related side effects is greatest in the first 3–6 months, providing an additional argument in support of early steroid withdrawal.

Unlike the bulk of late steroid withdrawal trials, widespread use of antibody induction is a common theme in the majority of early steroid withdrawal and steroid avoidance studies. A number of initial pilot studies employing early steroid withdrawal at ~5 days post-transplant showed favorable results in terms of graft survival and acute rejection rates.[22–25] Though not randomized, Matas et al.[26] published the largest to-date experience with early steroid withdrawal from a cohort of 589 low-risk patients. All patients received thymoglobulin induction for 5 days and had steroids withdrawn after 6 days post-transplant. Maintenance immunosuppression consisted of a CNI plus either MMF or SRL. Excellent outcomes were observed with actuarial 5-year patient survival at 91%, graft survival at 84%, and 1-year rejection-free graft survival at 89%. Compared to historical controls, this cohort experienced lower rates of CMV, avascular necrosis (AVN), post-transplant diabetes (PTDM), cataracts, bone fractures, and non-PTLD malignancy. Several other large single-center experiences of early steroid withdrawal protocols have also reported favorable results with alternative induction regimens and steroid withdrawal after 2 or 3 days.[27,28] Significantly less weight gain and PTDM were seen in the steroid withdrawal patients in the former study, supporting similar findings that were noted in the large observational cohort mentioned above.[26]

Recently, a large, multicenter, double-blind placebo-controlled *Astellas* study helped to clarify the potential risks and benefits of early steroid withdrawal.[29] This study documented 5-year outcomes of 397 low-risk patients that underwent antibody induction, tacrolimus/MMF maintenance immunosuppression, and steroid treatment that was either tapered to 5–10 mg at 6 months or withdrawn after 7 days. No significant difference was seen in the primary endpoint (a composite of death, graft loss, or moderate to severe acute rejection) or in any of the individual components. Renal function between the two cohorts was also similar at 5 years. However, there was a significantly higher rate of acute rejection in the steroid withdrawal group over 5 years (primarily noted in patients treated with IL-2 receptor antagonists rather than thymoglobulin) and a post hoc analysis of for-cause biopsies showed a significantly higher (4.8%) rate of chronic allograft nephropathy (CAN) ($p = 0.028$) in the steroid withdrawal group compared to control. Importantly, there was no difference in HDL, LDL, total cholesterol, blood pressure, mean weight change, or PTDM between groups, although triglyceride level and fracture rate were less in the steroid withdrawal arm.

Complete steroid avoidance has also been studied in a recent large multicenter trial. In the FREEDOM trial, 337 patients were randomized to undergo no steroid treatment at all, steroid withdrawal after 7 days, or standard chronic steroid use, all in the setting of induction with basiliximab and chronic immunosuppression with CsA and MMF. The three groups had a similar primary endpoint of GFR at 12 months;[30] however, the steroid avoidance cohort experienced a significantly higher amount of biopsy-proven acute rejection (31.5%) compared to the chronic steroid arm (14.7%). Of interest, a higher biopsy-proven acute rejection rate was reported in the steroid withdrawal arm (26.4%) compared to many of the early steroid withdrawal trials mentioned previously, possibly due in part to the open-label nature of this study leading to a significantly higher number of for-cause biopsies performed. While the de novo use of anti-hyperglycemic medications was significantly less in the steroid avoidance arm, significantly lower BMI and use of lipid-lowering medications were only seen in the early withdrawal arm, and no difference was detected in bone density or anti-hypertensive medication use between arms.

Corticosteroid Minimization: Summary

The untoward metabolic effects of chronic corticosteroid use have been apparent in kidney transplant recipients since they first became a mainstay in maintenance immunosuppression protocols over four decades ago. Strategies to reduce steroid exposure continue to gain interest as new immunosuppressive agents emerge. However, the potential metabolic benefits of reduced steroid exposure must be weighed carefully against the ongoing elevated risk of acute rejection and chronic graft nephropathy. Results from studies of steroid withdrawal at later time periods (>3 months) were disappointing, while studies of early withdrawal are more encouraging, particularly when performed in the setting of depleting antibody induction. The recent *Astellas* study and FREEDOM trials point toward caution, however, with higher rates of acute rejection and metabolic improvements that are not overwhelming.[29] Nevertheless, minimization of steroid exposure may be preferable for certain individuals at high risk for metabolic and/or cardiovascular complications. Clinicians must weigh the increased risk of acute rejection and potential for chronic allograft nephropathy vs. the patient's interest in avoiding the side effects of chronic steroid use when determining if steroid withdrawal is appropriate.

Calcineurin Inhibitor Minimization

Given the inherent nephrotoxicity as well as metabolic and cosmetic side effects common with CNI use, the elimination or withdrawal of CNI from the kidney transplant patient's regimen has been a growing practice. In 2004, 21% of patients were not taking CNI at 1 year following transplant. Similar to steroid withdrawal and avoidance, CNI minimization strategies can be segregated to CNI withdrawal/conversion at time points following early CNI use ("early" withdrawal/conversion, typically 3–6 months post-transplant, or "late" withdrawal/conversion, following identification of graft dysfunction) or CNI avoidance (Tables 10.3 and 10.4).

Early Calcineurin Inhibitor Withdrawal/Conversion

Reminiscent of the early steroid withdrawal trials, early studies of CNI withdrawal during the azathioprine era yielded disappointing results with unacceptably high rejection rates.[14] Newer agents such as MMF and SRL renewed enthusiasm for CNI withdrawal strategies[31,32] and led to a number of multicenter trials. With MMF as the antiproliferative agent, 536 patients in the large, prospective, multicenter *CEASAR* study on CsA, MMF, and prednisone maintenance were randomized to either undergo CsA withdrawal at 4 months, continue standard dose CsA (trough

Table 10.3 Summary of CNI withdrawal/conversion randomized controlled trials

Study	N	Intervention	Protocol	Results
Abramowitz (2005)	151	Early CNI w/d: 3 months	• CsA w/d vs. control • MMF + Pred maintenance	• Creatinine clearance and graft loss similar between groups at 5-year follow-up • AR higher in CsA w/d group (10%) vs. controls (1%)
Oberbauer (2005)	430	Early CNI w/d: 3 months	• CsA w/d vs. control • SRL + pred maintenance	• Improved graft survival, GFR, blood pressure in CsA w/d group at 4-year follow-up • Non-significant increased risk AR and death in CsA w/d group
Ekberg (2007) *"CAESAR"*	536	Early CNI w/d: 4 months	• CsA standard or low dose vs. w/d • MMF + pred maintenance	• Primary endpoint of GFR at 12 months similar between groups • AR higher in CsA w/d group (38%) vs. low dose (25%) or standard dose (27%) CsA groups
Dudley (2005) *"Creeping creatinine"*	143	Late CNI conversion: 5–6 years (worsening graft function)	• CsA converted to MMF vs. control • +/– Aza, +/– pred maintenance	• 58% responders (stabilization or improvement in serum creatinine) in CsA w/d group vs. 32% in controls • No acute rejection episodes in CsA w/d group
Brennen (2008) *"CONVERT"*	830	Late CNI conversion: 6–60 months	• CNI converted to SRL vs. control • MMF + pred maintenance	• No difference in GFR overall, worse proteinuria in SRL/MMF/pred arm • Improved renal function without increase AR at 2 years in patients with GFR > 40 cc/min and minimal baseline proteinuria

CsA, cyclosporine; MMF, mycophenolate mofetil; SRL, sirolimus; Aza, azathioprine; AR, acute rejection; w/d, withdrawal.

Table 10.4 Summary of CNI avoidance randomized controlled trials

Study	N	Protocol	Induction	Results
Asberg (2006)	54	CsA/MMF/pred vs. IL–2RA/MMF/pred	Dacluzimab for CsA avoidance arm	• Increased AR in avoidance arm (70%) vs. 30% in CsA arm • GFR 52 cc/min in avoidance arm vs. 69 cc/min in CsA arm
Flechner (2007)	61	CsA/MMF/pred vs. SRL/MMF/pred	Basiliximab	• Improved GFR in SRL arm (60 cc/min) vs. CsA arm (49 cc/min) • Non-significant AR increase in CsA arm (16%) vs. SRL arm (6%)
Larson (2006)	165	Tac/MMF/pred vs. SRL/MMF/pred	Thymoglobulin	• Similar AR and GFR between groups at 2 years • Higher discontinuation rate in SRL arm (38%) vs. Tac arm (16%)
Ekberg (2008) "*Elite-symphony*"	1645	Standard CsA/MMF/pred vs. Low-dose CsA/MMF/pred vs. Low-dose Tac/MMF/pred vs. SRL/MMF/pred	Dacluzimab except standard CsA arm	• Tac arm: lower AR, increased graft survival and GFR at 12 months compared to CsA or SRL arms • SRL arm: highest AR, lowest graft survival and GFR at 12 months compared to CNI arms

CsA, cyclosporine; MMF, mycophenolate mofetil; Tac, tacrolimus; SRL, sirolimus; IL–2RA, interleukin 2-receptor antagonist; AR, acute rejection; w/d, withdrawal.

150–300 ng/ml), or taper to low-dose CsA (trough 50–100 ng/ml). While no difference was seen in the primary endpoint of GFR at 12 months, significantly higher rejection rates were noted in the CsA withdrawal group (38%) compared to either of the CsA continuation groups (25–27%).[33] Single-center studies also report a higher rate of acute rejection when withdrawing CSA from a CSA/MMF/prednisone regimen which is associated with worse long-term graft survival rates[34] and a higher incidence of C4d staining on protocol biopsies.[35] With SRL as the antiproliferative agent, 430 patients in the multicenter "Rapamune Maintenance Regimen Trial" on CsA, SRL, and prednisone were randomized to CsA withdrawal and increased SRL target trough levels 3 months after transplant or remain on triple therapy. At 1, 3, and 5 years, GFR was significantly better in the CsA withdrawal arm, despite a nominally higher acute rejection rate.[36–38] Additional smaller studies of CNI withdrawal at 2–3 months post-transplant mirror these findings of improved GFR despite slightly higher acute rejection rates.[39–41] While SRL may be more effective than MMF in CNI withdrawal strategies in combination with prednisone, issues of tolerability may limit this approach. Ongoing clinical trials are investigating if the combination of lower dose SRL and MMF is effective and better tolerated in patients who undergo CNI discontinuation 1–3 months post-transplantation.

Later Calcineurin Inhibitor Withdrawal/Conversion

Frequently, clinicians will consider withdrawal of CNI when deterioration in GFR is noted or when biopsy findings suggest chronic nephrotoxicity and/or fibrosis. In the "Creeping Creatinine" study, the effect of removing CsA with MMF maintenance was compared to CsA maintenance (either alone or in combination with azathioprine or steroids) in 143 transplant recipients with deteriorating graft function. GFR stabilized without episodes of acute rejection in patients who underwent CsA discontinuation.[42] Another common CNI withdrawal strategy is conversion from CNI to SRL in patients on a CNI/MMF/prednisone regimen. Data from the multicenter randomized CONVERT trial, in which 830 patients 6–120 months post-kidney transplant were randomized 2:1 to SRL conversion vs. CNI maintenance, suggest that subjects with GFR > 40 ml/min and minimal proteinuria (urine protein/creatinine ratio <0.11) at baseline experienced improved renal function at 24 months following CNI conversion to SRL without increased acute rejection rates, while those with proteinuria or GFR < 40 ml/min did not derive benefit from the transition.[43] When data from the CONVERT trial are pooled in meta-analysis with other prospective trials converting CNI to SRL in CAN, improvements in renal function are noted, but issues of increased proteinuria and high rates of discontinuation of SRL due to adverse events remain common themes.[44] Proteinuria, GFR <30 ml/min, and moderate/severe interstitial fibrosis are factors that are associated with continued deterioration despite CNI withdrawal and limit the benefits of this strategy.

Calcineurin Inhibitor Avoidance

The rapid development of CNI nephrotoxicity has prompted efforts to completely eliminate exposure of CNIs from the outset of transplantation (Table 10.4). After a number of earlier trials suggested that MMF/prednisone was inadequate as initial immunosuppression due to unacceptably high acute rejection rates of 50–70%,[45,46] strategies using de novo SRL/MMF/prednisone gained a significant amount of attention.[47–52] In perhaps the two most clinically applicable single-center studies, Flechner et al. demonstrated better GFR with SRL when compared to a CsA-based regimen, while Larsen et al. did not show benefits with SRL vs. a tacrolimus-based regimen.[47,51,52] Induction therapy was different among these trials (basiliximab in the former, thymoglobulin in the latter), as were the target trough levels for SRL, which could explain a lack of benefit, a higher degree of medication intolerance, and a high incidence of impaired wound healing with SRL in the latter study. Registry data also support the findings of the latter study, with inferior graft survival and higher discontinuation rates in patients maintained on SRL/MMF compared to CNI/MMF combinations reported in a large retrospective analysis of >58,000 transplant recipients.[53]

The multicenter, randomized, controlled *Symphony* study is the largest comparison of CNI vs. SRL-based immunosuppression to date. A total of 1645 renal transplant recipients were prospectively randomized to receive either standard dose CsA (initial trough 150–300 ng/ml), low-dose CsA (trough 50–100 ng/ml), low-dose tacrolimus (trough 3–7 ng/ml), or CNI avoidance with SRL (trough 4–8 ng/ml). All patients were treated with MMF and steroids, and all patients except those in the standard dose CsA arm received induction therapy with dacluzimab. At 12 months of follow-up, the low-dose tacrolimus arm had a significantly higher GFR and graft survival rate with lower rate of acute rejection, while patients in the CNI avoidance SRL arm experienced worse outcomes in all primary and secondary endpoints compared to the other three groups.[54] Questions remain regarding the appropriateness of the SRL trough levels, but certainly these results have dampened enthusiasm for de novo CNI-free immunosuppression with SRL.

Conversely, a novel agent, beletacept (a costimulation blocker that inhibits T-cell proliferation) has been studied in a CNI-free regimen and compared favorably vs. a CsA-based regimen, with similar rejection rates, tolerability, and improved measured GFR at 12 months.[55] Further studies and FDA review are pending.

Calcineurin Inhibitor Minimization: Summary

Given the large registry data and multicenter trial results described, CNIs appropriately remain the standard of care in the de novo setting. Successful CNI withdrawal in the setting of graft dysfunction is unpredictable and appears to be influenced by the degree of chronic injury, particularly glomerular injury, clinically reflected by the degree of baseline proteinuria. Opportunities for CNI withdrawal appear most promising after a period of stability but prior to significant graft dysfunction. A number of newer agents including belatacept are in development and may prove to be more efficacious than our current immunosuppressive agents in CNI avoidance and/or withdrawal.

Optimizing Immunosuppression – Conclusions

CNI-based prednisone maintenance immunosuppression remains the standard immunosuppression regimen for the majority of patients. Strategies to minimize the untoward effects of these medications must be considered together with the patient's immunologic risk profile and potential for side effects, since most studies have been performed in low-risk patients. Novel agents will again permit the transplant community to continue to test strategies in order to optimize both graft survival and patient quality of life.

Acknowledgments   The authors wish to thank the Scientific Registry of Transplant Recipients for supplying data used to generate Fig. 10.1 within this chapter. The data and analyses reported in the 2007 Annual Report of the US Organ Procurement and Transplantation Network and the Scientific Registry of Transplant Recipients have been supplied by UNOS and Arbor Research under contract with HHS. The authors alone are responsible for reporting and interpreting these data.

References

1. Hariharan S et al. Improved graft survival after renal transplantation in the United States, 1988 to 1996. *N Engl J Med* 2000;342(9):605–612.
2. Meier-Kriesche HU et al. Lack of improvement in renal allograft survival despite a marked decrease in acute rejection rates over the most recent era. *Am J Transplant* 2004;4(3):378–383.
3. Nankivell BJ et al. The natural history of chronic allograft nephropathy. *N Engl J Med* 2003;349(24):2326–2333.
4. Meier-Kriesche HU et al. Immunosuppression: evolution in practice and trends, 1994–2004. *Am J Transplant* 2006;6(5 Pt 2):1111–1131.
5. Ojo AO et al. Chronic renal failure after transplantation of a nonrenal organ. *N Engl J Med* 2003;349(10):931–940.
6. Veenstra DL et al. Incidence and long-term cost of steroid-related side effects after renal transplantation. *Am J Kidney Dis* 1999;33(5):829–839.
7. Prasad GV et al. Renal transplant recipient attitudes toward steroid use and steroid withdrawal. *Clin Transplant* 2003;17(2):135–139.
8. Gonwa T et al. Randomized trial of tacrolimus + mycophenolate mofetil or azathioprine versus cyclosporine + mycophenolate mofetil after cadaveric kidney transplantation: results at three years. *Transplantation* 2003;75(12):2048–2053.
9. Kaplan B, Schold JD, Meier-Kriesche HU. Long-term graft survival with neoral and tacrolimus: a paired kidney analysis. *J Am Soc Nephrol* 2003;14(11):2980–2984.
10. Vincenti F et al. A long-term comparison of tacrolimus (FK506) and cyclosporine in kidney transplantation: evidence for improved allograft survival at five years. *Transplantation* 2002;73(5):775–782.
11. Schulak JA et al. A prospective randomized trial of prednisone versus no prednisone maintenance therapy in cyclosporine-treated and azathioprine-treated renal transplant patients. *Transplantation* 1990;49(2):327–332.

12. Hricik DE et al. Steroid-free immunosuppression in cyclosporine-treated renal transplant recipients: a meta-analysis. *J Am Soc Nephrol* 1993;4(6):1300–1305.
13. Sinclair NR. Low-dose steroid therapy in cyclosporine-treated renal transplant recipients with well-functioning grafts. The Canadian Multicentre Transplant Study Group. *CMAJ* 1992;147(5):645–657.
14. Kasiske BL et al. A meta-analysis of immunosuppression withdrawal trials in renal transplantation. *J Am Soc Nephrol* 2000;11(10):1910–1917.
15. Vanrenterghem Y et al. Double-blind comparison of two corticosteroid regimens plus mycophenolate mofetil and cyclosporine for prevention of acute renal allograft rejection. *Transplantation* 2000;70(9):1352–1359.
16. Ahsan N et al. Prednisone withdrawal in kidney transplant recipients on cyclosporine and mycophenolate mofetil – a prospective randomized study. Steroid Withdrawal Study Group. *Transplantation* 1999;68(12):1865–1874.
17. Sola E et al. Low-dose and rapid steroid withdrawal in renal transplant patients treated with tacrolimus and mycophenolate mofetil. *Transplant Proc* 2002;34(5):1689–1690.
18. Squifflet JP et al. Safe withdrawal of corticosteroids or mycophenolate mofetil: results of a large, prospective, multicenter, randomized study. *Transplant Proc* 2002;34(5):1584–1586.
19. Hricik DE et al. Long-term graft outcomes after steroid withdrawal in African American kidney transplant recipients receiving sirolimus and tacrolimus. *Transplantation* 2007;83(3): 277–281.
20. Pascual J et al. Steroid withdrawal in renal transplant patients on triple therapy with a calcineurin inhibitor and mycophenolate mofetil: a meta-analysis of randomized, controlled trials. *Transplantation* 2004;78(10):1548–1556.
21. Almawi WY, Melemedjian OK, Rieder MJ. An alternate mechanism of glucocorticoid anti-proliferative effect: promotion of a Th2 cytokine-secreting profile. *Clin Transplant* 1999;13(5):365–374.
22. Freise CE et al. Excellent short-term results with steroid-free maintenance immunosuppression in low-risk simultaneous pancreas-kidney transplantation. *Arch Surg* 2003;138(10): 1121–1125; discussion 1125–1126.
23. Kaufman DB et al. A prospective study of rapid corticosteroid elimination in simultaneous pancreas-kidney transplantation: comparison of two maintenance immunosuppression protocols: tacrolimus/mycophenolate mofetil versus tacrolimus/sirolimus. *Transplantation* 2002;73(2):169–177.
24. Khwaja K et al. Outcome at 3 years with a prednisone-free maintenance regimen: a single-center experience with 349 kidney transplant recipients. *Am J Transplant* 2004;4(6):980–987.
25. Vincenti F et al. Rapid steroid withdrawal versus standard steroid therapy in patients treated with basiliximab, cyclosporine, and mycophenolate mofetil for the prevention of acute rejection in renal transplantation. *Transplant Proc* 2001;33(1–2):1011–1012.
26. Matas AJ et al. Prednisone-free maintenance immunosuppression-a 5-year experience. *Am J Transplant* 2005;5(10):2473–2478.
27. Kaufman DB et al. Alemtuzumab induction and prednisone-free maintenance immunotherapy in kidney transplantation: comparison with basiliximab induction – long-term results. *Am J Transplant* 2005;5(10):2539–2548.
28. Kumar MS et al. Safety and efficacy of steroid withdrawal two days after kidney transplantation: analysis of results at three years. *Transplantation* 2006;81(6):832–839.
29. Woodle ES et al. A prospective, randomized, double-blind, placebo-controlled multicenter trial comparing early (7 day) corticosteroid cessation versus long-term, low-dose corticosteroid therapy. *Ann Surg* 2008;248(4):564–577.
30. Vincenti F et al. A randomized, multicenter study of steroid avoidance, early steroid withdrawal or standard steroid therapy in kidney transplant recipients. *Am J Transplant* 2008;8(2):307–316.
31. Abramowicz D et al. Cyclosporine withdrawal from a mycophenolate mofetil-containing immunosuppressive regimen in stable kidney transplant recipients: a randomized, controlled study. *Transplantation* 2002;74(12):1725–1734.

32. Smak Gregoor PJ et al. Withdrawal of cyclosporine or prednisone six months after kidney transplantation in patients on triple drug therapy: a randomized, prospective, multicenter study. *J Am Soc Nephrol* 2002;13(5):1365–1373.
33. Ekberg H et al. Cyclosporine sparing with mycophenolate mofetil, daclizumab and corticosteroids in renal allograft recipients: the CAESAR Study. *Am J Transplant* 2007;7(3):560–570.
34. Abramowicz D et al. Cyclosporine withdrawal from a mycophenolate mofetil-containing immunosuppressive regimen: results of a five-year, prospective, randomized study. *J Am Soc Nephrol* 2005;16(7):2234–2240.
35. Hazzan M et al. Assessment of the risk of chronic allograft dysfunction after renal transplantation in a randomized cyclosporine withdrawal trial. *Transplantation* 2006;82(5):657–662.
36. Johnson RW et al. Sirolimus allows early cyclosporine withdrawal in renal transplantation resulting in improved renal function and lower blood pressure. *Transplantation* 2001;72(5):777–786.
37. Kreis H et al. Long-term benefits with sirolimus-based therapy after early cyclosporine withdrawal. *J Am Soc Nephrol* 2004;15(3):809–817.
38. Oberbauer R et al. Early cyclosporine withdrawal from a sirolimus-based regimen results in better renal allograft survival and renal function at 48 months after transplantation. *Transpl Int* 2005;18(1):22–28.
39. Baboolal K. A phase III prospective, randomized study to evaluate concentration-controlled sirolimus (rapamune) with cyclosporine dose minimization or elimination at six months in de novo renal allograft recipients. *Transplantation* 2003;75(8):1404–1408.
40. Grinyo JM et al. Pilot randomized study of early tacrolimus withdrawal from a regimen with sirolimus plus tacrolimus in kidney transplantation. *Am J Transplant* 2004;4(8):1308–1314.
41. Stallone G et al. Early withdrawal of cyclosporine A improves 1-year kidney graft structure and function in sirolimus-treated patients. *Transplantation* 2003;75(7):998–1003.
42. Dudley C et al. Mycophenolate mofetil substitution for cyclosporine a in renal transplant recipients with chronic progressive allograft dysfunction: the "creeping creatinine" study. *Transplantation* 2005;79(4):466–475.
43. Schena FP et al. Conversion from calcineurin inhibitors to sirolimus maintenance therapy in renal allograft recipients: 24-month efficacy and safety results from the CONVERT trial. *Transplantation* 2009;87(2):233–242.
44. Mulay AV et al. Conversion from calcineurin inhibitors to sirolimus for chronic renal allograft dysfunction: a systematic review of the evidence. *Transplantation* 2006;82(9):1153–1162.
45. Vincenti F et al. Multicenter trial exploring calcineurin inhibitors avoidance in renal transplantation. *Transplantation* 2001;71(9):1282–1287.
46. Asberg A et al. Calcineurin inhibitor avoidance with daclizumab, mycophenolate mofetil, and prednisolone in DR-matched de novo kidney transplant recipients. *Transplantation* 2006;82(1):62–68.
47. Flechner SM et al. Kidney transplantation with sirolimus and mycophenolate mofetil-based immunosuppression: 5-year results of a randomized prospective trial compared to calcineurin inhibitor drugs. *Transplantation* 2007;83(7):883–892.
48. Groth CG et al. Sirolimus (rapamycin)-based therapy in human renal transplantation: similar efficacy and different toxicity compared with cyclosporine. Sirolimus European Renal Transplant Study Group. *Transplantation* 1999;67(7):1036–1042.
49. Kreis H et al. Sirolimus in association with mycophenolate mofetil induction for the prevention of acute graft rejection in renal allograft recipients. *Transplantation* 2000;69(7):1252–1260.
50. Morales JM et al. Sirolimus does not exhibit nephrotoxicity compared to cyclosporine in renal transplant recipients. *Am J Transplant* 2002;2(5):436–442.
51. Flechner SM et al. Kidney transplantation without calcineurin inhibitor drugs: a prospective, randomized trial of sirolimus versus cyclosporine. *Transplantation* 2002;74(8):1070–1076.
52. Larson TS et al. Complete avoidance of calcineurin inhibitors in renal transplantation: a randomized trial comparing sirolimus and tacrolimus. *Am J Transplant* 2006;6(3):514–522.

53. Srinivas TR et al. Mycophenolate mofetil/sirolimus compared to other common immunosuppressive regimens in kidney transplantation. *Am J Transplant* 2007;7(3):586–594.
54. Ekberg H et al. Reduced exposure to calcineurin inhibitors in renal transplantation. *N Engl J Med* 2007;357(25):2562–2575.
55. Vincenti F et al. Costimulation blockade with belatacept in renal transplantation. *N Engl J Med* 2005;353(8):770–781.

Chapter 11
Evaluation of Renal Allograft Dysfunction

Robert S. Gaston

Introduction

Measuring renal function to monitor the status of a kidney allograft dates back to the earliest days of transplantation.[1] Although numerous other techniques (including direct measurement of glomerular filtration rate [GFR], immunologic monitoring of blood or urine, gene expression, and surveillance biopsy) have been advanced as more accurate alternatives to detect allograft injury, serial measurement of serum creatinine levels remains the standard for assessing graft integrity. Each transplant center may have its own protocol for monitoring changes in renal function; Table 11.1 offers a sample schedule that originated as part of a clinical guideline.[1] Appropriate monitoring of allograft function also includes serial determination of urinary protein excretion.

Determinants of Allograft Function

Intercept: Establishing Baseline GFR

After successful kidney transplantation, most recipients establish a baseline GFR – usually between 40 and 70 ml/min – that is reflected in a serum creatinine value of 1–2 mg/dl. Several sources have indicated that baseline GFR has improved in recent years; Kasiske and colleagues document almost 20% greater baseline-estimated GFR (eGFR) in patients transplanted after 1999 compared to those transplanted before 1989 (55 vs. 46 ml/min, $p < 0.001$).[2] Determinants of baseline GFR include donor variables such as age, gender, body habitus, and preexisting hypertension; any preservation injury; recipient variables such as presensitization, gender, and

R.S. Gaston (✉)
Kidney and Pancreas Transplantation, Department of Medicine/Nephrology, University of Alabama at Birmingham, Birmingham, AL, USA
e-mail: rgaston@uab.edu

D.B. McKay, S.M. Steinberg (eds.), *Kidney Transplantation: A Guide to the Care of Kidney Transplant Recipients*, DOI 10.1007/978-1-4419-1690-7_11,
© Springer Science+Business Media, LLC 2010

Table 11.1 Recommendations for frequency of monitoring serum creatinine levels and urinary protein excretion in stable adult kidney transplant recipients[1]

Months posttransplant	Frequency of testing
1	Twice weekly
2	Weekly
3–4	Every 2 weeks
5–12	Monthly
13–24	Every 2 months
>24	Every 3–4 months

body habitus; immunosuppressant toxicities; and the residual impact of any early immunologic insult. Most would consider baseline renal function to be established on or before postoperative day 30, but by 3–6 months at the latest.

Baseline GFR is thought to be predictive of long-term graft survival. Kasiske and colleagues found higher baseline GFR (30 days) in patients who retained their grafts vs. those who subsequently died or lost their allografts and returned to dialysis.[2] Hariharan and colleagues found the serum creatinine 6 months posttransplant to be predictive of long-term graft survival.[3] Kaplan and coworkers, however, offered a different perspective: GFR does not predict, but rather correlates with, outcomes.[4] In a retrospective analysis of United States Renal Data System (USRDS) data for adult, first-transplant recipients, they confirmed each 1 mg/dl increase in serum creatinine to be associated with an increased risk of graft loss in subsequent years (see Table 11.2). However, analysis of the area under the receiver operating characteristic (ROC) curves indicated that a 1 mg/dl increase in serum creatinine correctly predicted graft outcome in approximately 62% of cases, only slightly better than the 50% expected on the basis of chance alone. Thus, excellent kidney function is a positive variable in achieving successful long-term outcomes, but graft failure may be the consequence of random additional insults to the kidney, superimposed on baseline allograft function.

Table 11.2 Relationship between increase in serum creatinine level and risk of allograft failure at 2 and 7 years after transplantation[4]

Follow-up (years)	Odds ratio (95% confidence interval)	AUC
2	2.22 (2.13–2.31)	0.627
7	2.40 (2.31–2.50)	0.624

1 mg/dl increase relative to 1-year posttransplant baseline level.
AUC indicates area under the receiver operating characteristic curve.

Predicting baseline GFR is difficult. Current criteria for expanded criteria donors (ECD) were based on characteristics predictive of graft survival, not renal dysfunction. Nonetheless, Sung and colleagues document lower baseline renal function in recipients of ECD kidneys.[5] Within the ECD category, kidneys with fewer than 5% of glomeruli sclerotic had greater eGFR at 1 year than those with more advanced glomerulosclerosis. Lopes and colleagues established a quantitative, histologic-based index that was predictive of GFR at 3 months posttransplant, with interstitial and vascular changes most informative.[6] In terms of individual variables, prolonged cold ischemia time is associated with compromised renal function. We previously documented lower baseline allograft function in recipients who were substantially larger than their deceased donors.[7] Gourishankar and colleagues found baseline GFR to be compromised among female donors and recipients, older donors and recipients, patients undergoing retransplantation, and patients experiencing early acute rejection.[8]

Slope: The Rate of Change of GFR

It has been assumed that kidney allograft function declines over time, as documented with aging and in several studies of chronic kidney disease. Indeed, data indicate that eGFR does decline over time after transplantation, with the rate of decline much greater in those destined to lose their allograft.[9] In recent years, the rate of decline has slowed appreciably, related at least in part to improved immunosuppression.[8] It now appears that the rate of decline of GFR in allografts (-1 to -1.7 ml/min/1.73 m^2/year) approximates that associated with aging and is much less than the decline of 2–10 ml/min/1.73 m^2/year that occurs with non-proteinuric kidney disease.[2,8]

Variables that impact slope are different than those affecting baseline GFR. For example, older donor age is associated with a reduced baseline GFR, but does not impact slope. Increasing MHC mismatch, deceased vs. living donor, and increased recipient size are associated with a greater rate of decline, but African American race is not. Finally, patients who have experienced moderate or severe acute rejection lose GFR faster than those who never rejected.

Although some might now advocate aggressive evaluation of any decline in GFR, it is rapid deterioration in kidney function that most often indicates reversible kidney injury. Both Hariharan and Kaplan noted that the risk of allograft failure was heralded most accurately by a rapid increase in serum creatinine: an increase of 0.3 mg/dl or greater during the interval from 6 months to 1 year posttransplant is linked to a 50% or greater reduction in projected allograft half-life. In an analysis of 7-year outcomes, a 30% decrease in inverse serum creatinine (1/SCr) level during the period from 6 months to 1 year posttransplant had a positive predictive value (PPV) of 69% and a negative predictive value (NPV) of 56%.[3,4]

Proteinuria

Appropriate monitoring of allograft function includes not only serial measurement of GFR but also urinary protein excretion.[1] A recent study of proteinuric patients receiving living donor allografts found daily urinary protein excretion to diminish to <200 mg at 4.5 weeks after transplantation, indicating that substantial proteinuria after the immediate posttransplant period is almost always of allograft rather than native kidney origin, and merits evaluation.[10]

Proteinuria (0.25–1.0 g/day) has been reported to occur in 26% of kidney transplant recipients at 6 months posttransplant.[11] Like an elevated serum creatinine level, proteinuria is associated with an increased risk for allograft loss (relative risk, 4.18).[11] In another study, Amer et al. found urinary protein excretion above 150 mg/24 h to be common (45% of recipients after 1 year posttransplant), often linked to glomerular pathology and/or sirolimus use, and associated with increased risk of graft failure (hazard ratio of 1.4).[12]

In management of CKD, it is becoming increasingly common to monitor urinary albumin, rather than total protein, excretion as a marker of kidney injury. Data are now emerging that albuminuria may be of similar significance in transplant recipients. Halimi and colleagues studied 616 French transplant recipients. Microalbuminuria defined a cohort at substantially greater risk (odds ratio 14.25) of graft failure than patients with no proteinuria; macroalbuminuria imparted an odds ratio of 16.41 vs. microalbuminuria. Both were also associated with significant increase in mortality risk.[13] Thus, even though relative risk may vary from report to report, it is increasingly clear that the presence of albuminuria or proteinuria defines an allograft at risk.

Measuring Renal Allograft Function

Because GFR cannot be measured directly, it is typically quantitated by evaluating the renal clearance of a known substance. Inulin is considered the ideal marker. However, the procedure for measuring inulin clearance requires continuous intravenous (IV) administration and is both time consuming and expensive, making it impractical for routine use. Similar limitations apply to other exogenous markers such as iothalamate and iohexol, although clearance of these agents is commonly used to measure GFR in clinical trials. Measurement of creatinine in blood and urine to calculate creatinine clearance as an approximation of GFR does not involve IV infusion, but does require timed urine collection. Improper collection of urine, as well as variability in creatinine metabolism and tubular secretion, often results in creatinine clearance values that do not accurately reflect the true GFR.[14,15] Some contend that measurement of another endogenous marker, cystatin C, is independent of such variables as age and muscle mass and reflects true GFR better than creatinine-based metrics.[16] However, cystatin C measurement is not widely available, can be expensive, and may not ultimately perform any better than creatinine-based metrics in kidney transplant recipients.[17,18]

Given the technical and physiologic limitations of these procedures, clinicians continue to use the serum creatinine as a proxy for GFR. It is widely available and reproducible. More recently, however, interpretation of the serum creatinine has been challenged as too dependent on extrarenal variables and insensitive to detect potentially important changes in GFR. In an attempt to improve precision of GFR estimates from serum creatinine levels, a number of formulae have been developed, usually based on a standardized serum creatinine level and incorporating biometric variables such as the patient's age, height, gender, and race. The utility of these formulae in transplant populations remains highly disputed.[14,15,19]

Gaspari et al. recently investigated the ability of 12 different equations to predict GFR in a group of kidney transplant recipients with normal to moderately impaired allograft function (mean serum creatinine 1.37 mg/dl).[14] Highly significant correlations ($p < 0.01$) were observed between the results produced by each equation and GFR as measured by iohexol clearance. However, all of the equations tended to overestimate the true GFR. The abbreviated Modification of Diet in Renal Disease (MDRD) equation and the Cockroft–Gault equation overestimated 58 and 75% of GFR predictions, respectively. The Nankivell equation, although developed specifically for predicting GFR in kidney transplant recipients, overestimated 81% of GFR predictions. These investigators also studied the ability of each equation to predict changes in allograft function over time and found each equation to predict a significantly higher rate of GFR decline than that determined by evaluation of iohexol clearance ($p < 0.05$ for each equation). Poggio and colleagues at the Cleveland Clinic found the MDRD equation to correlate best with measured GFR.[19] The deficiencies of each equation notwithstanding, most clinicians find eGFR to be a useful metric in monitoring kidney transplant recipients.

Surveillance Biopsy

Based on the experience of common usage of serial tissue examination in cardiac and hepatic transplantation, some have advocated timed surveillance biopsy of the renal allograft as a key component of monitoring.[20,21] Rush and colleagues, in an era of cyclosporine-based immunosuppression, found a significant number of patients with stable kidney function to have evidence of immunologic injury (subclinical rejection) on surveillance biopsies at 3, 6, and 12 months after transplantation.[22] Appropriate treatment seemed to improve graft survival. More recently, with use of current potent baseline immunosuppression (tacrolimus and mycophenolate) studies of surveillance biopsy have found subclinical rejection to be uncommon.[23] Currently, most see timed biopsy as outside usual care, though an important tool in investigation of the clinical course of allograft injury.

Evaluating Changes in Renal Allograft Function

After a baseline serum creatinine level has been established, a decline in GFR is thought to indicate a change in kidney allograft status that may lead to rapid graft failure unless appropriate intervention is provided. Although not universally accepted, a 10–25% decline in eGFR (or an increase in serum creatinine level of 25–30%) is thought to be significant enough to trigger evaluation. Likewise, new onset of proteinuria, with a threshold of perhaps 500 mg/24 h (or less given the recent data outlined above), should trigger evaluation.[1]

In general, allograft dysfunction in the kidney transplant recipient should be approached much as one would address acute renal insufficiency in any other patient. The new terminology of acute kidney injury (AKI) emphasizes the importance of prompt intervention in the face of declining GFR.[24] However, prompt intervention may be of even greater importance in the kidney transplant patient because of the potential reversibility of the injury, and the opportunity afforded by timely intervention to prevent ongoing insult to the graft and irreversible loss of allograft function. In most transplant centers, an elevated serum creatinine level will be investigated within a 24 to 72-h period, depending on the circumstances surrounding its detection.

The first step in evaluating allograft dysfunction is to eliminate the impact of potential conflicting variables. Prerenal azotemia is common among kidney transplant recipients, and its severity may be magnified by treatment with calcineurin inhibitors (CNIs) such as cyclosporine and tacrolimus.[25] It may be reasonable to reduce the dose of or withhold CNI for a brief period. Treatment with angiotensin-converting enzyme (ACE) inhibitors, angiotensin receptor blockers (ARB), and/or any other nephrotoxic drug may also be interrupted; intravascular volume should be optimized, with consideration for withholding diuretics as well.

In the absence of an obvious prerenal cause, the next step is to evaluate the patient for adequacy of urinary outflow, insuring no evidence of obstruction or urinary tract infection. This is best accomplished with urinalysis (with culture, if indicated) and diagnostic ultrasound. Is there pyuria? Is there hydronephrosis? In some circumstances, empiric antibiotic administration may be warranted while culture results are pending. Hydronephrosis indicates a high likelihood of urinary outflow obstruction as the cause of azotemia and should trigger urologic evaluation. In the early posttransplant period, fluid collections adjacent to the transplanted kidney are not uncommon and can adversely impact renal function.

If significant proteinuria is present, urinalysis indicates no evidence of infection, ultrasound findings are relatively normal, and/or renal function fails to improve with the interventions noted above, increasing serum creatinine levels probably indicate a problem with the allograft itself. At this point, some centers use radionuclide scintigraphy to aid in making the correct diagnosis. However, given the increasing complexity of correctly diagnosing the cause of kidney allograft dysfunction, percutaneous biopsy with histologic examination of renal cortical tissue is the gold standard. Worsening renal function without obvious cause, especially in the presence of proteinuria, should trigger a biopsy within 2–3 days, if not sooner.

Causes of Kidney Allograft Dysfunction

In the past, acute rejection and graft dysfunction were almost synonymous. Indeed, though much less frequent in recent years, acute rejection remains a common cause of allograft dysfunction and transplant failure.[26] However, the characteristics and underlying causes of kidney allograft dysfunction vary with time after transplantation (Table 11.3). In addition, individual patient variables, like presensitization, influence likelihood of each diagnostic entity. Thus, not all allograft dysfunction, especially beyond the first 6–12 months after transplantation, represents acute rejection. Empiric treatment of a rising creatinine with corticosteroids in the assumption that it represents acute rejection is no longer considered standard therapy. Prompt diagnosis is essential for proper therapy.

Table 11.3 Causes of kidney allograft dysfunction by time after transplantation

| Cause | Months posttransplant | | |
	1–3	3–12	>12
Delayed graft function	X		
Acute rejection	X	X	Less common except with nonadherence
CNI-related nephrotoxicity	X	X	X
Recurrent kidney disease	Uncommon, except in focal glomerulosclerosis	X	X
Chronic allograft nephropathy		X	X
Infection: Urinary tract	X	X	X
Sepsis	X	X	X
Cytomegalovirus	X	X	Uncommon
Obstruction	X	X	X
Polyomavirus type BK viremia/nephropathy		X	X

CNI, calcineurin inhibitor.

Delayed Graft Function

Delayed graft function (DGF) is a clinical event, namely the failure of a kidney transplant to function immediately after implantation. Its definition in most reports is likewise clinically based: the need for dialysis in the first postoperative week. National data from the Scientific Registry of Transplant Recipients (SRTR) indicate recipients of deceased donor kidneys with DGF have significantly lower 5-year kidney allograft survival rates than those without DGF (51% vs. 69%, $p < 0.001$).[27]

In an analysis of USRDS data for primary kidney allografts transplanted during 1985–1992, the incidence of DGF was 26%, while the incidence of early acute rejection was 25%.[28] Risk factors for DGF included cold ischemia time greater than 12 h (odds ratio [OR] 1.38–3.48; $p < 0.001$) and donor age greater than 40 years (OR 1.63–2.07, $p \leq 0.003$). DGF in recipients of living donor transplants is uncommon, but even more ominous in terms of outcome, as it reflects immunologic or technical injury rather than underlying organ quality or ischemic injury.[27]

Preimplantation biopsies may be of benefit in assessing risk for DGF. Factors noted to correlate with suboptimal posttransplant renal function include the presence of glomerulosclerosis and interstitial fibrosis. However, the strongest predictor of poor function in the recipient may be preexisting vascular disease in the donor.[29,30]

While DGF may reflect both organ quality and non-immunologic injury, at least a portion of its adverse impact on outcome is due to increased susceptibility of deceased-donor allografts to immunologic injury, and difficulty recognizing it.[31] Acute rejection is almost twice as common in patients with DGF (42% vs. 25%; $p < 0.001$). Without early rejection, 3-year graft survival was reduced from 82 to 71% for patients with DGF; with early rejection, DGF reduced 3-year graft survival from 63 to 54% ($p < 0.001$ for each comparison).[32] It is increasingly obvious that tissue injury related to age, ischemia, and preservation stimulates innate immunity, setting the stage for allospecific injury.[33] DGF is more common in sensitized than unsensitized recipients, also implying a role for immunologic injury in the process. In a transplant recipient with ongoing oliguric renal failure beyond the first 5–7 days, most would proceed with allograft biopsy; given our new appreciation for antibody-mediated injury, many would also examine sera for donor-specific reactivity.

Acute Rejection

Acute rejection remains an important cause of renal allograft dysfunction. In the current era of potent immunosuppressive therapy, the clinical presentation of acute rejection is highly variable. The classically described signs and symptoms are rarely present, especially early in the clinical course of acute rejection (Table 11.4). Allograft enlargement may or may not be evident on physical examination. Thus, while most patients continue to be taught the importance of watching for changes such as fever, graft tenderness, and a decline in urine output, most rejection episodes are diagnosed after a rise in serum creatinine-triggered allograft biopsy with confirmatory histologic findings. In general, for the practicing nephrologist, an increase in the serum creatinine level of ≥ 10–25% above baseline (or a corresponding decline in eGFR) should trigger referral back to the transplant center for evaluation that will likely include percutaneous biopsy.

Table 11.4 Signs and symptoms of acute rejection	Allograft pain and tenderness
	Fluid retention or sudden weight gain
	Sudden rise in blood pressure
	Decreased urine output
	Dyspnea
	Fever
	Flu-like symptoms (chills, nausea, malaise, headache, myalgia)

Meier-Kriesche et al. analyzed data from more than 62,000 adult first-transplant recipients and found that from 1995 to 2000, acute rejection rates fell from 36 to 15% in the first 6 months after transplant, from 21 to 6% in between 6 and 12 months posttransplant, and from 23 to 3% in the 12 to 24-month period.[34] In addition, our understanding of acute rejection has also evolved, related at least in part to the Banff process and its impact on understanding allograft histology, as well as growing appreciation of the role of anti-HLA antibody in allograft injury.[35] Now, discussion of acute rejection must be qualified further as cell mediated, antibody mediated (AMR), or both. (See Table 11.5)[36] Under current immunosuppression, and depending on the clinical scenario, AMR may be the more common variant, accounting for as many as two-thirds of rejection episodes.[37]

Table 11.5   Banff 97 diagnostic categories for acute rejection – Banff 2007 update[36]

1. Normal	
2. Acute antibody-mediated rejection: C4d+, presence of circulating antidonor antibodies	Type (grade) I. ATN-like minimal inflammation II. Capillary and/or glomerular inflammation and/or thromboses III. Arterial – v3
3. Borderline changes	"Suspicious" for acute T-cell-mediated rejection, no intimal arteritis, foci of tubulitis with minor interstitial infiltration, or interstitial infiltration with mild tubulitis
4. Acute T-cell-mediated rejection	Type (grade) IA. Interstitial inflammation (>25% of parenchyma) and foci of moderate tubulitis IB. Interstitial inflammation (>25% of parenchyma) and foci of severe tubulitis IIA. Mild-to-moderate intimal arteritis IIB. Severe intimal arteritis comprising >25% of luminal area III. Transmural arteritis and/or arterial fibrinoid change and necrosis of medial smooth muscle cells with accompanying lymphocytic inflammation

There is some uncertainty regarding the impact of acute rejection episodes on ultimate outcomes. Some would maintain that acute rejection is always a negative event in kidney transplantation, a position supported by the near uniform agreement that the best outcomes accrue to those patients never experiencing rejection.[38,39] Alternatively, others, including these same authors, have noted some rejections to be worse than others in terms of long-term impact (rejections occurring beyond 6 months after transplant, histologically severe rejections, and those that result in irreversible declines in eGFR) and that multiple rejection episodes are particularly detrimental to graft survival. In a recent study, overall 6-year graft survival rates were similar in patients without acute rejection and those who had acute rejection with near-complete recovery of baseline renal function (74 vs. 73%).[34] However, among patients who had acute rejection and less than complete recovery of baseline renal function, allograft survival rates were much lower, declining in proportion to the degree of impairment in renal function (Table 11.6). Most agree that antibody-mediated rejection also may be more likely to result in graft failure than classic cell-mediated rejection.[40]

Table 11.6 Overall 6-year allograft survival rates by acute rejection and recovery of baseline renal function[34]

Acute rejection during posttransplant months 6–12	Amount of baseline renal function recovered at 1 year posttransplant (%)	6-Year allograft survival (%)
No		74.4
Yes	95–100	72.7
	85–95	67.0
	75–85	50.2
	<75	38.0

Renal function as measured by Cockroft–Gault estimates of creatinine clearance; baseline renal function determined at 6 months posttransplant.

After acute rejection has been confirmed by biopsy, treatment will most often be initiated by the transplant center. In the past, it was common to prescribe high-dose corticosteroids as first-line therapy for almost all rejection episodes. Now, at many centers, biopsy findings guide therapy. Mild cellular rejection (Banff IA or less) typically responds to high-dose steroids; evidence of more severe cell-mediated injury may result in early use of antilymphocyte therapy. Evidence of AMR may result in a different approach to therapy, involving some combination of high-dose corticosteroids, plasmapheresis, anti-CD20 (rixtuximab) or other monoclonal antibodies, or intravenous immunoglobulin.[41] Most consider acute rejection indicative of inadequate immunosuppression, and many times intense anti-rejection therapy will be followed by increased doses of maintenance therapy.

Impact of Immunosuppressant Drugs on Renal Function

Although associated with significant improvement in risk of rejection and graft failure, cyclosporine and tacrolimus are clearly nephrotoxic, with adverse impact on kidney function as their major dose-limiting variable.[42] These agents are also associated with hypertension, hyperkalemia, hyperuricemia, and renal tubular acidosis. In general, clinical nephrotoxicity in kidney transplantation has been thought to be more severe with cyclosporine than tacrolimus.[43,44] More recently, sirolimus has been shown to potentiate the adverse impact of cyclosporine on renal function and to increase urinary albumin excretion in some patients.[45,46]

There appear to be two major patterns of CNI nephrotoxicity. The first is more acute and thought to reflect CNI-induced renal vasoconstriction, which in turn reduces GFR. This effect is typically reversible upon CNI dose reduction or discontinuation.[47] The second pattern is thought to be of longer duration, with a more gradual decline in GFR associated with histologic findings of progressive interstitial fibrosis, vascular sclerosis, and tubular atrophy.[48] While this latter scenario may also improve with CNI dose reduction, it is less amenable to altered therapy. Some, however, based on a variable clinical outcome, nonspecific histologic findings, and the fact that either nephrotoxicity or acute rejection can occur in the presence of both supratherapeutic and subtherapeutic drug levels, are now questioning the role of CNIs as etiologic agents in progressive fibrosis and atrophy.[49,50]

Typically, in the absence of urinary tract infection, evidence of urinary outflow obstruction, and biopsy evidence of other pathogenic processes, a trial of CNI dose reduction may be warranted, with an end point of improved eGFR. In some situations (e.g., failure of eGFR to improve with dose reduction, other non-renal CNI toxicities) conversion to a CNI-free regimen may be indicated, but only under the supervision of the transplant center.

Recurrent and De Novo Renal Disease

The pathogenesis of many renal diseases remains poorly understood, a factor that limits their prevention and treatment. After kidney transplantation, there are several native kidney diseases that can recur in the allograft, the most well described being focal glomerulosclerosis, IgA nephropathy, and diabetic nephropathy.[51] It is also possible for de novo diseases, such as hemolytic uremic syndrome secondary to cyclosporine, to develop after renal transplantation (Table 11.7).

Recurrence rates can be highly variable by disease entity and may be more prevalent in retransplanted patients who lost their initial allograft to recurrent disease. That said, recurrent disease does not necessarily lead to allograft failure. Treatment for recurrent or de novo renal diseases should be consistent with therapies utilized to treat the disease in native kidneys.

BK Virus Nephropathy

Renal dysfunction as a consequence of viral infection has long been recognized, particularly related to cytomegalovirus. BK, a polyoma virus, was first discovered in the 1970s, linked to urethral strictures in immunocompromised patients.[52] Since the introduction of tacrolimus and mycophenolate in the mid-1990s, BK nephropathy has become a relatively frequent cause of graft dysfunction. It is now recognized that BK viremia, usually arising from donor uroepithelium, occurs in 10–15% of recipients on potent immunosuppression, with overt nephropathy in as many as 3–5% of recipients.[53] A decade ago, most BK was diagnosed by kidney biopsy, relatively late in its course, with a high frequency of graft failure. Now thought to be a marker of overimmunosuppression, BK viremia or viruria is now detected by routine

Table 11.7 Recurrence of renal diseases after kidney transplantation[51]

Clinical classification

1. True recurrence: native and recurrent diseases are the same, confirmed by histology
2. Glomerulopathy in transplant with unknown primary disease: allograft biopsy confirming disease without native kidney biopsy
3. De novo disease: occurrence of new disease in transplanted kidney

Histologic classification

1. Recurrence of primary glomerulonephritides	Focal glomerulosclerosis
	Membranoproliferative GN
	IgA nephropathy
	Membranous Nephropathy
2. Recurrence of secondary glomerulonephritides	SLE
	Henoch–Schonlein purpura
	HUS/TTP
	Crescentic GN
	Anti-GBM disease
3. Recurrence of metabolic or systemic disease	Diabetic nephropathy
	Oxalosis
	Amyloidosis
	Fabry disease
	Scleroderma
	Cystinosis
	Fibrillary GN
4. De novo diseases	Anti-GBM disease in Alport's
	Membranous nephropathy in polycystic disease

screening of blood or urine, with correspondingly less graft dysfunction and failure as immunosuppressant dosing is adjusted to more appropriate levels.[54]

Chronic Allograft Nephropathy (CAN)

CAN, formerly called chronic rejection, is a nonspecific diagnosis applied to non-specific histologic findings and implying progressive loss of allograft function.[55] The current Banff schema refers to this entity descriptively as interstitial fibrosis/tubular atrophy, etiology not otherwise specified (IFTANOS) (Table 11.8). At our current level of understanding, CAN is indeed associated with progressive renal dysfunction (albeit at highly variable rates) and is not amenable to specific therapy. Currently, a great deal of attention is being devoted to better understanding the pathogenesis of CAN and defining entities that may be amenable to therapy.[56]

Treatment approaches to CAN include ensuring adequate immunosuppression and, in some cases, modification of CNI-based regimens.[57] Blood pressure control may slow the progression of CAN, much as it slows the progression of chronic kidney disease, and ACE inhibitors and/or angiotensin-receptor blockers may offer additional benefits including reduced urinary protein excretion.

Table 11.8 Banff 97 diagnostic categories for chronic injury in renal allograft biopsies – Banff 2007 update[36]

Chronic active antibody-mediated rejection	C4d+, presence of circulating antidonor antibodies, morphologic evidence of chronic tissue injury, such as glomerular double contours and/or peritubular capillary basement membrane multilayering and/or interstitial fibrosis/tubular atrophy and/or fibrous intimal thickening in arteries
Chronic active T-cell-mediated rejection	"Chronic allograft arteriopathy" (arterial intimal fibrosis with mononuclear cell infiltration in fibrosis, formation of neo-intima)
Interstitial fibrosis and tubular atrophy, no evidence of any specific etiology	Grade I. Mild interstitial fibrosis and tubular atrophy (<25% of cortical area) II. Moderate interstitial fibrosis and tubular atrophy (26–50% of cortical area) III. Severe interstitial fibrosis and tubular atrophy (>50% of cortical area)

Conclusion

As more kidney transplant recipients survive the early posttransplant period with excellent allograft function, greater emphasis is being placed on ensuring successful long-term outcomes. A key to achieving this goal is recognizing changes in allograft function and intervening quickly to prevent significant damage to the transplant. Periodic monitoring of serum creatinine, eGFR, and urinary protein excretion allows for early recognition of threats to the transplanted kidney. Timely evaluation of allograft dysfunction, many times including a kidney biopsy, usually results in a diagnosis that leads to institution of appropriate therapy. Presumably, implementation of appropriate therapy will contribute to long-term success of the graft.

References

1. Kasiske BL, Vazquez MA, Harmon WE, Brown RS, Danovitch GM, Gaston RS et al. Recommendations for the outpatient surveillance of renal transplant recipients. American Society of Transplantation. *J Am Soc Nephrol* 2000 Oct;11(Suppl 15):S1–S86.
2. Kasiske BL, Gaston RS, Gourishankar S, Halloran PF, Matas AJ, Jeffery J et al. Long-term deterioration of kidney allograft function. *Am J Transplant* 2005 Jun;5(6):1405–1414.
3. Hariharan S, McBride MA, Cherikh WS, Tolleris CB, Bresnahan BA, Johnson CP. Post-transplant renal function in the first year predicts long-term kidney transplant survival. *Kidney Int* 2002 Jul;62(1):311–318.
4. Kaplan B, Schold J, Meier-Kriesche HU. Poor predictive value of serum creatinine for renal allograft loss. *Am J Transplant* 2003 Dec;3(12):1560–1565.
5. Sung RS, Guidinger MK, Leichtman AB, Lake C, Metzger RA, Port FK et al. Impact of the expanded criteria donor allocation system on candidates for and recipients of expanded criteria donor kidneys. *Transplantation* 2007 Nov 15;84(9):1138–1144.

6. Lopes JA, Moreso F, Riera L, Carrera M, Ibernon M, Fulladosa X et al. Evaluation of pre-implantation kidney biopsies: comparison of Banff criteria to a morphometric approach. *Kidney Int* 2005 Apr;67(4):1595–1600.

7. Gaston RS, Hudson SL, Julian BA, Laskow DA, Deierhoi MH, Sanders CE et al. Impact of donor/recipient size matching on outcomes in renal transplantation. *Transplantation* 1996;61:383–388.

8. Gourishankar S, Hunsicker LG, Jhangri GS, Cockfield SM, Halloran PF. The stability of the glomerular filtration rate after renal transplantation is improving. *J Am Soc Nephrol* 2003 Sep;14(9):2387–2394.

9. Kasiske BL, Andany MA, Danielson B. A thirty percent chronic decline in inverse serum creatinine is an excellent predictor of late renal allograft failure. *Am J Kidney Dis* 2002 Apr;39(4):762–768.

10. D'Cunha PT, Parasuraman R, Venkat KK. Rapid resolution of proteinuria of native kidney origin following live donor renal transplantation. *Am J Transplant* 2005 Feb;5(2):351–355.

11. Reichel H, Zeier M, Ritz E. Proteinuria after renal transplantation: pathogenesis and management. *Nephrol Dial Transplant* 2004 Feb;19(2):301–305.

12. Amer H, Fidler ME, Myslak M, Morales P, Kremers WK, Larson TS et al. Proteinuria after kidney transplantation, relationship to allograft histology and survival. *Am J Transplant* 2007 Dec;7(12):2748–2756.

13. Halimi JM, Buchler M, Al-Najjar A, Laouad I, Chatelet V, Marliere JF et al. Urinary albumin excretion and the risk of graft loss and death in proteinuric and non-proteinuric renal transplant recipients. *Am J Transplant* 2007 Mar;7(3):618–625.

14. Gaspari F, Ferrari S, Stucchi N, Centemeri E, Carrara F, Pellegrino M et al. Performance of different prediction equations for estimating renal function in kidney transplantation. *Am J Transplant* 2004 Nov;4(11):1826–1835.

15. Poggio ED, Batty DS, Flechner SM. Evaluation of renal function in transplantation. *Transplantation* 2007;84:131–136.

16. Filler G, Bokenkamp A, Hofmann W, Le Bricon T, Martinez-Bru C, Grubb A. Cystatin C as a marker of GFR – history, indications, and future research. *Clin Biochem* 2005 Jan;38(1):1–8.

17. Poge U, Gerhardt T, Woitas RP. Calculation of glomerular filtration rate using serum cystatin C in kidney transplant recipients. *Kidney Int* 2006 Nov;70(10):1878; author reply – 1878–1879.

18. White C, Akbari A, Hussain N, Dinh L, Filler G, Lepage N et al. Estimating glomerular filtration rate in kidney transplantation: a comparison between serum creatinine and cystatin C-based methods. *J Am Soc Nephrol* 2005 Dec;16(12):3763–3770.

19. Poggio ED, Wang X, Weinstein DM, Issa N, Dennis VW, Braun WE et al. Assessing glomerular filtration rate by estimation equations in kidney transplant recipients. *Am J Transplant* 2006 Jan;6(1):100–108.

20. Mengel M, Chapman JR, Cosio FG, Cavaille-Coll MW, Haller H, Halloran PF et al. Protocol biopsies in renal transplantation: insights into patient management and pathogenesis. *Am J Transplant* 2007 Mar;7(3):512–517.

21. Rush D. Protocol transplant biopsies: an underutilized tool in kidney transplantation. *Clin J Am Soc Nephrol* 2006 Jan;1(1):138–143.

22. Rush D, Nickerson P, Gough J, McKenna R, Grimm P, Cheang M et al. Beneficial effects of treatment of early subclinical rejection: a randomized study. *J Am Soc Nephrol* 1998 Nov;9(11):2129–2134.

23. Rush D, Arlen D, Boucher A, Busque S, Cockfield SM, Girardin C et al. Lack of benefit of early protocol biopsies in renal transplant patients receiving TAC and MMF: a randomized study. *Am J Transplant* 2007 Nov;7(11):2538–2545.

24. Molitoris BA, Levin A, Warnock DG, Joannidis M, Mehta RL, Kellum JA et al. Improving outcomes from acute kidney injury. *J Am Soc Nephrol* 2007 Jul;18(7):1992–1994.

25. Laskow DA, Curtis JJ, Luke RG, Julian BA, Jones P, Deierhoi MH et al. Cyclosporine-induced changes in glomerular filtration rate and urea excretion. *Am J Med* 1990 May;88(5):497–502.

26. Cecka JM. The OPTN/UNOS renal transplant registry. In: Cecka JM, Terasaki PI, (eds.), Clinical Transplants 2004. Los Angeles, UCLA Tissue Typing Laboratory, 2005, pp. 1–15.
27. Gaston RS, Alveranga DY, Becker BN, Distant DA, Held PJ, Bragg-Gresham JL et al. Kidney and pancreas transplantation. *Am J Transplant* 2003;3(Suppl 4):64–77.
28. Ojo AO, Wolfe RA, Held PJ, Port FK, Schmouder RL. Delayed graft function: risk factors and implications for renal allograft survival. *Transplantation* 1997 Apr 15;63(7):968–974.
29. Kayler LK, Mohanka R, Basu A, Shapiro R, Randhawa PS. Correlation of histologic findings on preimplant biopsy with kidney graft survival. *Transpl Int* 2008 Sep;21(9):892–898.
30. Remuzzi G, Cravedi P, Perna A, Dimitrov BD, Turturro M, Locatelli G et al. Long-term outcome of renal transplantation from older donors. *N Engl J Med* 2006 Jan 26;354(4): 343–352.
31. Perico N, Cattaneo D, Sayegh MH, Remuzzi G. Delayed graft function in kidney transplantation. *Lancet* 2004;364:1814–1827.
32. Shoskes DA, Cecka JM. Deleterious effects of delayed graft function in cadaveric renal transplant recipients independent of acute rejection. *Transplantation* 1998 Dec 27;66(12): 1697–1701.
33. Kim IK, Bedi DS, Denecke C, Ge X, Tullius SG. Impact of innate and adaptive immunity on rejection and tolerance. *Transplantation* 2008 Oct 15;86(7):889–894.
34. Meier-Kriesche HU, Schold JD, Srinivas TR, Kaplan B. Lack of improvement in renal allograft survival despite a marked decrease in acute rejection rates over the most recent era. *Am J Transplant* 2004 Mar;4(3):378–383.
35. Halloran PF. The clinical importance of alloantibody-mediated rejection. *Am J Transplant* 2003 Jun;3(6):639–640.
36. Solez K, Colvin RB, Racusen LC, Haas M, Sis B, Mengel M et al. Banff 07 classification of renal allograft pathology: updates and future directions. *Am J Transplant* 2008 Apr;8(4): 753–760; Epub 2008 Feb 19.
37. Pascual J, Pirsch JD, Odorico JS, Torrealba JR, Djamali A, Becker YT et al. Alemtuzumab induction and antibody-mediated kidney rejection after simultaneous pancreas-kidney transplantation. *Transplantation* 2009 Jan 15;87(1):125–132.
38. Humar A, Payne WD, Sutherland DE, Matas AJ. Clinical determinants of multiple acute rejection episodes in kidney transplant recipients. *Transplantation* 2000 Jun 15;69(11): 2357–2360.
39. Matas AJ, Gillingham KJ, Humar A, Kandaswamy R, Sutherland DE, Payne WD et al. 2202 kidney transplant recipients with 10 years of graft function: what happens next? *Am J Transplant* 2008 Nov;8(11):2410–2419.
40. Crespo M, Pascual M, Tolkoff-Rubin N, Mauiyyedi S, Collins AB, Fitzpatrick D et al. Acute humoral rejection in renal allograft recipients: I. Incidence, serology and clinical characteristics. *Transplantation* 2001 Mar 15;71(5):652–658.
41. Gloor J, Cosio F, Lager DJ, Stegall MD. The spectrum of antibody-mediated renal allograft injury: implications for treatment. *Am J Transplant* 2008 Jul;8(7):1367–1373.
42. Halloran PF. Immunosuppressive drugs for kidney transplantation. *N Engl J Med* 2004 Dec 23;351(26):2715–2729.
43. Kaplan B, Schold JD, Meier-Kriesche HU. Long-term graft survival with neoral and tacrolimus: a paired kidney analysis. *J Am Soc Nephrol* 2003 Nov;14(11):2980–2984.
44. Vincenti F, Jensik SC, Filo RS, Miller J, Pirsch J. A long-term comparison of tacrolimus (FK506) and cyclosporine in kidney transplantation: evidence for improved allograft survival at five years. *Transplantation* 2002 Mar 15;73(5):775–782.
45. Grinyo JM, Cruzado JM. Mycophenolate mofetil and sirolimus combination in renal transplantation. *Am J Transplant* 2006 Sep;6(9):1991–1999.
46. Oberbauer R, Segoloni G, Campistol JM, Kreis H, Mota A, Lawen J et al. Early cyclosporine withdrawal from a sirolimus-based regimen results in better renal allograft survival and renal function at 48 months after transplantation. *Transpl Int* 2005 Jan;18(1):22–28.

47. Bobadilla NA, Gamba G. New insights into the pathophysiology of cyclosporine nephrotoxicity: a role of aldosterone. *Am J Physiol Renal Physiol* 2007 Jul;293(1):F2–F9.
48. Nankivell BJ, Borrows RJ, Fung CL, O'Connell PJ, Allen RD, Chapman JR. The natural history of chronic allograft nephropathy. *N Engl J Med* 2003 Dec 11;349(24):2326–2333.
49. Kandaswamy R, Humar A, Casingal V, Gillingham KJ, Ibrahim H, Matas AJ. Stable kidney function in the second decade after kidney transplantation while on cyclosporine-based immunosuppression. *Transplantation* 2007 Mar 27;83(6):722–726.
50. Naesens M, Lerut E, Damme BV, Vanrenterghem Y, Kuypers DR. Tacrolimus exposure and evolution of renal allograft histology in the first year after transplantation. *Am J Transplant* 2007 Sep;7(9):2114–2123.
51. Golgert WA, Appel GB, Hariharan S. Recurrent glomerulonephritis after renal transplantation: an unsolved problem. *Clin J Am Soc Nephrol* 2008 May;3(3):800–807.
52. Bohl DL, Brennan DC. BK virus nephropathy and kidney transplantation. *Clin J Am Soc Nephrol* 2007 Jul;2(Suppl 1):S36–S46.
53. Brennan DC, Agha I, Bohl DL, Schnitzler MA, Hardinger KL, Lockwood M et al. Incidence of BK with tacrolimus versus cyclosporine and impact of preemptive immunosuppression reduction. *Am J Transplant* 2005 Mar;5(3):582–594.
54. Ginevri F, Azzi A, Hirsch HH, Basso S, Fontana I, Cioni M et al. Prospective monitoring of polyomavirus BK replication and impact of pre-emptive intervention in pediatric kidney recipients. *Am J Transplant* 2007 Dec;7(12):2727–2735.
55. Halloran PF. Call for revolution: a new approach to describing allograft deterioration. *Am J Transplant* 2002 Mar;2(3):195–200.
56. El-Zoghby ZM, Stegall MD, Lager DJ, Kremers WK, Amer H, Gloor JM et al. Identifying specific causes of kidney allograft loss. *Am J Transplant* 2009 Mar;9(3):527–535; Epub 2008 Feb 3.
57. Jevnikar AM, Mannon RB. Late kidney allograft loss: what we know about it, and what we can do about it. *Clin J Am Soc Nephrol* 2008 Mar;3(Suppl 2):S56–S67.

Chapter 12
The Kidney Transplant Biopsy

Jose R. Torrealba and Milagros D. Samaniego

Introduction

The kidney transplant biopsy is an important tool for the diagnosis of kidney transplant dysfunction, and with advances in clinical kidney transplantation, biopsies are increasingly being used to help guide therapy and therapy choice. In addition to indication biopsies, they are also used for the following:

1. Surveillance of clinically stable transplants (i.e., protocol biopsies) for the diagnosis of subclinical acute and chronic rejection and chronic antigen-independent injury.
2. Evaluation of deceased donor organ quality and suitability for transplantation, particularly in expanded criteria and donors after cardiac death.
3. Assessment of immune activation through immunohistochemistry, genomic, and transcriptomic analysis.

Indication biopsies are performed in the setting of kidney allograft dysfunction as defined by a change in serum creatinine above a steady-state level or unexplained proteinuria. The most common histological diagnoses in transplant biopsy series are acute tubular necrosis, acute rejection, calcineurin inhibitor (CNI) toxicity, chronic allograft injury of immune or non-immune nature, recurrent/de novo glomerular disease, and – occasionally – post-transplant lymphoproliferative disorders having being commonly reported since the early CNI era. More recently, with increasing use of potent induction agents and immunosuppressants, viral infections of the allograft – primarily BK nephropathy – have been added to the etiologic spectrum of acute and chronic allograft dysfunction. In addition, with increasing numbers of sensitized kidney transplant recipients and the introduction of C4d

J.R. Torrealba (✉)
Pathology and Laboratory Medicine, University of Wisconsin Hospital and Clinics, Madison, WI, USA
e-mail: jrtorrea@wisc.edu

D.B. McKay, S.M. Steinberg (eds.), *Kidney Transplantation: A Guide to the Care of Kidney Transplant Recipients*, DOI 10.1007/978-1-4419-1690-7_12,
© Springer Science+Business Media, LLC 2010

staining, antibody-mediated rejection (AMR) has been identified as a common cause of dysfunction in acute and chronic stages of transplantation.

In this chapter we will review details of kidney transplant biopsies, including how to assure an adequate specimen, how biopsies are used for clinical decision-making, and we will review the histological features of the common causes of acute and chronic allograft dysfunction.

Kidney Transplant Biopsy: Specimen Adequacy

The first Banff Conference for Allograft Pathology in 1991 defined the criteria for biopsy specimen adequacy and minimization of sampling error with the main goal to avoid underestimation of the severity of lesions. According to the original criteria, adequate specimens for the diagnosis of kidney allograft pathology must include seven or more glomeruli with one artery. Marginal specimens were defined as having 1–6 glomeruli and 1 artery while unsatisfactory specimens had neither glomeruli nor arteries.[1]

Given the patchiness of early acute rejection, the Conference warned of a substantial false-negative rate if only a single core of tissue containing a small amount of cortex is examined and recommended the abandonment of frozen sections for diagnostic purposes.

These criteria were later changed in the 1997 Banff schema,[2] which defined an adequate specimen as that containing 10 or more glomeruli and at least two arteries, and a threshold of 7 glomeruli and 1 artery for minimal sample adequacy. Although the recommendations for the number of slides did not change (i.e., seven), Banff 1997 recommended the use of three slides stained with Periodic Acid Schiff or silver methenamine while keeping the same 1991 recommendation of staining three slides with hematoxylin–eosin and one slide with Masson trichrome.

In current practice, a minimum of two cores is submitted for light microscopy based on the fact that the sensitivity for transplant rejection with one core is 90% and rises to 99% with the addition of a second core. In centers in which immunofluorescence is used for C4d staining, a third core might be requested.

Any time during the life of the transplant that recurrence or de novo glomerular disease is suspected, as in native kidney biopsy, histological diagnosis would require electron microscopy in addition to light microscopy and immunostaining. In general, this full work-up is also recommended in biopsies performed beyond the first 6–12 months post-transplantation.

Utility of the Kidney Biopsy in the Assessment of Donor Quality and Transplant Outcomes

Time-zero biopsies obtained prior to implantation can be used to assess the viability of deceased donor kidneys and their suitability for transplantation. When used for assessment of donors, the frozen section is often used, yet the utility of this method is linked to the quality of the section produced. The 2007 Banff Conference of Renal Allograft Pathology recommends that time-zero biopsies be routinely scored using the same criteria as for protocol and indication biopsies, and the use of time-zero biopsies for tracking changes of individual lesions over time.[3]

In a landmark study, Remuzzi et al.[4] investigated in a prospective, multicenter, matched-cohort-controlled trial the impact of donor histopathological features in the clinical outcome of kidney transplants from older donors (i.e., older than 60 years). This study led to the Pirani histological score system, which evaluates vessels, glomeruli, tubules, and connective tissue in donors older than 60 years to define a global kidney score ranging from 0 (indicating absence of renal lesions) to 12 (indicating marked changes in renal parenchyma). Expanding on Remuzzi's study, a series of reports have evaluated the robustness of the Pirani score and the assessment of the donor vascular compartment as predictors of recipient outcomes. Anglicheau et al.[5] found that the highest performance in predicting low transplant function was achieved using a composite score that included serum creatinine and hypertension, and glomerulosclerosis (i.e., $\geq 10\%$ vs. $<10\%$). Woestenburg and colleagues[6] found that an intimal/media hyperplasia ratio >0.47 was considered diagnostic of vasculopathy at transplantation, and correlated with lower graft function beyond the first year post-transplantation.

Time-zero biopsies (i.e., pre-implantation biopsies) can also be used to assess the quality of living donor organs. Mancilla et al.[7] performed a retrospective analysis of 219 time-zero living donor kidney biopsies in which biopsies were evaluated for findings of chronic injury including interstitial fibrosis, tubular atrophy, arteriolar hyalinosis, mesangial matrix increase, and glomerulosclerosis. Surprisingly, 54.4% of biopsies of these relatively young living donors (i.e., mean age of 35.4 ± 10 years) selected on the basis of lack of clinical kidney dysfunction (i.e., mean eGFR 96 ± 16.6 ml/min and proteinuria 70.25 ± 62.8 mg/24 h) showed a substantial number of abnormalities. Interstitial fibrosis was found in 29%, tubular atrophy in 13%, mesangial matrix increase in 12%, arteriolar hyalinosis in 10%, and glomerulosclerosis in 10%. Of interest, tubular atrophy correlated with diastolic hypertension and proteinuria after donation, while changes in mesangial matrix increase correlated with a body mass index >27 kg/m^2 body surface area. Given the short period of follow-up, no conclusions could be made about the association of these findings and poor kidney outcomes post-donation.

Pathology of the Kidney Allograft

Graft dysfunction occurs in 30–60% of kidney transplants, and biopsy of the allograft still constitutes the gold standard to determine the etiology of graft dysfunction. Biopsies are particularly useful in separating rejection vs. non-rejection causes of kidney dysfunction and to guide the appropriate therapy.[8] On average, biopsy findings changed the clinical diagnosis in 36% of cases and therapy in almost 60%, while avoided unnecessary immunosuppression in approximately 20% of cases.[8-10] The sensitivity of the kidney biopsy depends on the biopsy size, number of cores, and percentage of cortex vs. medulla sampled on the biopsy. The reported sensitivity of two core biopsies is close to 99%.[11,12] For specimen adequacy at least seven non-sclerotic glomeruli and two cross-sections of arteries must be present for evaluation. However, the adequacy of the sample is relative to the underlying pathology. For instance, the finding of only one artery with intimal arteritis is sufficient for the diagnosis of acute vascular rejection. Similarly, the finding of acute crescentic glomerulonephritis in the only two non-sclerotic glomeruli present in the biopsy must suffice for adequate assessment.

In our institution two core biopsies are obtained from the allograft, a portion of which is processed in the cryostat for frozen sections and C4d immunolabeling by the immunoperoxidase technique. The remaining of the tissue is paraffin processed and eight levels are alternately stained with hematoxylin/eosin, periodic acid shift (PAS), trichrome, and silver staining (PAMM). Immunofluorescence for immunoglobulin/complement deposits and electron microscopic evaluations are not routinely performed in our center on kidney allograft biopsies and are indicated in selected cases of allograft recipients for the evaluation of significant proteinuria or when a glomerulopathy (recurrent or de novo) is highly suspected.

The kidney allograft can be the target of immune damage, both cellular and antibody-mediated, and therefore show signs of acute or chronic rejection (Table 12.1). In addition, there are a number of non-rejection-related causes of allograft injury that may affect the allograft at any time point. Immunosuppressive drugs, especially calcineurin inhibitors, can cause acute or chronic changes to the allograft. Viruses, including polyoma (BK) virus, cytomegalovirus, adenovirus, or Epstein–Barr may infect the allograft under appropriate conditions. Sometimes the kidney allograft will harbor changes related to recurrence of the primary glomerulopathy (i.e., focal and segmental glomerulosclerosis, IgA nephropathy, membranous glomerulopathy, membranoproliferative glomerulonephritis), or the primary disease process (lupus nephritis, diabetes mellitus), but sometimes the glomerulopathy appears as a "de novo" process without any prior history. Immunofluorescence and electron microscopic examination of the allograft biopsy is therefore relevant in those situations. More recently, it has been recognized that leukocytes may infiltrate allografts that are not necessarily related to rejection.[13,14] Hence, these unique cases belong to a new emerging category of "pathology" of the allograft tolerance.[13-15]

Traditionally, three major forms of rejection are recognized: hyperacute rejection, acute rejection, and chronic rejection. Acute rejection, either cellular or antibody-mediated, can happen in the allograft either separately or together, or even with changes of chronic allograft injury or findings not related to rejection resulting in a mixture of histopathological features. In order to standardize the diagnosis and reporting on allograft kidney biopsies a classification system known as "Banff" classification was developed through a combined effort between pathologists, transplant physicians, and researchers[1] in Banff, Canada. This system has gone through a number of significant revisions and modification over the years since it was first published in 1993, the most recent in 2007 in La Coruña, Spain, that led to the current revised Banff 07 classification (Table 12.2).[3]

Table 12.1 Pathologic classification of renal allograft diseases/conditions

I – Immunologic rejection
  – Antibody-mediated rejection
      Hyperacute rejection
      Acute humoral rejection
      Chronic humoral rejection
  – T-cell-mediated rejection
      Acute T-cell-mediated rejection
      Chronic T-cell-mediated rejection
II – Non-rejection injury
  – Acute tubular injury
  – Drug toxicity (calcineurin inhibitors, OKT3, rapamycin)
  – Infection (BK virus, CMV, adenovirus, EBV)
  – Acute tubulointerstitial nephritis
  – Interstitial fibrosis and tubular atrophy, no evidence of specific etiology
  – Post-transplant lymphoproliferative disorder
  – Artery/vein thrombosis or stenosis
  – Obstruction, urine leak
III – Recurrent primary disease
  – Focal and segmental glomerulosclerosis (FSGS)
  – IgA nephropathy
  – Membranoproliferative glomerulonephritis (MPGN)
  – Membranous nephropathy
  – Lupus nephritis
  – Diabetes mellitus
  – Amyloidosis
IV – Allo/autoantibody-mediated diseases
  – De novo glomerulopathies
  – Anti-GBM in Alport disease
  – Anti-TBM disease
  – Nephrotic syndrome in nephrin-deficient recipients
V – "Pathology" of allograft tolerance

CMV, cytomegalovirus; EBV, Epstein–Barr virus; GBM, glomerular basement membrane; TBM, tubular basement membrane

Antibody-Mediated Rejection

In the past decade thanks to new and more sensitive techniques to detect donor-specific antibodies in serum of transplanted patients and the development of C4d immunolabeling of kidney biopsies as a tissue marker of antibody-mediated rejection,[16–19] four forms of antibody-mediated graft injury have been defined: hyperacute rejection, acute humoral rejection (AHR), chronic humoral rejection (CHR), and accommodation[20] (Table 12.2 [category 2]).

Hyperacute Rejection

Hyperacute rejection by definition takes place within minutes to hours in the post-transplant period in presensitized patients who have circulating HLA, ABO, or other alloantibody-to-donor endothelial surface antigen and it is usually irreversible.[21]

Table 12.2 Banff 97 diagnostic categories for renal allograft biopsies – Banff 07 updates

1. Normal
2. Antibody-mediated changes
   – C4d deposition without morphologic evidence of active rejection
   C4d+, + circulating antidonor antibodies, no signs of acute or chronic AMR or TCMR
   – Acute antibody-mediated rejection
   C4d+, + circulating antidonor antibodies, morphologic evidence of acute tissue injury,
      such as
      I. ATN-like minimal inflammation
      II. Capillary and/or glomerular inflammation and/or thromboses
      III. Arterial (v3)
   – Chronic active antibody-mediated rejection
   C4d+, + circulating antidonor antibodies, morphologic evidence of chronic tissue injury,
      such as glomerular double contours and/or peritubular capillary basement membrane
      multilayering and/or interstitial fibrosis/tubular atrophy and/or fibrous intimal thickening
      in arteries
3. Borderline changes: "Suspicious" for acute T-cell-mediated rejection
   This category is used when no intimal arteritis is present, but there are foci of tubulitis with
      minor interstitial infiltration or interstitial infiltration with mild tubulitis
4. T-cell-mediated rejection
   – Acute T-cell-mediated rejection (type/grade)
      IA. Significant interstitial inflammation (>25% of parenchyma) and foci of moderate
         tubulitis
      IB. Significant interstitial inflammation (>25% of parenchyma) and foci of severe
         tubulitis
      IIA. Mild-to-moderate intimal arteritis
      IIB. Severe intimal arteritis comprising more than 25% of the luminal area
      III. Transmural arteritis and/or arterial fibrinoid change and necrosis of medial
         smooth muscle cells with accompanying lymphocytic inflammation
   – Chronic active T-cell-mediated rejection
   Chronic allograft arteriopathy. Arterial intimal fibrosis with mononuclear cell infiltration
      in fibrosis, formation of neointima
5. Interstitial fibrosis and tubular atrophy, no evidence of any specific etiology
   – Grade   I. Mild interstitial fibrosis and tubular atrophy (<25% of cortical area)
   – Grade   II. Moderate interstitial fibrosis and tubular atrophy (26–50% of cortical area)
   – Grade III. Severe interstitial fibrosis and tubular atrophy (>50% of cortical area)
6 – Other
   Changes not considered to be due to rejection, acute or chronic

Adapted from Solez K et al [3]

At implantation the kidney becomes dark, cyanotic, rapidly after establishing the renal artery anastomosis. If several hours or days have passed before the kidney is removed there may be complete hemorrhagic infarction of the kidney parenchyma. On light microscopic examination the earliest changes are swelling of vascular endothelial cells accompanied by neutrophil margination in glomerular and interstitial capillaries. Capillary fibrin thrombi of glomeruli and arterioles follow with subsequent widespread ischemic hemorrhagic necrosis and infarct of the renal parenchyma. In these circumstances, C4d immunolabeling usually shows diffusely positive peritubular capillaries. Early in the process, however, C4d may be negative presumably because of lack of access of C4 to the site (vasoconstriction) or enough time for sufficient amount of C4d to be produced.[20]

Acute Humoral Rejection (AHR)

Patients with AHR usually present with acute allograft dysfunction with elevation of serum creatinine and accompanied sometimes by reduced urine output and tenderness of the graft. It often arises within the first few weeks post-transplantation, but it can happen at any time, particularly if the immunosuppression is decreased due to non-compliance or medication dosage reduction. Presensitization to prior pregnancies, blood transfusions, or prior transplants are the major risk factors.

The diagnostic criteria for acute antibody-mediated rejection require the demonstration of each of the following:

(1) Morphologic evidence of acute tissue injury in the form of acute tubular injury, neutrophil margination, thrombotic microangiopathy, and/or arterial fibrinoid necrosis.
(2) The demonstration of C4d deposition in peritubular capillaries.
(3) Serologic evidence of circulating donor-specific HLA or other antidonor endothelial antigen.[3]

The recognition of only two of the three criteria is considered "suspicious" for acute antibody-mediated rejection. By light microscopy the earliest finding is neutrophil or leukocyte margination in dilated peritubular capillaries (Fig. 12.1). Peritubular capillaries is followed by endothelial injury and thrombosis of glomerular and interstitial capillaries in the most severe cases. Larger arteries may show transmural fibrinoid arteritis/necrosis with variable amount of leukocytic infiltrates in approximately 10–20% of cases.[20] The interstitium typically shows variable degree of edema and in some cases interstitial hemorrhages. If no concomitant acute cellular rejection is present, no significant interstitial mononuclear inflammation or tubulitis is detected.

In the current Banff classification[3] AHR class I corresponds to a biopsy with findings of acute tubular injury without significant inflammation. AHR class II is defined by capillary glomerulitis and/or capillary thromboses, and AHR class III is characterized by the transmural fibrinoid necrosis of small arteries (Fig. 12.1). Macrophages are recognized as a common intracapillary cell in AHR in the kidney.[22] Because of the short half-life of immunoglobulins and complement components, immunofluorescence usually does not reveal specific antibody or complement deposition. However, C4d, a stable degradation product of the C4 complement, binds covalently to tissue proteins and can stay in tissue for 7–10 days, therefore acting as a marker for acute antibody-mediated damage.[16–19]

The diagnostic pattern of C4d in immunolabeled kidney allograft biopsies with AHR corresponds to a strong, linear, smooth, and diffuse (>50%) staining of peritubular capillaries (Fig. 12.1). It is recommended to perform C4d immunolabeling on frozen preparations[20] because of the associated higher sensitivity with this

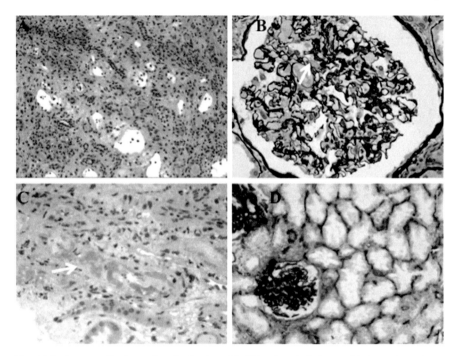

Fig. 12.1 Acute antibody-mediated rejection. (**a**) Dilated peritubular capillaries and moderate leukocyte margination, representing peritubular capillaries (H/E, 100X); (**b**) glomerulus with intracapillary fibrin thrombi (*arrows*), normal mesangial matrix, and cellularity and normal capillary wall thickness (PAMM, 400X); (**c**) acute vascular rejection with transmural arterial fibrinoid necrosis (*arrow*, H/E, 200X); (**d**) C4d immunolabeling of frozen section preparation depicts diffusely positive peritubular capillaries with a strong, smooth, and linear pattern of staining (C4d Immunohistochemistry, 100X)

technique. Immunohistochemistry on formalin-fixed paraffin-embedded tissue may be an option too in some circumstances.[23] C4d, however, may not be a reliable marker of acute antibody-mediated rejection in ABO-incompatible allograft, as over 80% of protocol biopsies without evidence of histologic injury in this setting have shown diffuse staining of peritubular capillaries.[24] C3d, a stable degradation product of C3 similar to C4d, may be a better marker of antibody-mediated rejection in ABO-incompatible grafts.[24] Others have reported more severe forms of antibody rejection in biopsies positive for C3d[25,26]

Chronic Humoral Rejection

After the elimination of the term chronic allograft nephropathy (CAN) by consensus of the Banff 05 meeting,[27] it is strongly recommended to pathologists to make any effort to identify the specific etiology when reporting biopsies with chronic allograft injury. The chronic injury may be rejection-related (antibody or cellular) or non-rejection related (chronic hypertension, chronic calcineurin inhibitor toxicity, chronic obstruction, bacterial pyelonephritis, viral infections, etc.). When no etiology is identified the biopsy could be classified as "interstitial fibrosis and tubular atrophy without evidence of any specific etiology" (Table 12.2, category 5).

Several groups have demonstrated that circulating anti-HLA class I or class II antibodies either donor-specific or non-donor specific are found in a significant number of renal allograft recipients with subsequent chronic allograft loss.[28–30] Pathologic findings usually associated with chronic alloimmune injury of the kidney allograft are transplant arteriopathy and transplant glomerulopathy. Transplant arteriopathy is characterized by progressive narrowing and occlusion of medium-sized and large caliber arteries by dense fibrointimal proliferation (Fig. 12.2). Transplant glomerulopathy is characterized by global duplication of the glomerular basement membrane, accompanied in many cases by mesangial expansion and intracapillary mononuclear cells accumulation, therefore resembling a membranoproliferative pattern of glomerular injury (Fig. 12.2). Patients with this glomerular injury often have significant proteinuria. We and others have shown that transplant glomerulopathy is significantly associated with the diffuse pattern of C4d labeling of peritubular

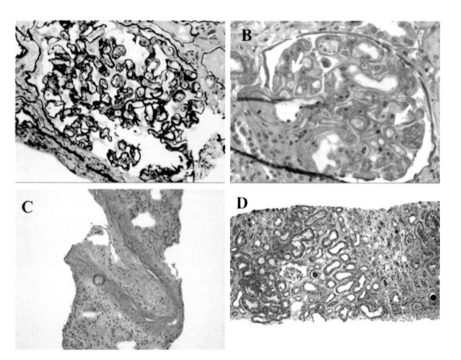

Fig. 12.2 Chronic allograft injury. (**a**) and (**b**) Transplant glomerulopathy. Both glomeruli show global duplication of capillary walls (*arrows*) with segmental intracapillary hypercellularity and cellular interposition, 400X, PAMM (**a**) and PAS (**b**). (**c**) Transplant arteriopathy. The artery depicted in the center of the biopsy reveals severe fibrointimal thickening and luminal narrowing (100X, HE). (**d**) Core kidney biopsy with patchy, severe interstitial fibrosis and tubular atrophy (trichrome, 100X)

capillaries.[16,31-34] Transplant glomerulopathy is strongly associated with circulating donor-specific HLA antibodies[17] and history of prior AHR[35] and usually portends a bad prognosis with a graft survival of approximately 50% 3 years after the diagnosis.[35]

Similar to AHR, the diagnostic criteria for CHR or chronic active antibody-mediated rejection of the Banff classification (Table 12.2, category 2) have been defined.[27,36] Three elements should be present:

(1) Histologic evidence of chronic injury (need 2 of 4) including arterial intimal fibrosis without elastosis, duplication of glomerular basement membrane, multilamination of peritubular capillaries basement membrane, and/or interstitial fibrosis with tubular atrophy.
(2) Evidence of antibody activation/deposition (C4d in peritubular capillaries).
(3) Serologic evidence of anti-HLA or other antidonor antibodies. Again, if only two of these criteria are present the diagnosis should be phrased as "suspicious" for chronic antibody rejection.

Accommodation

Protocol biopsies have shown C4d along the peritubular capillaries in 25–80% of ABO-incompatible renal allografts, with evidence of AHR in only 4–12%.[24,37] In these circumstances either the full complement pathway is not activated or the endothelium develops resistance to complement damage, therefore achieving an immunologic accommodation. C4d deposition also occurs in 2–26% of histologically normal ABO-compatible grafts, the higher frequency found in HLA-presensitized patients.[24,38] The finding of C4d alone does not warrant the diagnosis of acute antibody-mediated rejection in these biopsies and may indicate a form of accommodation. However, the long-term significance of C4d deposits in these cases is not completely clear. In a reported series, the 3-year graft loss was 32% in untreated C4d+ histologically normal biopsies compared to 0% in C4d+ histologically normal patients that were treated with increased immunosuppression.[39] Dr. Robert Colvin has suggested that accommodation may have different degrees of effectiveness and stability, ranging from none (hypercute rejection) to minimal (acute rejection), substantial (chronic rejection), or complete (stable accommodation).[20]

T-Cell-Mediated Rejection

Acute T-Cell-Mediated Rejection

Acute T-cell-mediated rejection is defined as the rapid loss (within days) of allograft function due to a T-cell-mediated (or cellular) rejection. It can happen at any time post-transplantation, even years after the transplant if the immunosuppression is reduced or stopped. T cells recognize donor histocompatibility antigens in the kidney, affecting all compartments with findings in glomeruli, tubules, interstitium, and vessels, separately or in combination. Glomeruli are characterized by increase in intracapillary cellularity, particularly mononuclear with or without associated endothelial swelling or damage. Tubulointerstitial rejection (type I Banff classification, Table 12.2) is characterized by interstitial infiltration by mononuclear cells, including lymphocytes and monocytes, accompanied by interstitial edema, acute tubular injury, and tubulitis. Tubulitis is defined by the invasion of tubules by mononuclear cells (lymphocytes or macrophages) across the tubular basement membrane (Fig. 12.3). Tubulitis is more significant and should be graded on non-atrophic tubules. A CD3 staining for T cells may be helpful in some cases to assess the degree of tubulitis. Type I cellular rejection requires the presence of more than 25% of interstitial inflammation accompanied at least with moderate tubulitis[3] (Table 12.2, category 4). Interstitial inflammation or tubulitis of lesser degree shall be classified as "suspicious" for acute T-cell-mediated rejection (Table 12.2, category 3). Vascular (type II) acute T-cell-mediated rejection is defined by the presence of mononuclear cells beneath the vascular endothelium (endarteritis, Fig. 12.3). The

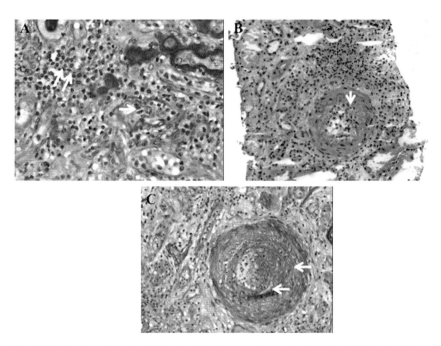

Fig. 12.3 T-cell-mediated rejection. (**a**) Tubulointerstitial acute T-cell-mediated rejection with severe tubulitis (*arrow*) and severe interstitial mononuclear inflammation (*double arrows*), PAS, 400X. (**b**) Endarteritis, mild to moderate. The artery depicted in the center of the biopsy reveals mild-to-moderate intimal mononuclear inflammatory infiltrate (*arrow*). Associated interstitial inflammation and tubulitis are also noted (H/E, 100X). (**c**) This artery reveals severe fibrointimal proliferation with luminal narrowing along with intimal mononuclear inflammation (*arrows*), representing an example of chronic active T-cell-mediated rejection. Interstitial fibrosis and chronic inflammation are also present (PAS, 200X)

finding of lymphocytes adhered to the endothelium or in the adventitia alone is not considered diagnostic of vascular cellular rejection. Likewise, venulitis is not included in the definition of vascular rejection.[21] One mononuclear cell under the arterial endothelium is considered by the Banff and the National Institute of Health Cooperative Clinical trials in Transplantation (CCTT) to be sufficient for the diagnosis of endarteritis.[2,11] In severe cases the intima of the vessels may be expanded by edema and fibrin deposition with endothelial swelling, proliferation, and degeneration. Transmural mononuclear infiltrate can be found affecting the media with focal myocyte necrosis, features that constitute type III vascular rejection (Table 12.2, category 4).

Chronic T-Cell-Mediated Rejection

Chronic T-cell-mediated rejection is a form of chronic graft injury due to ongoing T-cell-mediated (cellular) immunologic reaction to donor antigens. This process is active and progresses slowly (months to years). As for CHR, the criteria for chronic T-cell-mediated rejection would require the documentation of chronic structural changes (arterial intimal fibrosis, glomerular and/or peritubular capillary basement membrane duplication, and interstitial fibrosis and tubular atrophy) and the presence of T cells in sites of chronic damage (arterial intima, glomeruli, tubules, and interstitium).[21] The current Banff classification (Table 12.2, category 4) recognizes the category of "chronic active T-cell-mediated rejection" in those cases with arterial intimal fibrosis (transplant arteriopathy) with active mononuclear cell infiltration in areas of fibrosis (Fig. 12.3).

Calcineurin Inhibitor Nephrotoxicity

Calcineurin inhibitors (CNI), introduced in the early 1980s, revolutionized the field of organ transplantation for their high efficacy in preventing allograft rejection.[40-42] CNI nephrotoxicities occur in acute and chronic forms and can affect all the compartments in the kidney, including glomeruli, tubules, interstitium, and vessels. Acutely, CNIs may cause reductions in renal plasma flow and glomerular filtration rate without any structural damage (functional toxicity), may produce isometric vacuolization of tubules with dysmorphic nuclei and microcalcifications (toxic tubulopathy), or they may cause a form of thrombotic microangiopathy with fibrin thrombosis of small arteries, arterioles, and glomerular capillaries with or without vascular myocyte necrosis (acute arteriolopathy). Chronic CNI toxicity is characterized typically by nodular hyaline arteriolopathy and linear interstitial fibrosis and tubular atrophy ("striped" fibrosis)[41] (Fig. 12.4). Not all cases of chronic CNI toxicity, however, show these characteristic patterns and may reveal interstitial fibrosis, tubular atrophy, and hyaline arteriolosis indistinguishable of other etiologies. Given the low reproducibility of the Banff arteriolar hyaline thickening score, a new quantitative scoring system for CNI-arteriolopathy was proposed.[3] In this system the severity of hyaline arteriolopathy is quantified according to the presence of

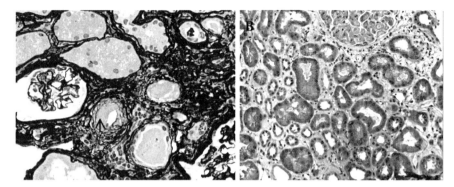

Fig. 12.4 Chronic calcineurin inhibitor toxicity. (**a**) Kidney core biopsy reveals severe interstitial fibrosis accompanied by nodular arteriolar hyalinosis (*arrow*) in a case of chronic CNI toxicity (200X, PAMM). (**b**) Severe interstitial fibrosis and tubular atrophy in a patient with chronic calcineurin inhibitor toxicity (100X, Trichrome)

circular or non-circular involvement and the number of involved arterioles. This system reportedly results in better interobserver reproducibility and is validated against graft function.[43] In some patients, due to the loss of nephrons and glomerulosclerosis related to chronic CNI toxicity, some of the remaining glomeruli may show secondary changes of focal and segmental glomerulosclerosis.

BK Virus Nephritis

BK virus, named after the initials of the first patient in whom it was described, is a member of the polyoma virus family and is related to both the JC and simian virus (SV) 40 viruses. It is an important and relatively common cause of tubulointerstitial inflammation (nephritis) of the kidney allograft due to reactivation of a latent infection in an immunosuppressed individual. The condition is characterized by prominent interstitial mononuclear infiltrate, including lymphocytes and plasma cells and foci of tubulitis. Given its resemblance to acute cellular rejection, it is crucial to accurately make the diagnosis on allograft biopsies in view of the opposed approaches to treatment, i.e., reduction of immunosuppression in BK-virus-positive biopsies vs. increase of immunosuppression in cases of rejection. The main features of the polyoma virus infection in the tubular epithelial cells are the presence of enlarged, atypical nuclei with smudgy, ground glass, basophilic inclusions that completely replace the nuclear chromatin (Fig. 12.5). The presence of the cytopathic virus could be confirmed by immunolabeling with antibodies for SV40 to detect the large T antigen (Fig. 12.5).

Acute Tubular Necrosis

Acute tubular necrosis in the kidney allograft is a common form of acute tubular injury that manifests more commonly in the immediate postoperative period and it

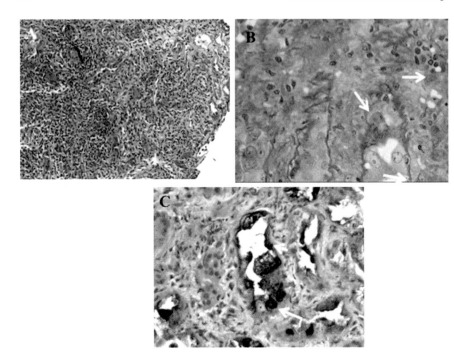

Fig. 12.5 BK (Polyoma) virus nephritis. (**a**) Acute tubulointerstitial nephritis, severe with dense mononuclear interstitial inflammation and tubulitis (PAS, 100X). (**b**) Higher magnification of biopsy in **a** shows atypical tubular epithelial cells with large nuclei, smudged chromatin, and nuclear inclusions of BK virus (*arrows*), PAS, 400X. (**c**) Immunoperoxidase using an anti-SV40 antibody confirms the intranuclear presence of the virus (*arrows*), 400X

is usually the result of prolong warm or cold ischemia.[44] It is a particularly common complication in allografts subjected to long cold or warm ischemia. As in native kidneys, ATN is characterized by flattening of tubular epithelial cells, loss of the brush border, focal epithelial coagulation necrosis and apoptosis, cytoplasmic basophilia, and evidence of epithelial regeneration manifested by prominent nucleoli and mitotic figures. There could be some interstitial edema, but interstitial inflammatory cells are usually sparse. Tubulitis and neutrophilic margination of peritubular capillaries are not findings of ATN. Peritubular capillaries are negative for C4d. The finding of diffusely positive peritubular capillaries for C4d in the setting of ATN is consistent with type I acute antibody-mediated rejection of the Banff 97 revised criteria (Table 12.2, category 2).

If transient dialysis is required during the first week post-transplantation, the term delayed graft function (DGF) is used. If the graft never made urine, the term "primary nonfunction" (PNF) is used instead. DGF has been reported to occur in 20–25% of deceased donor kidney allograft recipients[45] and is more common in those kidneys from asystolic donors (40–80%).[46,47] The average duration of DGF is 10–15 days. DGF is a clinical term that encompasses several possible pathologic processes in the allograft, including acute ischemic injury (acute tubular necrosis) related to cold and warm ischemia times, and other causes that may affect the allograft alone or in conjunction with acute ischemia, including drug toxicity (specially acute calcineurin inhibitors), acute cellular or antibody-mediated rejection, glomerular endothelial injury, and surgical complications at the anastomotic sites. In the immediate post-transplant period a biopsy is indicated if renal function does not recover and remains marginal. The biopsy is useful in this scenario to rule out rejection, drug toxicity, and other non-ischemic related injuries and to initiate appropriate therapy. In one series 18% of patients with DGF had acute rejection in biopsies taken within a week post-transplant.[48] Approximately 95–98% of grafts with DGF recover, 50% within 10 days and 83% within 20 days post-transplantation.[49]

Recurrent Glomerular Diseases

Recurrent glomerular disease is a significant problem in the kidney allograft, estimated to affect 1–8% of transplants. The diagnosis of recurrent disease requires that the primary kidney disease be appropriately identified and that the allograft biopsy undergo thorough adequate stainings, immunolabeling, and ultrastructural studies for diagnostic confirmation. Most recurrences occur within 6 months post-transplantation.

The most common glomerular disease that recurs in the allograft (95–100% rate of recurrence) is membranoproliferative glomerulonephritis type II (dense deposit disease), followed by membranoproliferative glomerulonephritis type I (40–70%), IgA nephropathy/Henoch–Schonlein purpura (30–50%), focal segmental glomerulosclerosis (30–40%), and hemolytic uremic syndrome (30%, non-epidemic form). Lower rates are reported for membranous glomerulopathy (10%), anti-GBM disease (5–10%), and lupus nephritis (less than 5%).[50] Systemic diseases that commonly recur in the allograft include diabetic nephropathy, amyloidosis, oxalosis, and Fabry's disease.

Recurrent glomerulopathies in the kidney allograft have the same light microscopy, immunofluorescence, and electron microscopic features as the disease occurring in the native kidney. In addition to the glomerulopathy, in the kidney allograft there may be additional evidence of acute or chronic rejection changes. Of particular interest is to render the adequate diagnosis of MPGN type I and to distinguish it from its look-alikes. Those include transplant glomerulopathy, calcineurin inhibitor-induced glomerulopathy, and other causes of chronic thrombotic microangiopathy. In contrast to MPGN type I the aforementioned lesions show less endocapillary and mesangial proliferation, less GBM duplication with cell interposition, and less crescent formation. In addition, immune deposits are usually absent or sparse in these conditions (Fig. 12.6).

Recurrent glomerulopathy may adversely affect the survival of the allograft. In one report, the 5-year survival of allografts with recurrence of FSGS was 34%

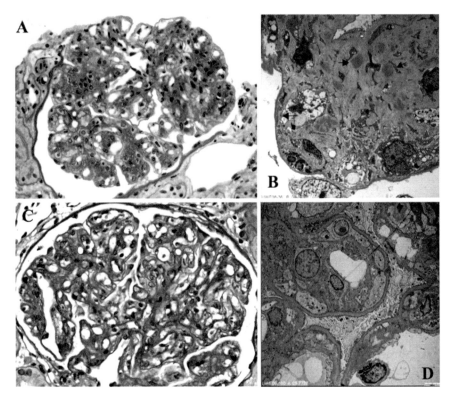

Fig. 12.6 Membranoproliferative glomerulonephritis. (**a**) Glomerulus reveals global increase in cellularity with lobular pattern, mesangial and endocapillary cellular proliferation. Thickening and reduplication of capillary walls are also noted (PAS, 400X). (**b**) On electron microscopy, capillary loops show marked increase in mesangial matrix and cellularity with intracapillary cellular proliferation. Cellular interposition and reduplication of glomerular basement membrane are also present. Mesangial and sub-endothelial electron dense immune deposits are present (*arrows*). (**c**) The recurrence of MPGN type I in the allograft must be distinguished from transplant glomerulopathy. In this example of transplant glomerulopathy, the glomerulus also shows increase in mesangial and endocapillary cellularity but to a somewhat lesser degree than MPGN type I. Duplication of glomerular basement membrane is seen in both conditions. However, very rare or practically no immune deposits are detected on immunofluorescence or electron microscopic (**d**) studies

compared to 67% in the control group.[51] Graft failure is common in patients with recurrent MPGN type I years (10–50%); the recurrence is higher in repeat grafts and if the native kidney had crescents.[52] Similarly, the recurrence of MPGN type II is related to the presence of crescents in the native kidney[52]; crescents in the allograft negatively correlates with graft survival. Recurrent HUS/TMA causes graft loss in most patients (70%)[53] and patient survival is reported to be only 50% at 3 years.[54] Recurrence of IgA nephropathy in general does not adversely affect the allograft survival and renal failure is uncommon.[55,56]

De Novo Glomerular Disease

A "de novo" glomerulopathy is diagnosed when the allograft develops a glomerular disease that is different from the original primary disease of the native kidney. Therefore, documentation of the original disease is necessary to rule out the possibility of a recurrent disease. As it is the case in the majority of "recurrent glomerulopathies," "de novo glomerulopathies" are diagnosed incidentally in biopsies obtained during rejection episodes or in the evaluation of newly diagnosed proteinuria or active urinary sediment.

Membranous glomerulopathy is the most common glomerular disease to occur de novo in the allograft with a reported incidence of 2–5%.[50] The patient typically presents in average 2 years after transplantation with proteinuria (sometime in the nephritic range). The diagnosis is usually established by typical granular capillary wall IgG and C3 deposits and the confirmation of small sub-epithelial deposits by electron microscopy. Repeat biopsies have shown persistence or progression of the deposits in most patients[57,58] and the long-term outcome of the allografts with membranous glomerulopathy does not seem to differ from those without it.

De novo antiglomerular basement membrane disease can develop in up to 15% of kidneys transplanted for end-stage hereditary nephritis.[59] An example of de novo antiglomerular basement membrane disease occurs in Alport's patients because their kidneys fail to express the autoantigen of Goodpasture's syndrome. Therefore patients with Alport's may lack self-tolerance to certain alpha chains of type IV collagen. The "donor" alpha chains can be recognized as a foreign antigen after transplantation and initiate an immune response. Some patients develop only linear IgG deposits in the allograft without evidence of nephritis, others develop severe crescentic glomerulonephritis with the exact morphology of anti-GBM disease in native kidneys, a condition that can lead to allograft failure.

De novo focal and segmental glomerulosclerosis (FSGS) in the allograft can occur in different settings: (1) as the result of hyperfiltration injury in longstanding grafts with loss of nephrons and fibrosis or in adult recipients of pediatric kidneys; (2) in grafts with severe vascular disease with glomerular hypoperfusion and secondary collapsing FSGS; (3) in kidney transplants with other glomerulopathies (i.e., transplant glomerulopathy); or (4) as a new onset primary disease (less common). The outcome is specially poor in those patients who develop collapsing variants of FSGS.[21]

Protocol Biopsies in Kidney Allografts

Protocol kidney allograft biopsies taken at the time of transplantation (time zero) and later (at specific time points) is the standard of care in some transplant centers[60–63] and have been shown to have the potential to influence clinical management and to better understand allograft pathogenetic mechanisms. A recent consensus report[61] concluded that protocol biopsies are safe and valuable means of detecting subclinical disease (immunologic and non-immunologic) that can benefit from modification of therapy. Moreover, protocol biopsies could be a source for molecular studies that may reveal evidence of activity or progression of diseases or conditions in the allograft that are not readily appreciated by histological techniques alone. In a large-scale study of over 900 protocol kidney biopsies, it was shown that histologic evidence of acute rejection in the absence of clinical suspicion (subclinical rejection, SCR) resulted in significant tubulointerstitial damage and preceded the development of chronic allograft injury.[64] Protocol biopsies taken 1 year post-transplantation showed persistence of SCR in 17% of biopsies.[64]

Early treatment of SCR with oral or IV steroids or increase in maintenance immunosuppression significantly decreased the 1-year prevalence of SCR and ameliorated the chronic inflammatory Banff scores.[65] Inflammation and glomerulopathy diagnosed in 1-year post-transplant protocol biopsies significantly predicted loss of graft function and graft failure in a group of 292 adult patients in a 4-year follow-up period.[66]

In a high-risk group of recipients of HLA incompatible transplants that underwent pre-transplant conditioning, 10 patients fulfilled the criteria for subclinical antibody-mediated rejection (SC-AMR), defined as patients with stable creatinine, diffuse C4d staining of peritubular capillaries, peritubular capillaritis, circulating donor-specific antibodies, and without concurrent acute cellular rejection.[67] The study demonstrated that biopsies with SC-AMR revealed higher chronic allograft injury (CAI) scores in follow-up biopsies compared to controls, suggesting that SC-AMR may contribute to the development of CAI.

Molecular studies of protocol biopsies have shown that biopsies from recipients with stable allograft function and normal histology can show higher expression of genes associated with T-cell activation compared to normal kidneys.[68] Protocol kidney allograft biopsies therefore may be valuable in the diagnosis and management of sub-clinical rejection or sub-clinical diseases (non-rejection related) with the likely potential to prevent or ameliorate chronic allograft injury if early detected and treated. There is a need, however, for more studies on protocol biopsy to validate it as a surrogate marker of graft survival.[61]

References

1. Solez K, Axelsen RA, Benediktsson H, Burdick JF, Cohen AH, Colvin RB, Croker BP, Droz D, Dunnill MS, Halloran PF et al. . International standardization of criteria for the histologic diagnosis of renal allograft rejection: the Banff working classification of kidney transplant pathology. *Kidney Int* 1993;44:411.
2. Racusen LC, Solez K, Colvin RB, Bonsib SM, Castro MC, Cavallo T, Croker BP, Demetris AJ, Drachenberg CB, Fogo AB, Furness P, Gaber LW, Gibson IW, Glotz D, Goldberg JC, Grande J, Halloran PF, Hansen HE, Hartley B, Hayry PJ, Hill CM, Hoffman EO, Hunsicker LG, Lindblad AS, Yamaguchi Y et al. . The Banff 97 working classification of renal allograft pathology. *Kidney Int* 1999;55:713.
3. Solez K, Colvin RB, Racusen LC, Haas M, Sis B, Mengel M, Halloran PF, Baldwin W, Banfi G, Collins AB, Cosio F, David DS, Drachenberg C, Einecke G, Fogo AB, Gibson IW, Glotz D, Iskandar SS, Kraus E, Lerut E, Mannon RB, Mihatsch M, Nankivell BJ, Nickeleit V, Papadimitriou JC, Randhawa P, Regele H, Renaudin K, Roberts I, Seron D, Smith RN,

Valente M. Banff 07 classification of renal allograft pathology: updates and future directions. *Am J Transplant* 2008;8:753.

4. Remuzzi G, Grinyo J, Ruggenenti P, Beatini M, Cole EH, Milford EL, Brenner BM. Early experience with dual kidney transplantation in adults using expanded donor criteria. Double Kidney Transplant Group (DKG). *J Am Soc Nephrol* 1999;10:2591.

5. Anglicheau D, Loupy A, Lefaucheur C, Pessione F, Letourneau I, Cote I, Gaha K, Noel LH, Patey N, Droz D, Martinez F, Zuber J, Glotz D, Thervet E, Legendre C. A simple clinico-histopathological composite scoring system is highly predictive of graft outcomes in marginal donors. *Am J Transplant* 2008;8:2325.

6. Woestenburg AT, Verpooten GA, Ysebaert DK, Van Marck EA, Verbeelen D, Bosmans JL. Fibrous intimal thickening at implantation adversely affects long-term kidney allograft function. *Transplantation* 2009;87:72.

7. Mancilla E, Avila-Casado C, Uribe-Uribe N, Morales-Buenrostro LE, Rodriguez F, Vilatoba M, Gabilondo B, Aburto S, Rodriguez RM, Magana S, Magana F, Alberu J. Time-zero renal biopsy in living kidney transplantation: a valuable opportunity to correlate predonation clinical data with histological abnormalities. *Transplantation* 2008;86:1684.

8. Waltzer WC, Miller F, Arnold A, Jao S, Anaise D, Rapaport FT. Value of percutaneous core needle biopsy in the differential diagnosis of renal transplant dysfunction. *J Urol* 1987;137:1117.

9. Al-Awwa IA, Hariharan S, First MR. Importance of allograft biopsy in renal transplant recipients: correlation between clinical and histological diagnosis. *Am J Kidney Dis* 1998; *31:S15.*

10. Matas AJ, Tellis VA, Sablay L, Quinn T, Soberman R, Veith FJ. The value of needle renal allograft biopsy. III. A prospective study. *Surgery* 1985;98:922.

11. Colvin RB, Cohen AH, Saiontz C, Bonsib S, Buick M, Burke B, Carter S, Cavallo T, Haas M, Lindblad A, Manivel JC, Nast CC, Salomon D, Weaver C, Weiss M. Evaluation of pathologic criteria for acute renal allograft rejection: reproducibility, sensitivity, and clinical correlation. *J Am Soc Nephrol* 1997;8:1930.

12. Sorof JM, Vartanian RK, Olson JL, Tomlanovich SJ, Vincenti FG, Amend WJ. Histopathological concordance of paired renal allograft biopsy cores. Effect on the diagnosis and management of acute rejection. *Transplantation* 1995;60:1215.

13. Torrealba JR, Katayama M, Fechner JH Jr., Jankowska-Gan E, Kusaka S, Xu Q, Schultz JM, Oberley TD, Hu H, Hamawy MM, Jonker M, Wubben J, Doxiadis G, Bontrop R, Burlingham WJ, Knechtle SJ. Metastable tolerance to rhesus monkey renal transplants is correlated with allograft TGF-beta 1+CD4+ T regulatory cell infiltrates. *J Immunol* 2004; 172:5753.

14. Xu Q, Lee J, Jankowska-Gan E, Schultz J, Roenneburg DA, Haynes LD, Kusaka S, Sollinger HW, Knechtle SJ, VanBuskirk AM, Torrealba JR, Burlingham WJ. Human CD4+CD25 low adaptive T regulatory cells suppress delayed-type hypersensitivity during transplant tolerance. *J Immunol* 2007;178:3983.

15. Torrealba J, Burlingham W. Transforming Growth factor Beta and the immunopathologic assessment of tolerance. *Curr Opin Organ Transplant* 2004;9:241.

16. Mauiyyedi S, Crespo M, Collins AB, Schneeberger EE, Pascual MA, Saidman SL, Tolkoff-Rubin NE, Williams WW, Delmonico FL, Cosimi AB, Colvin RB. Acute humoral rejection in kidney transplantation: II. Morphology, immunopathology, and pathologic classification. *J Am Soc Nephrol* 2002;13:779.

17. Mauiyyedi S, Pelle PD, Saidman S, Collins AB, Pascual M, Tolkoff-Rubin NE, Williams WW, Cosimi AA, Schneeberger EE, Colvin RB. Chronic humoral rejection: identification of antibody-mediated chronic renal allograft rejection by C4d deposits in peritubular capillaries. *J Am Soc Nephrol* 2001;12:574.

18. Collins AB, Schneeberger EE, Pascual MA, Saidman SL, Williams WW, Tolkoff-Rubin N, Cosimi AB, Colvin RB. Complement activation in acute humoral renal allograft rejection: diagnostic significance of C4d deposits in peritubular capillaries. *J Am Soc Nephrol* 1999;10:2208.

19. Racusen LC, Colvin RB, Solez K, Mihatsch MJ, Halloran PF, Campbell PM, Cecka MJ, Cosyns JP, Demetris AJ, Fishbein MC, Fogo A, Furness P, Gibson IW, Glotz D, Hayry P, Hunsickern L, Kashgarian M, Kerman R, Magil AJ, Montgomery R, Morozumi K, Nickeleit V, Randhawa P, Regele H, Seron D, Seshan S, Sund S, Trpkov K. Antibody-mediated rejection criteria - an addition to the Banff 97 classification of renal allograft rejection. *Am J Transplant* 2003;3:708.
20. Colvin RB. Antibody-mediated renal allograft rejection: diagnosis and pathogenesis. *J Am Soc Nephrol* 2007;18:1046.
21. Colvin RRenal transplant pathology. In *Heptinstall's Pathology of the Kidney*. Jennette JC, Olson JL, Schwartz MM, Silva FG, (eds.), 6th Ed., Vol. II. Lippincott-Raven, Philadelphia, p. 1347, 2006.
22. Tinckam KJ, Djurdjev O, Magil AB. Glomerular monocytes predict worse outcomes after acute renal allograft rejection independent of C4d status. *Kidney Int* 2005;68:1866.
23. Lorenz M, Regele H, Schillinger M, Exner M, Rasoul-Rockenschaub S, Wahrmann M, Kletzmayr J, Silberhumer G, Horl WH, Bohmig GA. Risk factors for capillary C4d deposition in kidney allografts: evaluation of a large study cohort. *Transplantation* 2004;78:447.
24. Haas M, Rahman MH, Racusen LC, Kraus ES, Bagnasco SM, Segev DL, Simpkins CE, Warren DS, King KE, Zachary AA, Montgomery RA. C4d and C3d staining in biopsies of ABO- and HLA-incompatible renal allografts: correlation with histologic findings. *Am J Transplant* 2006;6:1829.
25. Sund S, Hovig T, Reisaeter AV, Scott H, Bentdal O, Mollnes TE. Complement activation in early protocol kidney graft biopsies after living-donor transplantation. *Transplantation* 2003;75:1204.
26. Kuypers DR, Lerut E, Evenepoel P, Maes B, Vanrenterghem Y, Van Damme B. C3D deposition in peritubular capillaries indicates a variant of acute renal allograft rejection characterized by a worse clinical outcome. *Transplantation* 2003;76:102.
27. Solez K, Colvin RB, Racusen LC, Sis B, Halloran PF, Birk PE, Campbell PM, Cascalho M, Collins AB, Demetris AJ, Drachenberg CB, Gibson IW, Grimm PC, Haas M, Lerut E, Liapis H, Mannon RB, Marcus PB, Mengel M, Mihatsch MJ, Nankivell BJ, Nickeleit V, Papadimitriou JC, Platt JL, Randhawa P, Roberts I, Salinas-Madriga L, Salomon DR, Seron D, Sheaff M, Weening JJ. Banff '05 Meeting Report: differential diagnosis of chronic allograft injury and elimination of chronic allograft nephropathy ('CAN'). *Am J Transplant* 2007;7:518.
28. Worthington JE, Martin S, Al-Husseini DM, Dyer PA, Johnson RW. Posttransplantation production of donor HLA-specific antibodies as a predictor of renal transplant outcome. *Transplantation* 2003;75:1034.
29. Hourmant M, Cesbron-Gautier A, Terasaki PI, Mizutani K, Moreau A, Meurette A, Dantal J, Giral M, Blancho G, Cantarovich D, Karam G, Follea G, Soulillou JP, Bignon JD. Frequency and clinical implications of development of donor-specific and non-donor-specific HLA antibodies after kidney transplantation. *J Am Soc Nephrol* 2005;16:2804.
30. Terasaki PI, Ozawa M. Predictive value of HLA antibodies and serum creatinine in chronic rejection: results of a 2-year prospective trial. *Transplantation* 2005;80:1194.
31. Torrealba J, Lopez F, Djamali A, Knechtle S, Sollinger S, Pirsch J, Samaniego M. Histopathologic parameters of acute allograft rejection in kidney biopsies associated with the development of chronic allograft injury. *Am Soc Transplant* 2008;8:1. Am J Transplan.
32. Regele H, Bohmig GA, Habicht A, Gollowitzer D, Schillinger M, Rockenschaub S, Watschinger B, Kerjaschki D, Exner M. Capillary deposition of complement split product C4d in renal allografts is associated with basement membrane injury in peritubular and glomerular capillaries: a contribution of humoral immunity to chronic allograft rejection. *J Am Soc Nephrol* 2002;13:2371.
33. Vongwiwatana A, Gourishankar S, Campbell PM, Solez K, Halloran PF. Peritubular capillary changes and C4d deposits are associated with transplant glomerulopathy but not IgA nephropathy. *Am J Transplant* 2004;4:124.

34. Sijpkens YW, Joosten SA, Wong MC, Dekker FW, Benediktsson H, Bajema IM, Bruijn JA, Paul LC. Immunologic risk factors and glomerular C4d deposits in chronic transplant glomerulopathy. *Kidney Int* 2004;65:2409.

35. Gloor JM, Cosio FG, Rea DJ, Wadei HM, Winters JL, Moore SB, DeGoey SR, Lager DJ, Grande JP, Stegall MD. Histologic findings one year after positive crossmatch or ABO blood group incompatible living donor kidney transplantation. *Am J Transplant* 2006; 6:1841.

36. Takemoto SK, Zeevi A, Feng S, Colvin RB, Jordan S, Kobashigawa J, Kupiec-Weglinski J, Matas A, Montgomery RA, Nickerson P, Platt JL, Rabb H, Thistlethwaite R, Tyan D, Delmonico FL. National conference to assess antibody-mediated rejection in solid organ transplantation. *Am J Transplant* 2004;4:1033.

37. Fidler ME, Gloor JM, Lager DJ, Larson TS, Griffin MD, Textor SC, Schwab TR, Prieto M, Nyberg SL, Ishitani MB, Grande JP, Kay PA, Stegall MD. Histologic findings of antibody-mediated rejection in ABO blood-group-incompatible living-donor kidney transplantation. *Am J Transplant* 2004;4:101.

38. Mengel M, Bogers J, Bosmans JL, Seron D, Moreso F, Carrera M, Gwinner W, Schwarz A, De Broe M, Kreipe H, Haller H. Incidence of C4d stain in protocol biopsies from renal allografts: results from a multicenter trial. *Am J Transplant* 2005;5:1050.

39. Dickenmann M, Steiger J, Descoeudres B, Mihatsch M, Nickeleit V. The fate of C4d positive kidney allografts lacking histological signs of acute rejection. *Clin Nephrol* 2006;65:173.

40. D'Agati VD. Morphologic features of cyclosporine nephrotoxicity. *Contrib Nephrol* 1995;114:84.

41. Mihatsch MJ, Thiel G, Ryffel B. Morphologic diagnosis of cyclosporine nephrotoxicity. *Semin Diagn Pathol* 1988;5:104.

42. Mihatsch MJ, Thiel G, Ryffel B. Histopathology of cyclosporine nephrotoxicity. *Transplant Proc* 1988;20:759.

43. Sis B, Dadras F, Khoshjou F, Cockfield S, Mihatsch MJ, Solez K. Reproducibility studies on arteriolar hyaline thickening scoring in calcineurin inhibitor-treated renal allograft recipients. *Am J Transplant* 2006;6:1444.

44. Olsen S, Burdick JF, Keown PA, Wallace AC, Racusen LC, Solez K. Primary acute renal failure ("acute tubular necrosis") in the transplanted kidney: morphology and pathogenesis. *Medicine (Baltimore)* 1989;68:173.

45. Troppmann C, Gillingham KJ, Gruessner RW, Dunn DL, Payne WD, Najarian JS, Matas AJ. Delayed graft function in the absence of rejection has no long-term impact. A study of cadaver kidney recipients with good graft function at 1 year after transplantation. *Transplantation* 1996;61:1331.

46. Renkens JJ, Rouflart MM, Christiaans MH, van den Berg-Loonen EM, van Hooff JP, van Heurn LW. Outcome of nonheart-beating donor kidneys with prolonged delayed graft function after transplantation. *Am J Transplant* 2005;5:2704.

47. Rudich SM, Kaplan B, Magee JC, Arenas JD, Punch JD, Kayler LK, Merion RM, Meier-Kriesche HU. Renal transplantations performed using non-heart-beating organ donors: going back to the future? *Transplantation* 2002;74:1715.

48. Jain S, Curwood V, White SA, Furness PN, Nicholson ML. Sub-clinical acute rejection detected using protocol biopsies in patients with delayed graft function. *Transpl Int* 2000; 13(Suppl 1):S52.

49. Perico N, Cattaneo D, Sayegh MH, Remuzzi G. Delayed graft function in kidney transplantation. *Lancet* 2004;364:1814.

50. Vivette DD'A, Jennette JC, Silva FG. 2005. Pathology of Renal Transplantation. *In Atlas of Nontumor Pathology. Non-Neoplastic Kidney Disease. AFIP:667.*

51. Hariharan S, Adams MB, Brennan DC, Davis CL, First MR, Johnson CP, Ouseph R, Peddi VR, Pelz C, Roza AM, Vincenti F, George V. Recurrent and de novo glomerular disease after renal transplantation: a report from renal allograft disease registry. *Transplant Proc* 1999;31:223.

52. Little MA, Dupont P, Campbell E, Dorman A, Walshe JJ. Severity of primary MPGN, rather than MPGN type, determines renal survival and post-transplantation recurrence risk. *Kidney Int* 2006;69:504.
53. Hebert D, Kim EM, Sibley RK, Mauer MS. Post-transplantation outcome of patients with hemolytic-uremic syndrome: update. *Pediatr Nephrol* 1991;5:162.
54. Reynolds JC, Agodoa LY, Yuan CM, Abbott KC. Thrombotic microangiopathy after renal transplantation in the United States. *Am J Kidney Dis* 2003;42:1058.
55. Ponticelli C, Traversi L, Feliciani A, Cesana BM, Banfi G, Tarantino A. Kidney transplantation in patients with IgA mesangial glomerulonephritis. *Kidney Int* 2001;60:1948.
56. Ponticelli C, Traversi L, Banfi G. Renal transplantation in patients with IgA mesangial glomerulonephritis. *Pediatr Transplant* 2004;8:334.
57. Antignac C, Hinglais N, Gubler MC, Gagnadoux MF, Broyer M, Habib R. De novo membranous glomerulonephritis in renal allografts in children. *Clin Nephrol* 1988;30:1.
58. Monga G, Mazzucco G, Basolo B, Quaranta S, Motta M, Segoloni G, Amoroso A. Membranous glomerulonephritis (MGN) in transplanted kidneys: morphologic investigation on 256 renal allografts. *Mod Pathol* 1993;6:249.
59. Gobel J, Olbricht CJ, Offner G, Helmchen U, Repp H, Koch KM, Frei U. Kidney transplantation in Alport's syndrome: long-term outcome and allograft anti-GBM nephritis. *Clin Nephrol* 1992;38:299.
60. Nankivell BJ, Chapman JR. The significance of subclinical rejection and the value of protocol biopsies. *Am J Transplant* 2006;6:2006.
61. Mengel M, Chapman JR, Cosio FG, Cavaille-Coll MW, Haller H, Halloran PF, Kirk AD, Mihatsch MJ, Nankivell BJ, Racusen LC, Roberts IS, Rush DN, Schwarz A, Seron D, Stegall MD, Colvin RB. Protocol biopsies in renal transplantation: insights into patient management and pathogenesis. *Am J Transplant* 2007;7:512.
62. Colvin RB. Eye of the needle. *Am J Transplant* 2007;7:267.
63. Karpinski J, Lajoie G, Cattran D, Fenton S, Zaltzman J, Cardella C, Cole E. Outcome of kidney transplantation from high-risk donors is determined by both structure and function. *Transplantation* 1999;67:1162.
64. Nankivell BJ, Borrows RJ, Fung CL, O'Connell PJ, Allen RD, Chapman JR. Natural history, risk factors, and impact of subclinical rejection in kidney transplantation. *Transplantation* 2004;78:242.
65. Kee TY, Chapman JR, O'Connell PJ, Fung CL, Allen RD, Kable K, Vitalone MJ, Nankivell BJ. Treatment of subclinical rejection diagnosed by protocol biopsy of kidney transplants. *Transplantation* 2006;82:36.
66. Cosio FG, Grande JP, Wadei H, Larson TS, Griffin MD, Stegall MD. Predicting subsequent decline in kidney allograft function from early surveillance biopsies. *Am J Transplant* 2005;5:2464.
67. Haas M, Montgomery RA, Segev DL, Rahman MH, Racusen LC, Bagnasco SM, Simpkins CE, Warren DS, Lepley D, Zachary AA, Kraus ES. Subclinical acute antibody-mediated rejection in positive crossmatch renal allografts. *Am J Transplant* 2007;7:576.
68. Hoffmann SC, Hale DA, Kleiner DE, Mannon RB, Kampen RL, Jacobson LM, Cendales LC, Swanson SJ, Becker BN, Kirk AD. Functionally significant renal allograft rejection is defined by transcriptional criteria. *Am J Transplant* 2005;5:573.

Chapter 13
Evaluation of the Kidney Transplant Candidate and Follow-Up of the Listed Patient

Roy D. Bloom and Alden M. Doyle

The Pre-transplant Evaluation and Follow-Up of the Listed Patient

The most fundamental aspect of the entire transplant course is the pre-transplant evaluation of the potential kidney recipient. The pre-transplant evaluation is the initial step that triggers a sequence of events and actions, resulting in the wait-listing and eventual transplantation of patients, with the primary outcome goals of enhancing quality of life and/or prolonging life expectancy. In this chapter, we shall provide an overview of the process involved in getting transplant candidates through their evaluation onto the waiting list and their subsequent transplant center-relevant management until they are transplanted.

Introduction

The purpose of the transplant evaluation is to identify, educate, and prepare suitable candidates for transplantation. It is increasingly important for physicians who care for patients with kidney disease to be familiar with the evaluation process so that they can help their patients make the best informed medical decisions. For example, awareness of the minimum criteria for listing and transplantation should trigger opportune discussions between nephrologists and their patients, followed by referral for a transplant evaluation in a time frame that anticipates listing for a kidney as soon as the patient is eligible. This is particularly true as the average waiting times for deceased donor kidneys have continued to grow, reflective of the burgeoning disparity between organ demand and supply. Long wait times for these organs have, in turn, driven the development of new strategies to increase the supply of suitable organs and better match these organs with potential recipients. The pre-transplant

R.D. Bloom (✉)
Kidney Transplant Program, Hospital of the University of Pennsylvania, Philadelphia, PA, USA
e-mail: rdbloom@mail.med.upenn.edu

D.B. McKay, S.M. Steinberg (eds.), *Kidney Transplantation: A Guide to the Care of Kidney Transplant Recipients*, DOI 10.1007/978-1-4419-1690-7_13,
© Springer Science+Business Media, LLC 2010

evaluation should be recognized as a dynamic phase of the transplant process that is continually revised to incorporate relevant material for educating and identifying potentially suitable candidates for these emerging new transplant strategies.

Although not every person is an acceptable transplant candidate, the range of potential kidney recipients is wide and still broadening as evidence demonstrating the benefits of transplantation over dialysis continues to emerge. Growing recognition of these benefits has brought about a surge in the number of referrals for kidney transplantation, resulting in expansion of the waiting list of patients wanting an organ and a lengthening of waiting times for listed candidates, as well as an increase in the age and comorbid conditions among this population.[1] At the present time, UNOS regulations dictate that patient can be listed for kidney transplant when they have a measured or estimated glomerular filtration rate of 20 ml/min or less.

There are several phases that kidney recipients go through to reach the point of transplantation (see Fig. 13.1). This process commences in their local nephrologist's office when education for kidney replacement therapy preparation is first initiated. Following referral to the transplant center, the *Evaluation Phase* starts with a formal patient assessment that typically consists of a minimum standard evaluation required for all potential candidates. Patients may be accepted as candidates with no need for additional evaluation, turned down at the initial visit, or required by the

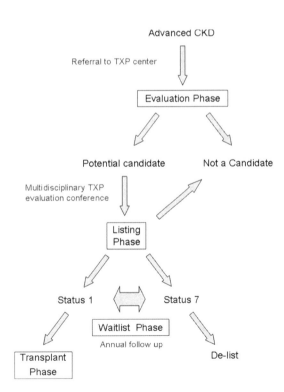

Fig. 13.1 Transplant evaluation process

transplant center to undergo additional testing and consultation on a case-by-case basis to assist in the determination of their candidacy. Acceptable transplant candidates next enter the *Waitlist Phase* when they are placed on the waiting list. Unsuitable candidates do not enter the Waitlist Phase and should be formally notified of the decision, so that they have the option of seeking a transplant evaluation elsewhere should they desire. The Waitlist Phase terminates when patients are either transplanted (*Transplant Phase*) or removed from the waiting list because intervening medical or psychosocial issues contraindicate future transplantation.

The Evaluation Phase

The basic function of the transplant evaluation is to identify and adequately treat comorbid conditions that may lead to post-transplant complications and jeopardize either patient or graft survival. The evaluation is a process that requires the multidisciplinary participation and coordination of professionals of several disciplines. At a minimum, this includes an assessment by transplant surgery, transplant nephrology, a nurse coordinator, social worker, a financial coordinator, and a dietician. Additional subspecialty consultants such as cardiologists or psychiatrists are frequently called upon on a case-by-case basis. The evaluation process goes beyond a preoperative risk assessment and necessarily involves active involvement from patients, their families, and frequently their referring physicians as well. At its best, these parties should also receive comprehensive education and counseling through their participation to become acquainted with the major life-altering events that accompany transplantation. The foremost goal is to try to ensure that harm is minimized and benefit is maximized so that the optimal use of the organs can be assured.

Education of the Kidney Transplant Candidate

The education of transplant candidates occurs at many levels and should continue to take place throughout the entire process starting in the office of the referring nephrologist. As patients are confronted with an enormous amount of complex information, the importance of ongoing edification cannot be overemphasized. This educational reinforcement also allows for the vital opportunity to set realistic expectations concerning the transplant process and its potential impact on their future health and well-being.

Within the evaluation process itself, complementary educational input is typically provided during initial evaluation by all the members of the transplant team. The forum may be any combination of a one-on-one interaction, group lecture, question and answer session, or provision to the patient of relevant literature, publications, and brochures. Regardless of the method, we believe that it is the responsibility of the transplant center to provide comprehensive patient-level education in all aspects of kidney transplantation. This should include in-depth information pertaining to the transplant evaluation process and should, at a minimum, include the following: (1) the pre-transplant testing required, (2) the benefits and risks of kidney transplantation compared to dialysis, (3) details regarding the transplant surgery itself, (4) instruction regarding optimal health maintenance and adherence while on the waiting list and after the surgery, (5) the advantages of living donor and preemptive transplantation,[1] (6) a review of the types of deceased donor kidneys that can be transplanted, the risk of recurrence of native kidney disease, and (7) a review of possible post-transplant complications with an emphasis on immunosuppression side effects. For kidney transplant candidates with type 1 diabetes mellitus, a discussion about possible simultaneous pancreas–kidney transplantation may be appropriate as well. At all times, the transplant center has an obligation to provide objective information that is both relevant and in the best interest of the potential transplant candidate. For example, a 24-year-old otherwise healthy patient with stage 4 CKD secondary to IgA nephropathy and not yet on dialysis should not be advised to accept a kidney from an extended criteria donor (ECD).

In addition to these above avenues of education, instructive information regarding transplantation is widely disseminated over the Internet at a multitude of well-respected websites (e.g., those of American Society of Transplantation (www.a-s-t.org), United Network for Organ Sharing (www.UNOS.org)). Transplant recipient-directed initiatives have also fostered growth of patient support groups in some communities that provide opportunity for first-hand dissemination of information in this regard.

Medical Evaluation

This aspect of the evaluation is structured to determine whether patients are medically suitable candidates for transplantation. The medical evaluation is "coordinated" by transplant coordinators, who have the responsibility of overseeing pre-transplant-related management of candidates at all phases of the evaluation and waiting list process. Transplant coordinators are usually registered nurses or nurse practitioners with expertise in kidney transplantation and/or kidney disease and dialysis. They typically have the most contact with the patient undergoing evaluation and on the waiting list. Transplant coordinators are fundamental to all aspects of the evaluation, serving as central conduits for education and communication between the various entities involved.

Medical contraindications to transplantation center around four primary lines of analysis: (1) Does the candidate have a reasonable expected survival? (2) Can the perioperative risk be reasonably managed? (3) Does the patient have a condition or conditions that will worsen with the transplant surgery and/or immunosuppression required? (4) Is the surgery technically feasible? In order to make these determinations, both the transplant nephrologist and the transplant surgeon need to perform a comprehensive evaluation that encompasses medical, surgical, psychiatric, and social history, accompanied by a careful examination of all the major systems. Specific emphasis should be placed on examination of the abdomen as well as the peripheral arterial system (e.g., femoral bruits, absent pedal pulses), in the context of (i) assuring an acceptable location and vascular anatomy for placement of a future allograft and (ii) being able to apprise the transplant candidate of future operative risk (e.g., in the case of abdominal obesity). Access to prior medical records of potential candidates can often be extremely helpful to the transplant physician in assessing the transplantability of patients. Since cardiovascular disease is the major CKD comorbidity, pertinent records relating to prior stress testing, echocardiography, carotid artery evaluations, and coronary angiography are of particular importance. In many situations, consultation with other medical specialists is frequently required in order to assist the transplant medical staff determine the candidacy of potential transplant recipients.

With medical advancement over the past half-century, kidney transplantation has progressed to the point where it is now absolutely contraindicated in very few situations (Table 13.1). Such circumstances include either intractable malignancy or chronic illness associated with a very short life expectancy, uncontrolled psychosis, active substance abuse, and untreated current active infection.[2] Often, appropriate and effective therapy of any of these conditions (e.g., treatment of active infection) may subsequently render patients suitable transplant candidates.

In the context of the foregoing, generally accepted standard evaluation testing (Table 13.2) includes blood work assessing nutritional status (e.g., albumin), liver injury, complete blood count, as well as serologic evidence of prior exposure to (or infection with) hepatitis B or C viruses, human immunodeficiency virus, cytomegalovirus, and syphilis.[3] A baseline chest X-ray and ECG are also recommended. Many transplant centers also insist on age- and gender-appropriate screening such as mammography, pap smears, prostate-specific antigen, and colonoscopy. Finally, in order to be placed on the waiting list, patients are required to have HLA testing, a panel reactive antibody (PRA) assay to detect prior sensitization as well as blood typing performed in duplicate.[3]

Special Situations

There are several clinical scenarios that may warrant additional concern in the consideration of patients for kidney transplantation:

i. *Obesity.* This is a condition that is highly prevalent in patients with CKD and is associated with decreased post-transplant patient and graft survival. Obese patients also have a higher incidence of wound infections and other postoperative complications but generally still enjoy a quality and quantity of life benefit from successful transplantation. Many centers use a BMI cutoff of 40, although

Table 13.1 Potential contraindications for kidney transplantation

Potential contraindication for TXP	Center-specific
Cardiovascular disease	Prohibitive rarely – only when severe and inoperable
Peripheral arterial disease	Can diminish candidacy if blood flow to the extremities threatened or extensive calcifications of arterial walls prevent surgical anastamosis
Liver disease	Generally requires liver biopsy. While mild disease not prohibitive, patients with decompensated cirrhosis are not candidates without receiving a concomitant liver transplant
Lung disease	Should be evaluated by pulmonary specialist. Can be contraindication if severe
Psychiatric disease	Usually contraindicated if unstable; steroid minimization/avoidance considered if history of psychosis
Non-adherence	Assessment for transplantability requires comprehensive psychosocial clearance
Substance abuse	If active, patients must be referred for counseling and detoxification and are only candidates when no longer actively using
Active infection	Active infections must be cleared by the time of transplant. Pockets of infection including infected hardware and stones must be removed before patients are candidates
HIV	No longer considered a contraindication. Most patients on stable HAART therapy with undetectable viral loads. Most HIV+ patients transplanted in context of clinical trials
Obesity	While obese patients are counseled to lose weight and have higher rates of complication, they still derive benefit from transplantation. Morbid obesity is considered a contraindication in some centers if BMIs are greater than 40 in some centers

this remains a matter of some debate.[4] Current guidelines recommend that ideally patients employ exercise and diet to achieve and maintain a BMI of 30 or less.

ii. *Malignancy.* Some malignancies can be worsened with immunosuppression, while others carry a high rate of recurrence and are associated with a prohibitively short survival. Depending on the specific histologic and patient characteristics, most malignancies require a 2- to 5-year disease-free interval in order for patients to be eligible for transplantation.[2] During this interval, if the malignancy is deemed to have a high likelihood of cure or if it is anticipated that the patient will be transplanted after the waiting period, potential candidates may be eligible for waitlisting in an inactive status.

iii. *Cardiovascular disease.* As the leading cause of death in kidney recipients, this common CKD comorbidity is considered a contraindication to transplantation only when it is deemed inoperable, such that the perioperative mortality or expected post-transplant survival is prohibitively poor. The optimal cardiovascular disease screening strategy in kidney transplant candidates is unknown,

Table 13.2 Transplant evaluation testing

Required	Center-specific	Case-specific
1. Medical H&P	1. PSA	1. Cardiac catheterization
2. Chemistry panel	2. Colonoscopy	2. Echocardiography
3. Complete blood count	3. Mammography	3. SPEP/UPEP
4. PT/PTT	4. Stress test	4. Disease serologies (anti-dsDNA, ANCA, anti-GBM Ab, ESR)
5. Blood type (in duplicate)	5. PPD	
6. HepBsAg, hepatitis C Ab, RPR, HIV, HSV, CMV Ab	6. HSV, EBV, VZV	5. Voiding cystourethrogram
7. Pelvic exam/pap smear		6. Carotid duplex
8. Tissue typing		7. ABI/toe pressures and/or arteriogram of lower extremities
9. Chest X-ray		
10. ECG		

based on the limited predictive value of non-invasive testing in this population. Although cardiovascular disease testing in transplant candidates is widely performed, the exact approach appears to be center-specific according to individual practice style and experience. The approach in our center has been to employ a low threshold for stress testing if the potential transplant candidate has additional Framingham cardiovascular risk factors beyond their advanced kidney disease, especially if the patient has underlying diabetes or known peripheral vascular disease. We generally obtain nuclear stress testing over exercise treadmill tests, as the diminished exercise capacity commonly observed among kidney candidates limits the utility and interpretability of the latter type of study. Patients with positive stress tests are referred for cardiology evaluation and then coronary angiography is typically performed. Peripheral arterial disease is initially assessed clinically and, if indicated, ABI/toe pressure measurements and additional radiological studies of the femoral and abdominal vasculature are obtained.

iv. *Pulmonary disease.* Very little data exists regarding pulmonary evaluation in kidney transplant candidates. Generally, kidney transplantation is contraindicated in the setting of restrictive or obstructive lung disease advanced enough to confer increased perioperative morbidity or mortality. Severe pulmonary hypertension may similarly, render patients not transplantable. This decision is usually made in conjunction with a pulmonary specialist consultation.

v. *Liver disease.* Patients with known liver disease are carefully evaluated. It is recommended that patients with active liver disease, including detectable hepatitis B or C viremia, consult with a hepatologist and undergo a liver biopsy as part of their evaluation. Efforts to treat these viral infections should be undertaken prior to transplantation as a way of reducing related post-transplant morbidity. Decompensated cirrhosis is associated with prohibitively high perioperative mortality and is considered an absolute contraindication to kidney transplantation alone unless in the setting of a simultaneous liver transplant.[5]

vi. *Advancing age.* The upper age limit for kidney transplantation is increasing and the decision to consider transplantation is now more likely to be based on patient comorbidities rather than age specifically. Although the life-expectancy advantage of kidney transplantation compared to remaining on dialysis is shorter for older than younger recipients, many elderly patients still derive a significant quality-of-life benefit. Consequently, the ageing population is contributing to the growth in the waitlist in an incremental manner. In response to the greater demand, many transplant centers attempt to separate the biological age from the chronological age, allowing for greater latitude in age limits when potential recipients have minimal comorbidities and have maintained themselves in good physical shape. The evaluation process should take into account blood type, availability of potential living donors, and average wait times in the organ procurement organizations (OPOs) because the patient's age and possible level of health at time of listing will be different to that at transplantation. The evaluation process should also address the willingness of the potential elderly recipient to accept ECD kidneys, where the trade-off for receiving a lesser quality organ can be offset by shorter wait times, a greater proportion of remaining life-years being free of dialysis, and a reduction in the likelihood of dying while awaiting a kidney.[6]

vii. *Urological issues.* Issues related to the genitourinary tract should be evaluated thoroughly prior to transplant surgery. Whenever possible, the lower genitourinary tract should be made functional. All men of appropriate age should be screened for prostate cancer and treated as appropriate. Patients must be free of active urinary tract infection. Infected hardware and infected stones need to be removed and the urine sterilized before patients can be considered transplantable. If there is any doubt or if there is concern about infected or bleeding kidneys, pre-transplant nephrectomies may be indicated. Benign prostatic hypertrophy often becomes more evident with the increased urine output that follows successful kidney transplantation. Other factors that may compromise bladder function and/or complete bladder emptying should also be considered as relatively small amounts of urinary post-void residual in transplant patients pose a risk for decreased allograft function and recurrent urinary tract infections.

viii. *Recurrence of native kidney disease.* Several native kidney diseases may recur in the post-transplant setting (Table 13.3). Glomerular diseases such as membranoproliferative glomerulonephritis, focal segmental glomerulosclerosis, and fibrillary glomerulonephritis recur frequently and, when they do, they may be associated with shortened allograft survival.[7] However, no primary kidney disease specifically contraindicates an effort at kidney transplantation for at least two reasons. First, it is not possible to accurately identify patients

Table 13.3 Risk and consequence of recurrent kidney disease after transplantation

Kidney disease	Rate of recurrence (%)	Rate of graft loss (%)
FSGS	20–50	13–20
IgA nephropathy	12–53	1–16
SLE	2–9	2–4
Membranous nephropathy	10–30	10–15
MPGN	20–80[a]	15–30[a]
ANCA-associated glomerulonephritis	17	8
Diabetes	90+[b]	Uncommon

[a] MPGN recurrence and graft loss rates dependent on type, with type II substantially worse in each case.
[b] Prevalence refers to functional lifespan of allograft; it is felt that most if not all allografts will eventually demonstrate DM histology.

in whom recurrence in their first transplant will develop. Second, if the recurrence is associated with an insidious decline in allograft function, patients are in many cases still better off transplanted than remaining on dialysis. It is widely recognized that the risk of recurrence in a second or subsequent transplant is almost invariable if the first allograft was lost from this mechanism. In this situation, many transplant centers may be very reluctant to re-transplant patients who experienced rapid failure of their first allograft on this basis. On the other hand, a transplant lost due to recurrence after several years of function does not preclude re-transplantation. An effort to ascertain the primary kidney disease is therefore important in order to avail patients of the risks and potential consequences of recurrence after transplantation. Some diseases, such as IgA nephropathy, frequently recur, though seldom impact on allograft survival.[8] For patients whose native kidneys failed in the setting of systemic diseases (e.g., Wegener's granulomatosis, Goodpasture's syndrome, systemic lupus erythematosus), it is generally recommended to proceed with transplantation when the disease is quiescent, based on clinical and occasionally serological (e.g., anti-GBM titers) criteria.Patients with autosomal dominant polycystic kidney disease generally do well with transplantation but do require careful assessment to ensure that they will have enough space in the abdomen for placement of an allograft in the setting of large kidneys and liver. Patients with persistent headaches or a family history of aneurysms should have their cerebral vasculature screened. Patients should be informed of the increased risk for bouts of diverticulitis.

ix. *Combined and sequential multi-organ transplantation.* There are increasing numbers of patients who have received either a simultaneous or sequential combination of transplanted organs where a kidney is one of the organs. The expansion of transplantation of sequential kidneys after prior solid organs is attributable to a number of factors that include a substantial improvement in post-transplant survival following transplantation of these non-renal organs and the association with increased rates of progressive chronic kidney disease in this setting.[9] Carefully selected non-renal organ recipients can be successfully transplanted with a sequential kidney although the renal outcomes may not be quite as favorable as observed in recipients of primary kidney transplants. The evaluation of such patients must take into account the function of the non-renal organ as well as the immunosuppressive burden that the patient has been exposed to with that transplant. There has also been a rise in simultaneous multiple-organ transplantation involving kidneys, largely associated with the introduction of the MELD system for liver allocation. The evaluation process in these settings is generally driven by the non-renal organ. The criteria for using a kidney as part of a multi-organ transplant are not yet uniformly agreed upon although consensus opinion is starting to emerge.[5] A comprehensive discussion of these criteria is beyond the scope of this chapter.

Psychosocial Evaluation

An assessment by a dedicated social worker is undertaken that aims to evaluate the support systems available to potential recipients and screen for untreated or unstable psychiatric disease as well as substance abuse issues. The social worker will also try to proactively identify problems that may arise in the post-transplant period and for which solutions can be strategized in advance.

Candidates are evaluated on their ability to care for both the transplanted organ and themselves. Facets of this evaluation include the ability to be compliant with follow-up and complex medical regimens. Non-adherence has been definitively associated with higher rates of rejection and increased graft loss.[10,11] Dialogue between the transplant center and the patient's physicians (and, often, the dialysis center) is routinely needed to assess this risk. Sometimes a trial period with objective targets (such as compliance with dialysis treatments) can be utilized following a discussion of these issues with the potential transplant candidate. As the social context in which the patient operates can have a profound influence on the potential candidate's ability to maintain compliance, the family, professional, and social network circumstances are assessed by the social work team in detail. Active substance abuse may impact on post-transplant health and adherence and every effort should be made to ensure it is sufficiently addressed and treated before transplantation. Most transplant programs require a period of documented abstinence before activation on the waiting list and periodic screening thereafter. American Society of Transplantation clinical practice guidelines recommend that all patients with mental illness undergo appropriate evaluation, counseling, and treatment prior to transplantation.[2] Mental illness is also not an absolute contraindication to transplantation but should be evaluated and deemed to be stable at the time of transplant. When appropriate, psychiatrists may be involved to complete these evaluations and initiate treatment plans and/or counseling. The effect of the surgery, the hospitalization, and the transplant medications (especially glucocorticoids) on the stability of the patient's psychiatric conditions should also be taken into account and discussed at the time of evaluation.

Financial Evaluation

A financial coordinator performs a financial and insurance assessment in order to make certain that patients have suitable coverage for the (often expensive) long-term medications that will be required to maintain the health of the patient and the transplanted organ following the transplant surgery.

Dietary Evaluation

Transplant dieticians are involved in performing nutritional assessments of patients and counseling on appropriate dietary recommendations. This evaluation may focus on issues of pre-transplant weight loss, in the case of a morbidly obese patient who may not meet listing criteria, or counseling candidates about post-transplant nutritional issues and risk of weight gain.

All studies and consultations are reviewed in conjunction with input from the various members of the transplant team at a regularly conducted transplant patient selection committee meeting that represents all the disciplines involved in the evaluation. Final decisions about status changes, patient candidacy, or the requirement for additional testing or consultation are made at this forum.

The Waitlist Phase

How Does Kidney Listing Work?

The United Network for Organ Sharing (UNOS) is a privately administered, non-profit scientific and educational organization that is contracted to the federal government to oversee on a national level the allocation of deceased donor organs for transplantation. The topic of UNOS and organ allocation is discussed in depth in Chapter 5. The United States is geographically divided into 58 federally funded contiguous semi-autonomous *organ procurement organizations* (OPOs) that are responsible for recovering deceased donor organs and arranging their distribution at a local level in accordance with UNOS policies. Some OPOs contain only a single transplant center, while other OPOs may be comprised of several centers. Patients get on the waiting list in the OPO in which their transplant center is found. Some patients list at transplant centers in multiple different OPOs in order to try and increase their access to kidney offers.

Patients are listed according to blood type, which is the primary criterion by which deceased donor kidneys are allocated. The average wait times vary significantly by blood type and by OPO. National data suggest that potential recipients whose HLA antigens share no mismatches with any of the prospective deceased donor HLA antigens (*zero-mismatch*) have superior allograft outcomes and are prioritized for transplantation independent of accumulated wait time. Public policy changes have recently gone into effect that restrict the importation of these *zero-mismatched* kidneys from one region of the country to another to sensitized patients.

Although there are variances across OPOs, kidney allocation for most patients is based on a system of points. Points are allocated to transplant candidates according to duration of time on the waiting list, the degree of HLA-DR mismatch, as well as a panel reactive antibody (PRA) titer of greater than 80%. Under consideration at the present time is national policy that gives points to sensitized patients according to a percent PRA sliding scale with the recognition that there is a roughly linear relationship between magnitude of sensitization and increased average wait times. To help address the extremely deleterious effect advanced kidney disease has on growth of young children, points are awarded for younger age. Points (but not immediate priority) are also given to prior kidney donors in the United States who subsequently develop advanced CKD and have the misfortune of requiring a kidney transplant themselves. Finally, points may be assigned on the grounds of medical urgency on an individualized basis. Points allocation on this basis typically occurs at a local level and involves a cooperative medical decision by the transplant centers within the OPO.

Waitlist Status

Patients on the kidney transplant waiting list can be listed in one of two status categories. Patients are listed *status 1* where there have been deemed suitable transplant candidates that are ready to receive kidney offers. *Status 7* listing represents an "on-hold" status where candidates accrue time on the wait list but are not ready for transplant surgery and therefore do not receive any organ offers. There are a variety of reasons that patients can be made status 7 including intercurrent illness or hospitalization, lack of availability due to travel, mandatory disease-free wait times after treatment for cancer, or waiting to achieve weight loss or medical compliance targets. Patients can be moved between status 1 and status 7 many times while on the wait list according to interim events and can also be removed from the list altogether if changes in circumstances are felt to irreversibly impair their transplant candidacy. It is essential for patients and referring physicians to understand how the waiting list works and how the various factors such as blood type, sensitization (PRA titer), and willingness to accept ECD kidneys may affect wait times, testing, and possibly clinical decision making.

Once patients are felt to be suitable candidates during the evaluation phase, they are placed on the waiting list, where their status is determined by the transplant center according to whether or not the prescribed criteria outlined by the transplant center are met (e.g., weight loss, improved compliance). Once listed, patients begin to accumulate wait list time, which under current guidelines remains the principal determinant of the patient's access to organ offers. Patients who are *status 7* accumulate wait time (and therefore "move up the list") at the same rate as patients who are *status 1*.

Management of the Patient on the Waiting List (*Wait List Maintenance Phase*)

Patients on the waitlist require active management. This process includes an ongoing open bi-directional dialogue between the referring nephrologist and the transplant center. Intermittent periodic reevaluation by the transplant center is also recommended as new medical issues often arise that may affect candidacy and/or require additional testing or treatment. The waitlisted patient will also need to ensure that they send blood to the HLA laboratory of the transplant center that can be used to perform a *crossmatch* with serum from the potential donor just prior to the scheduled transplant. This blood, the *current sample*, is sent by the patient or the dialysis unit on a monthly basis. The acquisition and delivery of the current samples is managed in different ways by different centers but in all cases requires a high degree of organization and ongoing communication between the transplant programs, the patients, and dialysis centers.

In addition, guidelines issued by a National Consensus Conference on management of waitlisted patients, held earlier this decade, recommended periodic surveillance of candidates by the transplant center for certain infections. This surveillance includes annual testing for HCV in previously uninfected patients and annual HIV screening in patients with high-risk behavior for this infection. Immunization with hepatitis B vaccine in unexposed patients (or boosters in cases of patients with declining titers) was also recommended.[12] Although repeat cardiovascular screening has been proposed for patients on the waiting list, there is no agreement on who should be tested or the type or frequency of testing.[12] Our own practice is to do annual non-invasive stress testing in high-risk patients (e.g., history of long-standing diabetes or known coronary artery disease). Lower risk patients are tested every 2–3 years depending on their perceived risk. Patients are asked to keep their age- and gender-appropriate screening up to date and to forward all testing and relevant medical records to the transplant center for review.

Strategies to Reduce Waiting Time for Listed Patients

Strategies have begun to be implemented that increase organ supply in an effort to decrease wait times for listed patients. Patients should be counseled about these options at the time of evaluation, and reiteration should occur at times of reevaluation as well. Community nephrologists should also be aware of these evolving strategies, as part of the decision-making process of their patients may be based on discussion with their providers. One example of this is the segregation of sub-optimal deceased donors into a separate *expanded criteria* pool. Donors considered expanded criteria are defined as those of at least 60 years of age or those over 50 years with two of the following: history of hypertension, elevated creatinine, or death from a cerebrovascular accident.[13] Although the outcomes in recipients of these kidneys are inferior to those observed with patients transplanted with kidneys from standard criteria donors (SCD), they may be associated with a shorter average wait time to a kidney transplant. ECD kidneys are therefore a reasonable option for waitlisted candidates with a high mortality risk on dialysis, such as patients who are older, sicker, diabetic, or running out of dialysis access.[6] An additional source of deceased donor kidneys derive from donors who were known to have social behaviors that placed them at an increased risk for viral infectious diseases such as HIV, hepatitis B, or hepatitis C. Such donors, termed *CDC high-risk donors*, test negative for these viruses at the time of procurement, but still carry a small risk of having acquired one of these viral infections just prior to death at a point preceding their discovery. The risk of transmission has been estimated to range (depending upon the type of virus (HIV vs. hepatitis C) and specific social situation) from 0.02 to 1.28%.[14]

Another emerging strategy is the transplantation of patients across traditional immunological barriers, e.g., ABO blood type or crossmatch-incompatible barriers. In each of these cases a regimen of preoperative intensive immunosuppression is utilized to diminish the humoral immune responses that normally render patients incompatible with their potential donors. Not all centers offer such programs at this time, but the commitment by the waitlisted patient is significantly greater than is required for conventional transplantation. Paired kidney exchange is another novel approach that can be facilitated when two or more incompatible recipient–donor pairings are found to share compatibility with one another's donors and the donor kidneys are exchanged between recipients. These exchanges can be brokered as simple exchanges or as part of a larger multi-pairing system. A very recent trend has seen several centers collaborating to pool their incompatible recipient–donor pairings in the hopes of increasing the likelihood of finding compatible pairs through the exchange mechanism.

Conclusions

Transplantation has evolved from a specialty niche, with kidneys offered to only the most pristine candidates, to one where it has been established as the treatment of choice for late stage 4 and stage 5 chronic kidney disease (CKD). Advancements on several fronts have resulted in improved patient and allograft survival over the past decades. Kidney transplantation has become a victim of its success and the demand for organs has been fuelled. The ability to meet or even improve on these transplant outcomes is likely to become a mounting challenge as the age limits and medical complexity of potential kidney recipients continue to be upwardly redefined. In this context, coupled with ongoing organ shortage, appropriate selection of patients for kidney transplantation is paramount. The importance of thorough evaluation by the transplant center accompanied by vigorous waitlist management, often in conjunction with the referring nephrologist, is critical to achieving these goals.

References

1. Wolfe RA, Ashby VB, Milford EL, Ojo AO, Ettenger RE, Agodoa LY, Held PJ, Port FK. Comparison of mortality in all patients on dialysis, patients on dialysis awaiting transplantation, and recipients of a first cadaveric transplant. *N Engl J Med* 1999 Dec 2;341(23):1725–1730.
2. Kasiske BL, Cangro CB, Hariharan S, Hricik DE, Kerman RH, Roth D, Rush DN, Vazquez MA, Weir MR. American Society of Transplantation. The evaluation of renal transplantation candidates: clinical practice guidelines. *Am J Transplant* 2001;1(Suppl 2):3–95.
3. Danovitch GM, Hariharan S, Pirsch JD, Rush D, Roth D, Ramos E, Starling RC, Cangro C, Weir MR. Clinical Practice Guidelines Committee of the American Society of Transplantation. Management of the Waiting List for Cadaveric Kidney Transplants: Report of a Survey and Recommendations by the Clinical Practice Guidelines Committee of the American Society of Transplantation. *J Am Soc Nephrol* 2002;13: 528–535.
4. Glanton CW, Kao TC, Cruess D, Agodoa LY, Abbott KC. Impact of renal transplantation on survival in end-stage renal disease patients with elevated body mass index. *Kidney Int* 2003 Feb;63(2):647–653.
5. Eason JD, Gonwa TA, Davis CL, Sung RS, Gerber D, Bloom RD. Proceedings of Consensus Conference on Simultaneous Liver Kidney Transplantation (SLK). *Am J Transplant* 2008 Nov;8(11):2243–2251. Epub 2008 Sep 19.
6. Ojo AO, Hanson JA, Meier-Kriesche H, Okechukwu CN, Wolfe RA, Leichtman AB, Agodoa LY, Kaplan B, Port FK. Survival in recipients of marginal cadaveric donor kidneys compared with other recipients and wait-listed transplant candidates. *J Am Soc Nephrol* 2001 Mar;12(3):589–597.
7. Hariharan S, Adams MB, Brennan DC, Davis CL, First MR, Johnson CP, Ouseph R, Peddi VR, Pelz CJ, Roza AM, Vincenti F, George V. Recurrent and de novo glomerular disease after renal transplantation: a report from Renal Allograft Disease Registry (RADR). *Transplantation* 1999 Sep 15;68(5):635–641.
8. Choy BY, Chan TM, Lai KN. Recurrent glomerulonephritis after kidney transplantation. *Am J Transplant* 2006 Nov;6(11):2535–2542.
9. Ojo AO, Held PJ, Port FK, Wolfe RA, Leichtman AB, Young EW, Arndorfer J, Christensen L, Merion RM. Chronic renal failure after transplantation of a nonrenal organ. *N Engl J Med* 2003 Sep 4;349(10):931–940.
10. de Geest S, Borgermans L, Gemoets H, Abraham I, Vlaminck H, Evers G, Vanrenterghem Y. Incidence, determinants, and consequences of subclinical noncompliance with immunosuppressive therapy in renal transplant recipients. *Transplantation* 1995 Feb 15;59(3): 340–347.
11. Jindel RM, Joseph JT, Morris MC, Santella RN, Baines LS. Noncompliance after kidney transplantation; a systematic review. *Transplant Proc* 2003 Dec;35(8):2868–2872.
12. Gaston RS, Danovitch GM, Adams PL, Wynn JJ, Merion RM, Deierhoi MH, Metzger RA, Cecka JM, Harmon WE, Leichtman AB, Spital A, Blumberg E, Herzog CA, Wolfe RA, Tyan DB, Roberts J, Rohrer R, Port FK, Delmonico FL. The report of a national conference on the wait list for kidney transplantation. *Am J Transplant* 2003 Jul;3(7):775–785.

13. Merion RM, Ashby VB, Wolfe RA, Distant DA, Hulbert-Shearon TE, Metzger RA, Ojo AO, Port FK. Deceased-donor characteristics and the survival benefit of kidney transplantation. *JAMA* 2005 Dec 7;294(21):2726–2733.
14. Schweitzer EJ, Perencevich EN, Philosophe B, Bartlett ST. Estimated benefits of transplantation of kidneys from donors at increased risk for HIV or hepatitis C infection. *Am J Transplant* 2007 Jun;7(6):1515–1525.

Chapter 14
The Acute Care of the Transplant Recipient

Phuong-Thu T. Pham, Phuong-Chi T. Pham, and Gabriel M. Danovitch

Introduction

Early post-transplant factors including delayed graft function (DGF), acute rejection episodes, nephrotoxic agents, post-transplant hypertension, dyslipidemia, and new onset diabetes mellitus after transplantation (NODAT) have all been implicated in worsening both short- and long-term morbidity and mortality after renal transplantation. Optimal management of the transplant recipient begins in the immediate postoperative period. This chapter provides a stepwise approach to the medical and urological management of the transplant recipient in the first 3 months after transplantation. The management of transplant recipients can be divided into three periods: immediate postoperative period, first week post-transplant, and first 3 months post-transplant. Immunosuppressive therapy is discussed in Chapter 9.

Immediate Postoperative Period

Patients should be evaluated immediately upon arrival to the recovery room, preferably by a combined medical surgical team. The initial assessment is similar to that following any major surgical procedure and attention should be paid to cardiovascular and respiratory stability. Most patients are successfully extubated and awake, and pain should be assessed and promptly controlled. Additional evaluation includes a full electrolyte panel including sodium, potassium, creatinine, glucose, calcium, phosphorous, magnesium, complete blood count with platelets, chest x-ray, and an electrocardiogram (EKG). Intraoperative anesthetic record, blood loss, volume replacement, and operative report should also be reviewed to identify intraoperative events or complications with potentially adverse sequelae.

P.-T.T. Pham (✉)
Division of Nephrology, Department of Medicine, Kidney and Pancreas Transplant Program, David Geffen School of Medicine at UCLA, Los Angeles, CA, USA
e-mail: ppham@mednet.ucla.edu

D.B. McKay, S.M. Steinberg (eds.), *Kidney Transplantation: A Guide to the Care of Kidney Transplant Recipients*, DOI 10.1007/978-1-4419-1690-7_14,
© Springer Science+Business Media, LLC 2010

In general, it is possible to anticipate early graft function based on pre- and postoperative characteristics of the donor and the recipient as well as the intraoperative perfusion characteristics of the kidney allograft. In patients with minimal residual urine output, an immediate postoperative increase in urine output may serve as an indicator of early graft function. A brisk large volume diuresis following graft revascularization may be due to preoperative volume overload, osmotic diuresis in previously uremic patients, intraoperative mannitol or furosemide, or excessive intraoperative intravenous crystalloid or colloid fluid administration. Total fluid intake and output should be monitored on an hourly basis. If dopamine is used intraoperatively, it can be promptly discontinued in polyuric patients. Suggested maintenance and urine replacement fluids are given in Table 14.1.

Table 14.1 Maintenance and replacement fluid

Maintenance fluid: D5 $\frac{1}{2}$ NS
Replacement fluid
• For urine output ≤ 200 cc/h, replace cc per cc with D5 $\frac{1}{2}$ NS[a]
• For urine output > 200 cc/h, give 200 cc + $\frac{1}{2}$ cc for each cc > 200
• For urine output > 300 cc for 4 consecutive hours, hold replacement fluid and reassess in 2 h
• For urine output > 500 cc/h for 2 consecutive hours, hold replacement fluid and reassess in 2 h
• For urine output < 50 cc/h, check for Foley catheter patency, reassess hemodynamic status. Volume challenge and/or high-dose diuretics as clinically indicated. Imaging studies if no response
• Other fluid and electrolyte replacement will be determined appropriately for each individual patient after clinical assessment of volume status

[a]Consider $\frac{1}{2}$ NS for diabetic transplant recipients

An abrupt cessation or significant reduction in urine output should prompt immediate investigation. Irrigation of the Foley catheter to check for patency should be performed. In a persistently anuric patient, Doppler ultrasound or radioisotope flow scan to ensure ongoing blood flow to the allograft and to exclude surgical complications should be done in the recovery room. The absence of blood flow to the allograft requires urgent evaluation by the surgical team for possible re-exploration. The length of time a patient remains in the recovery room is variable. A stable patient may typically be transferred to the general transplant care unit within 1–2 h. Intensive care unit observation is usually not required except under special circumstances involving postoperative EKG changes or high cardiac risk patients with known cardiomyopathy and/or a low preoperative ejection fraction (EF ≤ 40%) who are at risk for perioperative congestive heart failure. In these patients, intraoperative Swan–Ganz placement for continuous monitoring of cardiovascular and volume status is advisable. For those with known coronary artery disease or those with multiple risk factors, perioperative administration of a beta-blocker is recommended.

The First Postoperative Week

In general, stable patients should be encouraged to ambulate within 24–48 h. A liquid diet may be started when bowel function recovers, typically on the first postoperative day. Patients with slow return of bowel function or severe diabetic gastroparesis may require fasting for a longer time period at the discretion of the clinician. Intravenous fluid can generally be discontinued when the patient is able to tolerate solid food diet. Electrolyte abnormalities are not uncommon in the early postoperative period and laboratory evaluation should initially be performed every 6 h, then daily. Suggested postoperative orders on transfer to the transplant care unit are shown in Table 14.2.

Table 14.2 Postrenal transplant orders

Nursing Care
  Vital signs q 1 × 12 h, q 2 × 8 h, then q 4 h
  Fluid input and output q 1 h
  Daily weight
  Turn, cough, and deep breathe q 1 h, encourage incentive spirometry q 1 h while awake
  Out of bed first postoperative day, ambulate q.i.d. thereafter
  Elevate head of bed 30°
  Change dressing q.d. and p.r.n.
  Check dialysis access for function q 4 h and record
  No blood pressure checks or venipunctures in extremity with dialysis access
  Foley catheter to drainage, irrigate gently with 30 cc normal saline p.r.n. for clots or no urine
    flow
  Catheter care q 8 h
  N.P.O. until diet is changed by surgical team

Laboratory orders
  Complete blood count with platelets, electrolytes, creatinine, glucose q 6 × 3, then daily[a]
  Alkaline phosphatase, total bilirubin, calcium, phosphorus, SGOT, SGPT, LDH, urine
    culture and sensitivity twice a week
  Cyclosporine or tacrolimus level every morning
  Sirolimus level 3–5 days after dosage change at the discretion of the clinician

[a]For diabetic transplant recipients monitor fingerstick blood glucose before meals and at bedtime

Specific management of patients in the first postoperative week depends on the immediate functional status of the graft, which may be categorized as immediate graft function, slow recovery of graft function, and delayed graft function (DGF).

Patients with Immediate Graft Function

For patients who have immediate graft function, the first postoperative week is generally characterized by gradual improvement in the patient's general sense of well-being. Serum creatinine commonly decreases by 1.0 to >4.0 mg/dL daily. Patients with immediate graft function can usually be discharged on postoperative day 4 or 5 following successful Foley catheter removal and voiding trial. Patients with a small bladder capacity (<100 ml) may go home with an indwelling Foley catheter and the latter can be removed after 7–14 days.

Patients with Slow Recovery of Graft Function

Patients who have slow recovery of graft function are generally non-oliguric and experience a slow decline in serum creatinine. The level typically decreases by 0.2–1.0 mg/dL daily. These patients usually do not require dialysis support unless complicated by hyperkalemia, fluid overload, or severe anemia requiring blood product administration. Great care must be given to fluid management. Volume depletion must be avoided to prevent precipitation of acute tubular necrosis. An initial reduction in urine output may be challenged with intravenous fluid infusion and/or furosemide after careful assessment of the patient's volume status. If there is no response to these therapeutic trials, Doppler ultrasound or nuclear imaging studies should be obtained to assess renal blood flow and to rule out obstruction or urine leak. The serum creatinine of patients with slow graft function generally does not normalize within the first postoperative week. Nevertheless, most patients can be discharged on postoperative day 5–10 with close outpatient follow-up. In patients who are at high risk for obstruction such as diabetics with neurogenic bladder or male patients with benign prostatic hypertrophy and a high postvoid residual >125–150 ml, it is advisable to leave the Foley catheter in place or to instruct the patient to perform self-catheterization prior to discharge. In addition, these patients may benefit from pharmacological therapy. Two classes of drugs are typically used including α-1-blocker and 5-α-reductase inhibitor. The former acts against the dynamic component of bladder outlet obstruction (prostate relaxant). Commonly used α-1-blockers include tamsulosin, terazosin, and doxazosin. The second class of drug acts by reducing the size of the prostate and includes finasteride, dutasteride, and alfuzosin. In patients at risk for developing a urine leak or rupture at the ureterovesical junction in the presence of a high urine volume such as those with a small contracted bladder (bladder capacity <100 ml), it is also wise to leave the Foley catheter in place for a more prolonged period (7–14 days).

Patients with Delayed Graft Function

The incidence of delayed graft function (DGF) may range from 10 to 60% and can often be anticipated based on both recipient and donor factors[1–5] (Table 14.3). Unless these patients have adequate residual urine output from the native kidneys, most will require temporary dialysis support for volume, hyperkalemia, or uremia. Although peritoneal dialysis may be performed in patients with a functioning

Table 14.3 Donor and recipients factors for DGF due to acute tubular necrosis

Donor factors	Recipient factors
Premorbid factors	*Premorbid factors*
Age (<10 or >50)	Age
Donor hypertension	African Americans (compared to Caucasians)
Donor macrovascular or microvascular disease	Peripheral vascular disease
Cause of death (cerebrovascular vs. traumatic)	Hemodialysis (compared with peritoneal dialysis)
	Duration of dialysis before transplant
	Presensitization (PRA > 50)
	Reallograft transplant
	Body mass index > 30 kg/m^2
	Hypercoagulability state[a]
Preoperative donor characteristics	*Perioperative and postoperative factors*
Brain-death stress	
Hypotension, shock	
Prolonged used of vasopressors	Recipient volume contraction
Preprocurement ATN	Early high-dose calcineurin
Donation after cardiac death (DCD)	Inhibitors
Nephrotoxic agents	Sirolimus[b]
	± Early OKT3 use
Organ procurement surgery	
Hypotension prior to cross-clamping of aorta	
Traction on renal vasculatures antiphospholipid	
Cold storage flushing solutions	
Kidney preservation	
Prolonged warm ischemia time	
(± Contraindication to transplantation)	
Prolonged cold ischemia time	
Cold storage vs. machine perfusion	
Intraoperative factors	
Intraoperative hemodynamic instability	
Prolonged rewarm time (anastomotic time)	

[a]Such as presence of factor V Leiden mutation or antibodies.
[b]May prolong the duration of DGF.

peritoneal catheter in place, hemodialysis may be more effective in the early postoperative period when severe hyperkalemia is present or prolonged absence of bowel function is a problem. The differential diagnoses of DGF are shown in Table 14.4. A systematic approach to the evaluation of DGF may be divided into prerenal (or preglomerular type), intrinsic, and postrenal. Although uncommon, vascular causes of DGF must be excluded, particularly in the early postoperative period.

Table 14.4 Differential diagnosis of DGF

Prerenal (or preglomerular type)
  Volume contraction
  Nephrotoxic drugs (see text)

  Vascular complications
    Arterial or venous thrombosis
    Renal artery stenosis

Intrinsic renal
  Acute tubular necrosis
  Accelerated acute or acute rejection
  Thrombotic microangiopathy
  Recurrence of primary glomerular disease (particularly FSGS)

Post-renal
  Catheter obstruction
  Perinephric fluid collection (lymphocele, urine leak, hematoma)
  Ureteral obstruction:
    Intrinsic (blood clots, poor re-implantation, ureteral slough, ureteral fibrosis, polyoma BK
      virus)
    Extrinsic (ureteral kinking, periureteral fibrosis)
    Neurogenic bladder
  Benign prostatic hypertrophy
  Stones
  Malignancy

Prerenal Causes of DGF

Intravascular Volume Depletion and Nephrotoxic Drugs

Severe intravascular volume depletion or significant fall in blood pressure is usually suggested by a careful review of patients' preoperative history and intraoperative report. Knowing patients' dialysis dry weight and preoperative weight may be invaluable in the assessment of their volume status in the immediate postoperative period. Intraoperative Swan–Ganz placement for continuous monitoring of central venous or pulmonary wedge pressure may be useful in assessing the volume status of patients with cardiomyopathy and/or coronary artery disease.

Both calcineurin inhibitors (CNI) cyclosporine and, to a lesser extent, tacrolimus have been shown to cause a dose-related reversible afferent arteriolar vasoconstriction and "preglomerular type" allograft dysfunction that manifests clinically as delayed recovery of allograft function. Intraoperative direct injection of the calcium channel blocker verapamil into the renal artery has been suggested to reduce capillary spasm and improve renal blood flow.[6,7] A thorough chart review should focus on the recent use of nephrotoxic medications and perioperative blood pressure curves. Angiotensin-converting enzyme inhibitors or angiotensin receptor blockers, amphotericin B, nonsteroidal anti-inflammatory drugs (NSAIDS), and radiocontrast dye are commonly used drugs that may potentially precipitate or exacerbate acute preglomerular type allograft dysfunction.

Vascular Complications

Graft Thrombosis

Arterial or venous thrombosis generally occurs within the first 2–3 postoperative days but may occur as long as 2 months post-transplant. In most series reported, the incidence of graft thrombosis ranges from 0.5% to as high as 8% with arterial accounting for one-third and venous thrombosis for two-thirds of cases.[8,9] Thrombosis occurring early after transplantation is most often due to technical surgical complications, whereas later onset is generally due to acute rejection.[8] In patients with initial good allograft function, thrombosis is generally heralded by the acute onset of oliguria or anuria associated with deterioration of allograft function. Abnormal laboratory findings may include thrombocytopenia, hyperkalemia, and a rising lactate dehydrogenase level. Clinically, the patient may present with graft swelling or tenderness, and/or gross hematuria. In patients with DGF and good residual urine output from the native kidneys, overt signs or symptoms may be absent and the diagnosis must be based on clinical suspicion and prompt imaging studies. The diagnosis can be made with a Doppler ultrasound or isotope flow scan. Confirmed arterial or venous thrombosis typically necessitates allograft nephrectomy. In recipients of kidneys with multiple arteries, thrombosis may occur in a single branch, and depending on the extent of renal parenchymal supplied, adequate functioning tissue may remain.

Suggested predisposing factors for vascular thrombosis include arteriosclerotic involvement of the donor or recipient vessels, intimal injury of graft vessels, kidneys with multiple arteries, history of recurrent thrombosis, thrombocytosis, younger recipient and/or donor age, and the presence of antiphospholipid antibody (anticardiolipin antibody and/or lupus anticoagulant).[10] There has been no consensus on the optimal management of recipients with abnormal hypercoagulability profile including abnormal activated protein C resistance ratio or factor V Leiden mutation, antiphospholipid antibody positivity, protein C, or protein S deficiency and antithrombin III deficiency. However, unless contraindicated, perioperative and/or postoperative prophylactic anticoagulation should be considered, particularly in patients with a prior history of recurrent thrombotic events. Transplant of pediatric en bloc kidneys into adult recipient with a history of thrombosis should probably be avoided. The duration of anticoagulation has not been well defined, but lifelong anticoagulation should be considered in high-risk candidates.[10]

Renal Artery Stenosis

Transplant renal artery stenosis may occur as early as the first week, but it is usually a late complication occurring 3 months to 2 years post-transplant with a reported prevalence of 1–23%.[10,11] Clinically, patients may present with new onset or accelerated hypertension, acute deterioration of graft function, severe hypotension associated with the use of angiotensin-converting enzyme inhibitors (ACEI), recurrent pulmonary edema or refractory edema in the absence of heavy proteinuria, and/or erythrocytosis. The latter, when associated with hypertension and impaired graft function should raise the suspicion of renal artery stenosis (i.e., triad: erythrocytosis, hypertension, elevated serum creatinine). The presence of a bruit over the allograft is neither sensitive nor specific for the diagnosis of graft renovascular disease. However, a change in the intensity of the bruit or the detection of new bruits warrants an evaluation. Although noninvasive, radionuclide scan with and without captopril is neither sufficiently sensitive nor specific for detecting transplant renal artery stenosis (sensitivity and specificity: 75 and 67%, respectively). Color Doppler ultrasound is highly sensitive and serves well as an initial noninvasive assessment of the transplant vessels. It should be noted, however, that color Doppler ultrasound is limited by its relatively low specificity. CO_2 angiography avoids nephrotoxic contrast agents but its use is not without limitations. Overestimation of the degree of stenosis, bowel gas artifact, and/or patients' intolerance has been reported with the use of CO_2 angiogram[12] Although gadolinium-enhanced MR angiography has been suggested to be an alternative non-nephrotoxic method in identifying transplant renal artery stenosis, its use should be avoided in those with allograft dysfunction due to the association between gadolinium and the development of nephrogenic fibrosing dermopathy (NFD) and systemic fibrosis (NSF).[13] Although invasive, renal angiography remains the gold standard for establishing the diagnosis of RAS.

Intrinsic Renal Causes of DGF

Intrinsic renal causes of DGF typically include acute tubular necrosis, acute rejection, thrombotic microangiopathy (TMA), or recurrence of the glomerular disease affecting the native kidneys.

Acute Tubular Necrosis

Post-transplant acute tubular necrosis is the most common cause of DGF. The two terms are often used interchangeably, although not all cases of DGF are caused by ATN. The incidence of ATN varies widely among centers and has been reported to occur in 20–25% of patients (range 2–60%).[1–5,14,15] The difference in the incidence reported may, in part, be due to the more liberal use of organs from marginal donors by some centers but not by others, the difference in the criteria used to define DGF, or both. Unless an allograft biopsy is performed, post-transplant ATN should be a diagnosis of exclusion. In the absence of superimposed acute rejection, ATN typically resolves over several days but may occasionally require several weeks (4–6 weeks), particularly in recipients of older donor kidneys. Recovery of ATN is usually heralded by a steady increase in urine output associated with a decrease in interdialytic increase in serum creatinine and eventual dialysis independence. Prolonged DGF should prompt a diagnostic allograft biopsy. Some centers perform serial biopsies in patients with prolonged DGF to exclude covert acute rejection or other intrinsic causes of allograft dysfunction. Both donor and recipient factors are important determinant(s) of early allograft function. ATN is exceptional in living-donor renal transplants while it may occur in 20–50% of deceased donor renal transplants. Potential risk factors for DGF secondary to ATN are shown in Table 14.3.

Management of Delayed Graft Function

The differential diagnosis of DGF (see Table 14.4) must be considered before a patient is labeled with post-transplant ATN. Most patients with DGF are oliguric or anuric. Knowledge of the patient's native urine output is critical to assess the origin of the early post-transplant urine output. From the previous discussion of the etiology of DGF, it is clear that information about the donor kidney itself is critical. When the transplant is from a living donor, postoperative oliguria is rare because of the short ischemia time. Nonetheless, if postoperative oliguria does occur, complications with allograft vascularization must be immediately considered. In contrast, when a patient receives a deceased donor kidney from a non-ideal donor, DGF may be anticipated. The mate kidney from a deceased donor often behaves in a similar manner, and information on its function can be useful.[16]

Anuria refers to negligible urine production. Oliguria in the peri-transplant period typically refers to a urine output of less than 500 ml/day. Before the patient is submitted to a full evaluation for poor urine output, his or her volume status and fluid balance as well as patency of the Foley catheter must be assessed. If clots are present, the catheter should be removed while gentle suction is applied in an attempt to capture the offending clot. Thereafter, replacement with a larger catheter may be required. If the Foley catheter is patent and the patient is clearly hypervolemic, up to 200 mg of furosemide may be given intravenously. If the patient is judged to be hypovolemic or if a confident clinical assessment cannot be made, a judicious trial of isotonic saline infusion may be given, with or without subsequent administration of furosemide as dictated by the patient's response to saline infusion alone. A suggested algorithmic approach to postoperative fluid management in an oliguric patient is shown in Fig. 14.1.

Indications for dialysis in the transplant recipient with DGF are essentially the same as in any non-transplant patient with renal dysfunction and typically include hyperkalemia, volume overload, uremic symptoms, and severe metabolic acidosis in patients with insufficient urine output to tolerate the intravenous administration of large volume of sodium bicarbonate.

Patients with DGF often become volume overloaded in the early post-transplant period because they are frequently subjected to repeated volume challenges. It is not infrequent for such patients to gain several kilograms of fluid over their dialysis dry weight. Ultrafiltration with or without dialysis may be required depending on concomitant electrolyte abnormalities. When dialyzing post-transplantation patients

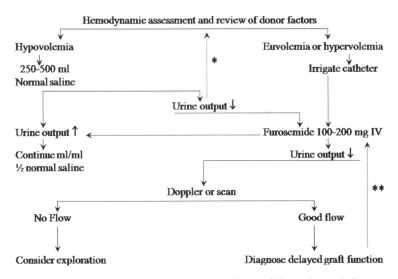

Fig. 14.1 Algorithmic approach to post-transplant oliguria. *The volume challenge can be repeated, but only after careful reassessment of the volume status and fluid balance. **Repeated doses of intravenous furosemide or furosemide "drips" may be valuable in patients whose urine output fluctuates. Persistent oliguria will usually not respond to a repeat dose. (Modified from Amend et al.[64])

with DGF, care must be taken to avoid the precipitation of hypotensive episodes to prevent added injury to the allograft. Where indicated, priming the patient with normal saline at dialysis initiation or infusion of blood products may be considered. A bicarbonate dialysate and biocompatible dialyzer should be used. In patients with established DGF, the dialysis requirement should be assessed daily until graft function improves sufficiently.

Diagnostic Studies in Persistent Oliguria or Anuria

Failure to respond to volume challenge and furosemide administration warrants further evaluation with diagnostic imaging studies to determine the cause of the early post-transplant oliguric state. The urgency of this evaluation partially depends on specific clinical circumstances. If diuresis is expected following uncomplicated living-donor kidney transplantation and oliguria occurs, diagnostic studies should be performed immediately—in the recovery room if necessary. In contrast, if oliguria is anticipated following ECD kidney transplantation, studies can usually be safely delayed by several hours.

Diagnostic studies are used to confirm the presence of blood flow to the graft and the absence of a urine leak or obstruction. Blood flow studies are performed scintigraphically or by Doppler ultrasound.[17] The typical scintigraphic finding in ATN is relatively good flow to the graft in association with poor excretion. If the flow study reveals no demonstrable blood flow, a prompt surgical re-exploration is necessary to repair any vascular technical problem and diagnose hyperacute rejection. These kidneys are usually not salvageable, however, and are typically removed during the second surgery. If adequate blood flow is visible in the scintiscan or Doppler studies, the possibility of ureteral obstruction or urinary leak should be evaluated by the same imaging studies. In the first 24 h after transplantation, when the Foley catheter has already provided good bladder drainage, any obstruction or leak present is almost always at the ureterovesical junction and represents a technical problem that needs surgical correction.[8]

Acute Rejection

While hyperacute or accelerated acute rejection due to presensitization may occur immediately or several days after transplantation, classic cell-mediated acute rejection or antibody-mediated acute rejection is typically seen after the first post-transplant week (discussed in further details under the first 3 post-transplant months). Studies suggest that there is an interactive effect between ATN and acute rejection. Ischemia-reperfusion injury has been shown to cause upregulation of multiple cytokines and growth factors within the allograft including IL-1, IL-2, IL-6, TNF, IFN-α, and transforming growth factor β among others. The proinflammatory cytokine response may, in turn, trigger acute allograft rejection through upregulation of various costimulatory and adhesion molecules as well as through increased expression of major histocompatibility complex class I and class II antigens. It is, therefore, prudent to perform a diagnostic allograft biopsy in the presence of prolonged ATN.

Thrombotic Microangiopathy

Although uncommon, the use of cyclosporine and tacrolimus and the proliferation signal inhibitors (sirolimus and everolimus) has been shown to be associated with thrombotic microangiopathy. The concomitant presence of strong peritubular capillary staining for C4d on biopsy should raise the suspicion of acute antibody-mediated rejection.

TMA may develop as early as 4 days postoperative to as late as 6 years posttransplantation. It may be evident clinically by virtue of the typical laboratory findings of intravascular coagulation (e.g., thrombocytopenia, distorted erythrocytes, elevated lactate dehydrogenase levels) accompanied by an arteriolopathy and intravascular thrombi on transplant biopsy. Unlike the primary form of thrombotic thrombocytopenic purpura or hemolytic-uremic syndrome, however, cyclosporine-to tacrolimus-associated TMA may be covert, and the laboratory findings may be inconsistent. In recipients of renal allograft, renal dysfunction is the most common manifestation. Thrombocytopenia and microangiopathic hemolysis are often mild or absent and the diagnosis is often made from graft biopsies performed to determine the cause of DGF.[18] Although there have been no controlled trials comparing the different treatment modalities of this condition, dose reduction or discontinuation of the most likely offending agent appears to be pivotal. Adjunctive plasmapheresis with fresh frozen plasma replacement may offer survival advantages. In transplant recipients with cyclosporine-associated TMA, successful use of tacrolimus immunosuppression has been reported. However, recurrence of TMA in renal transplant recipients treated sequentially with cyclosporine and tacrolimus has been described.[18] In patients with calcineurin inhibitor-associated TMA, successful conversion to sirolimus-based immunosuppression in a CNI-free regimen has been reported. With the increasing use of sirolimus in solid organ transplantation, sirolimus-induced TMA has also been recognized.[19] Indeed, clinicians must remain vigilant for signs and symptoms of TMA recurrence in patients who are switched from cyclosporine to tacrolimus or vice versa or in those who are switched from a CNI to sirolimus or vice versa. The use of the monoclonal muromonab-CD3 OKT3 has also been associated with the development of post-transplant TMA, although infrequently.

Other potential causative factors of post-transplant-associated TMA include the presence of lupus anticoagulant and/or anticardiolipin antibody, cytomegalovirus infection, and less frequently, systemic viral infection with parvovirus B19 or influenza A virus.[18] An increased incidence of TMA has been described in a subset of renal allograft recipients with concurrent hepatitis C virus infection and anticardiolipin antibody positivity.[20]

Recurrence of Glomerular Disease of the Native Kidneys

Recurrence of glomerular disease is the third most common cause of graft loss after chronic allograft nephropathy and death with a functioning graft. Currently available data on the incidence of recurrent disease and resultant graft loss are heterogenous due to different study design, follow-up durations, and patient samples. The reported incidence of recurrent renal disease after renal transplantation and the risk of graft loss from disease recurrence are shown in Table 14.5. The clinical course and impact on graft survival vary between different types of glomerulonephritis. Nonetheless, with the exception of FSGS, recurrent glomerular disease is usually a late complication after transplantation. The following section discusses the clinical course of recurrent FSGS, its potential pathogenic mechanism(s), and suggested management of disease recurrence. For a detailed discussion of recurrence of other glomerular disease of the native kidneys readers are referred to the review by Choy et al.[21]

Recurrent Focal Segmental Glomerulosclerosis (FSGS)

Recurrent FSGS typically occurs within the first post-transplant month and is usually heralded by heavy proteinuria and graft dysfunction. A circulating permeability factor has been suggested to play an important role in disease

Table 14.5 Incidence of disease recurrence and risk of graft loss

	Recurrence rates (%)[a]	Graft loss from disease recurrence (%)[b]
FSGS	30–50	50
IgA nephropathy	30–60	10–30
MPGN I	15–50	30–35
MPGN II	80–100	10–20
Membranous GN	3–30	30
HUS	10–40	10–40
Anti-GBM disease	10	<5
SLE	3–10	<5

FSGS, focal segmental glomerulosclerosis; MPGN, membranoproliferative glomerulonephritis; GN, glomerulonephropathy; HUS, hemolytic uremic syndrome; SLE, systemic lupus erythematosus.
[a]Only selected renal diseases are listed. For a more extensive list of estimated rates of recurrence of primary and secondary glomerulopathies, readers are referred to Sharma et al.[22]
[b]Rates reported vary widely among studies.

recurrence. A single injection of human FSGS factor has been shown to increase glomerular albumin permeability and transient albuminuria and proteinuria in rats.[22] The permeability factor is bound to immunoglobulin and is removed by plasma exchange or immunoadsorption. No predictive characteristics have been observed that would identify patients who will respond to therapy. Nonetheless, plasmapheresis should be initiated early because the effectiveness of treatment decreases with more glomerular damage.[21] Disease remission has been reported to occur in the majority of patients who receive treatment within 2 weeks of recurrence. Some centers advocate the concomitant use of cyclophosphamide while others only add cyclophosphamide therapy in those with an incomplete response or disease relapse following cessation of plasmapheresis. Rituximab has been used in adult and pediatric patients with recurrent FSGS refractory to conventional therapy with variable success. Discussion is beyond the scope of this chapter. Anecdotal reports suggest that sirolimus can cause de novo or recurrent FSGS and its use should be avoided in these patients.[21] Adjunctive therapy includes ACEI or ARB and mycophenolate mofetil or azathioprine. Suggested risk factors for disease recurrence include less than 15 years of age, heavy proteinuria, and aggressive clinical course of the original disease with the interval from diagnosis to end-stage renal failure of less than 3 years, diffuse mesangial proliferation on native kidney biopsies, and history of previous graft loss due to recurrence. The beneficial effect of pre-emptive pre-transplantation plasmapheresis in preventing disease recurrence in high-risk transplant recipients has not been consistently demonstrated.

Postrenal Causes of DGF

Postrenal DGF is generally due to obstruction and may occur anywhere from the intrarenal collecting system to the level of the bladder–catheter drainage system.

The latter is generally due to blood clots and can often be managed by flushing the catheter. Nursing care orders should routinely include irrigation of the Foley catheter as needed for clots or no urine flow. In patients with persistent gross hematuria, continuous bladder irrigation may be helpful. However, potential serious complications such as bleeding from vascular anastomoses or graft thrombosis should first be excluded. Table 14.4 summarizes the possible causative factors of postrenal causes of DGF. Obstruction secondary to urological complications is discussed under urological complications.

The First Three Post-transplant Months

The first post-transplant month involves the transition from inpatient to outpatient care. The frequency of clinic visits may vary between centers. However, patients should be seen two to three times a week for the first 2 weeks, twice a week for the next 2 weeks, and weekly for the next month. After the first 2 months, the frequency of outpatient visits largely depends on the complexity of the patient's early postoperative course. Most patients with stable graft function and an uneventful postoperative course can return to work and/or their regular daily activities 2–3 months post-transplant. Laboratory assessment during the first 1–2 months should include a complete blood count with platelets, urinalysis, serum creatinine, immunosuppressive drug concentration, electrolyte, and metabolic panel including potassium, calcium, phosphorous, and glucose. Liver enzymes and cholesterol should also be monitored regularly. Management of post-transplant infectious complications, cardiovascular disease, and new onset diabetes mellitus after transplantation is discussed elsewhere.

Acute Allograft Dysfunction

An increase of 10–20% in serum creatinine from baseline commonly represents laboratory variability and can be rechecked within 48–72 h at the clinician's discretion. However, a 25% or greater increase in serum creatinine should prompt further evaluation. Prerenal azotemia is usually evident through obtaining a medical history and/or physical exam. The presence of fever, graft tenderness, and/or pyuria suggests pyelonephritis. In the era of potent immunosuppression, fever and graft tenderness are usually absent during acute allograft rejection periods. Accurate diagnosis necessitates an allograft biopsy. All medications must be reviewed to exclude any drug-induced nephrotoxicity. Deteriorating allograft function associated with markedly elevated cyclosporine or tacrolimus concentrations may be managed expectantly by dose reduction. Acute CNI toxicity typically improves within 24–48 h after dosage adjustment. Hence, a persistently elevated serum creatinine warrants further evaluation.

In contrast, acute allograft dysfunction in the face of persistently low cyclosporine or tacrolimus concentrations, high pre-transplant panel reactive antibody (PRA), and/or retransplantation raises the possibility of acute rejection and requires aggressive diagnostic and/or therapeutic intervention. Initial evaluation with Doppler ultrasound to exclude vascular complications and to rule out hydronephrosis, or perinephric fluid collection (due to lymphocele, hematoma, or urine leak) is appropriate. If copious drainage remains through the incision, the fluid should be sent for measurement of creatinine. Elevated fluid creatinine concentration to more than one and a half times over that of plasma suggests urine leak and appropriate steps should be taken. Diagnostic imaging studies and management of urological complications are discussed under urological complications. A diagnostic allograft biopsy can be performed after vascular and urological causes of graft dysfunction have been excluded. In patients with high risks for complications (those who are anticoagulated, or those in whom an allograft biopsy may be difficult due to overlying bowels or obesity), it may be appropriate to proceed with pulse corticosteroid therapy without biopsy confirmation particularly when there is a high clinical suspicion of acute rejection.

Acute Allograft Rejection

Acute rejections occur, most typically, between the first weeks and months after transplantation. In unsensitized patients with low levels of preformed antibodies, acute rejection rarely occurs in the first week, while very early rejection or accelerated acute rejection may occur in sensitized patients. In recent years, various desensitization protocols have allowed successful transplantation in highly sensitized renal transplant candidates (discussion is beyond the scope of this chapter). On the basis of the underlying immunopathogenic mechanisms, acute rejection can be divided into cell mediated and antibody mediated. Approximately 90% of all acute rejection episodes are predominantly cell mediated, whereas 12–37% of all acute rejection episodes have a humoral component.[23,24] The histopathologic findings of acute cellular rejection and acute antibody-mediated rejection may occur in a renal biopsy simultaneously and are discussed in more detail in Chapter 12. In a National Conference to assess antibody-mediated rejection (AMR) in solid organ transplantation, it has been suggested by experts in the field that the diagnosis of acute AMR should require graft dysfunction to distinguish clinical from subclinical rejection, a criterion not specified in the 2001 Banff criteria for AMR.[25] AMR may occur with or without the features of ACR. The histopathological diagnostic criteria of AMR include detection of the complement component C4d in peritubular capillaries and evidence of acute tissue injury (Table 14.6). A definitive diagnosis requires demonstration of serologic evidence of antidonor (either anti-HLA or anti-ABO) antibody.

Table 14.6 Diagnostic criteria for acute antibody-mediated rejection (adapted fromTakemoto[65])

Clinical evidence of graft dysfunction	
Histologic evidence of tissue injury	*ATN/macrophages/thrombi in capillaries +/or fibrinoid necrosis +/or acute tubular injury*
Immunopathologic evidence for antibody action	*C4d in PTC or Ig/C3 in arteries*
Serologic evidence of anti-HLA or other antidonor antibody at the time of biopsy	

Treatment of Acute Cellular Rejection

Pulse Corticosteroid

Pulse corticosteroid is appropriate for the initial treatment of biopsy-proven first episode of acute cellular rejection with mild-to-moderate allograft dysfunction and without evidence of vascular involvement. There is no standardized "pulse steroid" protocol and it has been suggested that an oral pulse with prednisone or prednisolone at a dose of 125–250 mg a day may not necessarily be less effective than higher-dose intravenous methylprednisolone pulse. Nonetheless, most centers favor an intravenous methylprednisolone pulse which can be given at a dose of 5 mg/kg of body weight or at a fixed dose of 250–500 mg daily for 3–5 days. After completion of steroid therapy, prednisone can be gradually tapered over a 1–2 week period to its previous level (steroid recycle) or be immediately resumed at its previous dose. Steroid resistant, defined as failure of the serum creatinine to decrease or a continuing increase in serum creatinine after 3–5 days of therapy, usually necessitates antibody salvage treatment. Renal biopsy (or repeat biopsy) may be helpful but should be individualized and biopsy is mandatory for those without a previous biopsy particularly if antibody treatment is given.

Antilymphocyte Antibody Therapy

The monoclonal antibody OKT3 and the polyclonal antibodies ATGAM and thymoglobulin are highly effective antirejection therapy. Their use as induction therapy is discussed elsewhere. Although the choice and duration of antilymphocyte antibody treatment may differ among centers, the common indications for antibody treatment include steroid-resistant first rejection, biopsy-confirmed cellular and/or vascular rejection (Banff grade II or III), second episodes of rejection, severe allograft dysfunction at presentation, or rapid deterioration of allograft function despite steroid therapy. During antibody treatment, cyclosporine or tacrolimus should be withheld or dose reduced to avoid over-immunosuppression while oral prednisone is replaced by intravenous methylprednisolone. Mycophenolate formulations are withheld during treatment with thymoglobulin. Studies comparing monoclonal to polyclonal antilymphocyte antibody preparations have generally been inconclusive, although rabbit antithymocyte globulin (Thymoglobulin) has been suggested to be superior to the equine preparation (ATGAM) in reversing acute rejection and preventing recurrent rejection episodes.[26] Thymoglobulin is given at a dose of 1.5 mg/kg of body weight infused over 4–8 h through a central venous catheter or into the venous limb of an arteriovenous fistula. Administration of thymoglobulin through a peripheral vein may cause vein thrombosis or thrombophlebitis and should be avoided. ATGAM is given at 10–15 mg/kg body weight infused over 4 h, and similar to thymoglobulin, should be given through a central catheter or an arterovenous fistula. Premedication with intravenous methylprednisolone, diphenhydramine hydrochloride, and acetaminophen should be given prior to commencement of antilymphocyte antibody therapy. ATGAM has now largely been replaced by thymoglobulin whereas the use of OKT3 has drastically declined over the last half decade. Similar to OKT3, the polyclonal antibodies are xenogeneic proteins and can induce a number of side effects including fevers, chills, and arthralgia. ATG, however, does not cause the severe first-dose cytokine-mediated reactions seen with OKT3.

Acute Antibody-Mediated Rejection

Acute antibody-mediated rejection frequently presents with severe allograft dysfunction refractory to conventional antirejection therapy including antilymphocyte antibody and is associated with a high risk of graft loss. The mainstay of treatment includes removal of donor-specific antidonor antibodies (DSA) and inhibition of further antibody synthesis. Multiple therapeutic approaches have been used with variable success including high-dose intravenous immunoglobulin (IVIg), immunoadsorption, plasmapheresis with or without low-dose CytoGam®, or a combination of therapeutic modalities.[27,28] Rituximab, an anti-CD20 antibody targeting B cells, has also been shown to reduce antidonor antibody production. Nonetheless, it should be noted that the majority of plasma cells lack CD20 and are unaffected by rituximab. The cancer drug, bortezomib (Velcade®) has recently shown promise in AMR although the studies are still early. The addition of agents targeting against cell-mediated rejection such as antilymphocyte antibody has been reported to be beneficial in a subset of patients.[29] These therapies have been suggested to downregulate B-cell response through a decrease in the activity of helper T cells. Cyclosporine to tacrolimus conversion therapy and mycophenolate mofetil adjunctive therapy have also been reported to be beneficial.

Urological Complications

Ureteral Obstruction

Ureteral obstruction occurs in 2–10% of renal transplants[30] and often manifests itself as painless impairment of graft function due to the lack of innervation of the engrafted kidney. Hydronephrosis may be minimal or absent in early obstruction, whereas low-grade dilatation of the collecting system secondary to edema at the ureterovesical anastomosis may be seen early post-transplantation and does not necessarily indicate obstruction. A full bladder may also cause mild calyceal dilatation due to ureteral reflux and repeat ultrasound with an empty bladder should be carried out. Persistent or increasing hydronephrosis on repeat ultrasound examinations is highly suggestive of obstruction. Renal scan with furosemide washout may help support the diagnosis, but it does not provide anatomic details. Confirmation of the obstruction can be made by retrograde pyelogram but the ureteral orifice may be difficult to catheterize. Although invasive, percutaneous nephrostomy tube placement with antegrade nephrostogram is the most effective way to visualize the collecting system and can be of both diagnostic and therapeutic value.

Blood clots, technically poor reimplant, and ureteral sloughing are common causes of early acute obstruction after transplantation.[8,31] Ureteral fibrosis secondary to either ischemia or rejection can cause intrinsic obstruction. The distal ureter close to the ureterovesical junction is particularly vulnerable to ischemic damage due to its remote location from the renal artery, hence compromised blood supply. Although uncommon, ureteral fibrosis associated with polyoma BK virus in the setting of renal transplantation has been well-described.[32] Ureteral kinking, lymphocele, pelvic hematoma or abscess, and malignancy are potential causes of extrinsic obstruction. Calculi are uncommon causes of ureteral obstruction.[8]

Definitive treatment of ureteral obstruction due to ureteral strictures consists of either endourologic techniques or open surgery. Intrinsic ureteral scars can be treated effectively by endourologic techniques in an antegrade or retrograde approach. An indwelling stent may be placed to bypass the ureteral obstruction and removed cystoscopically after 2–6 weeks.[33] An antegrade nephrostogram should be performed to confirm that the urinary tract is unobstructed prior to nephrostomy tube removal. Routine ureteral stent placement at the time of transplantation has been suggested to be associated with a lower incidence of early postoperative obstruction.[33] Extrinsic strictures, strictures that are longer than 2 cm, or those that have failed endourologic incision, are less likely to be amenable to percutaneous techniques and are more likely to require surgical intervention.[33] Obstructing calculi can be managed by endourologic techniques or by extracorporeal shock wave lithotripsy.

Perinephric Fluid Collections

Symptomatic perinephric fluid collections in the early postoperative period can be due to lymphoceles, hematoma, urinoma, or abscesses. Lymphoceles are collections of lymph caused by leakage from severed lymphatics. They typically develop within weeks after transplantation. Most lymphoceles are small and asymptomatic. Generally, the larger the lymphocele, the more likely it is to produce symptoms and require treatment. However, small but strategically positioned lymphoceles may cause unilateral obstruction and necessitate therapeutic intervention. Lymphoceles can also cause compression of the iliac vein leading to ipsilateral leg swelling or deep vein thrombosis, or even urinary incontinence due to bladder compression.[8]

Lymphoceles are usually detected by ultrasound. They appear as a roundish, sonolucent, septated mass[17] that may be distinguished from other types of perinephric fluid collections such as hematoma or urine leak. Hydronephrosis may be present with or without a visible compressed adjacent ureter. Needle aspiration yields a clear fluid with a creatinine concentration similar to that of the serum.

No therapy is necessary for the common, small, asymptomatic lymphocele. Percutaneous aspiration should be performed if a ureteral leak, obstruction, or infection is suspected. The most common indication for treatment is ureteral obstruction. If the cause of the obstruction is simple compression resulting from a mass effect of the lymphocele, percutaneous drainage alone usually resolves the problem. Repeated percutaneous aspirations in resistant cases are not advised because they seldom lead to eventual dissolution of the lymphocele and often result in infection. Lymphoceles can also be marsupialized into the peritoneal cavity where the fluid is reabsorbed or intraluminally instilled with sclerosing agents such as povidone–iodine, tetracycline, or fibrin-glue. Infected or obstructing lymphoceles can be drained externally. Not uncommonly, the ureter is narrowed due to its inflammatory response to the adjacent lymphocele wall and require re-implantation.

An obstructed hematoma is best managed by surgical evacuation. Urinoma or evidence of a urine leak should be treated without delay. A small leak can be managed expectantly with insertion of a Foley catheter to reduce intravesical pressure. This maneuver may occasionally reduce or stop the leak altogether. Persistent allograft dysfunction, particularly in a symptomatic patient, often necessitates early surgical exploration and repair. Infected perinephric fluid collections should be treated by external drainage or open surgery in conjunction with systemic antibiotics.

Common Laboratory Abnormalities

Hematologic Abnormalities

Anemia

Severe anemia is uncommon in the era of erythropoietin therapy. Mild anemia, however, is common in the early post-transplant period when erythropoietin therapy is typically discontinued, but it generally improves within several weeks to months. Assessment of baseline iron stores at the time of transplantation may be invaluable as iron deficiency is not uncommon in the dialysis population. Profound iron deficiency should be treated with intravenous iron as tolerated. Erythropoietin therapy is generally effective in patients who have impaired allograft function and adequate iron stores. Refractory or severe anemia mandates aggressive evaluation to exclude the possibility of surgical postoperative bleeding particularly in those with a rapid fall in hemoglobin and hematocrit levels. Other possibilities include gastrointestinal bleed, tertiary hyperparathyroidism, underlying inflammatory conditions, or parvovirus B19 infection. Sirolimus and other commonly used drugs including angiotensin-converting enzyme inhibitors (ACEI) and angiotensin receptor blockers (ARB) may cause or exacerbate anemia and should not be overlooked.[34] Anemia secondary to sirolimus may respond to a short course of erythropoietin although higher doses may be required. Erythropoietin-resistant anemia has been described in patients receiving sirolimus immunosuppression. Recent studies demonstrated that in stable kidney transplant recipients conversion from sirolimus to enteric-coated mycophenolate sodium led to an increase in hemoglobin and a decrease in erythropoietin resistance independent of renal functional changes or changes in iron sequestration. Of interest, conversion was complicated by post-transplant erythrocytosis in two patients (2/25 patients).[35]

Leukopenia and Thrombocytopenia

Leukopenia and thrombocytopenia are not uncommon in transplant recipients and are most commonly related to adverse drug effects including azathioprine (which has been replaced by mycophenolate mofetil by most centers), mycophenolate mofetil, antilymphocyte antibody treatment, sirolimus,[36,37] and trimethoprim–sulfamethoxazole among others. Withholding the offending agent or dose reduction generally corrects these hematologic abnormalities. Severe leukopenia may be safely treated with granulocyte-stimulating factor (Neupogen). Potential medical complications such as thrombotic microangiopathy or cytomegalovirus infection should be excluded. Parvovirus B19 infection may present with refractory anemia, pancytopenia, and thrombotic microangiopathy.[38] More recently, an increase in the incidence of leukopenia was found in kidney and pancreas transplant recipients receiving alemtuzumab induction.[39]

Erythrocytosis

Renal artery stenosis, polycystic kidney disease, renal cell carcinoma, hepatocellular carcinoma, cerebellar hemangioblastoma, or chronic hypoxia in heavy tobacco users are potential causes of secondary erythrocytosis and should be excluded as clinically indicated.[10,11]

Post-transplant erythrocytosis (PTE) of varying degrees has been reported to occur in 20–25% of transplant recipients within the first 2 years. Risk factors for PTE include the presence of native kidneys, male gender, excellent graft function and the absence of rejection episodes, high baseline hemoglobin pre-transplant, smoking, hypertension, and diabetes mellitus. Transplant renal artery stenosis has been shown to be a risk factor for PTE in some.[40,41] but not all studies.[42] Suggested pathogenic mechanism(s) include defective feedback regulation of erythropoietin metabolism, direct stimulation of erythroid precursors by angiotensin II, and/or abnormalities in circulating insulin-like growth factor-1 (IGF-1) levels.[43,44] Erythropoietin level has been shown to be inconsistently elevated.[45] Treatment is generally recommended for hemoglobin (Hb) level $\geq$ 17–18 g/dl or hematocrit level $\geq$ 52–55% due to the associated risk of thromboembolic complications, hypertension, and headaches. The use of either ACEI or ARB is often sufficiently effective, although phlebotomy may occasionally be necessary. A negative association between the use of sirolimus and PTE has been reported[40] – whether sirolimus might prove to be beneficial in the prevention and treatment of PTE remains to be studied.[35]

Hyperkalemia

Mild hyperkalemia is commonly encountered in renal transplant recipients particularly in the early post-transplant period when relatively high-dose calcineurin inhibitor is given. It is often associated with mild hyperchloremic acidosis, a clinical presentation reminiscent of type IV renal tubular acidosis. Suggested mechanism(s) of calcineurin inhibitor-induced hyperkalemia include hyporeninism hypoaldosteronism, aldosterone resistance, end-organ defect in potassium secretion, or inhibition of cortical collecting duct potassium secretory channels.[46] In patients receiving cyclosporine or tacrolimus immunosuppression, a potassium level in the range of 5.2–5.5 mmol/L is typically seen and generally does not require treatment. However, dietary potassium restriction is recommended (2,000 mg/day). Higher potassium levels, especially in the presence of concomitant use of drugs that may exacerbate hyperkalemia such as ACEI, ARB, or β-blockers, may require treatment at the clinicians' discretion. Caution should be made when potassium-containing phosphorus supplement is prescribed. Although trimethoprim can cause hyperkalemia via an amiloride-like effect, the routine use of low-dose trimethoprim-sulfamethoxazole (Bactrim) for PCP and urinary tract infections prophylaxis is rarely the cause of severe or refractory hyperkalemia in recipients of renal allograft transplant.

Depending on the severity and/or acuteness of hyperkalemia and associated EKG changes, treatment may include diuretics and potassium exchange resin (sodium polystyrene or kayexalate) for mild-to-moderate hyperkalemia and the addition of insulin with glucose and calcium gluconate for more severe hyperkalemia. Of note, sodium polystyrene sulfonate (kayexalate) should not be administered rectally in the early post-transplant period because it may induce colonic dilatation and predispose to perforation.[47] Diuretics are usually effective in mild-to-moderate hyperkalemia and are appropriate therapy for those patients who are also volume overloaded. Treatment of constipation, when present, should not be overlooked to improve gastrointestinal potassium secretion and alleviate hyperkalemia. In life-threatening hyperkalemia, inhaled β-agonist may be added in patients with low cardiovascular risks and urgent hemodialysis may be required especially for those with poor allograft function.

Hypokalemia

Unlike cyclosporine or tacrolimus, sirolimus has been suggested to be associated with hypokalemia. In an early European phase II trial in which sirolimus was compared directly to cyclosporine in renal transplantation (in a triple therapy regimen consisting of either cyclosporine or sirolimus, azathioprine, and steroid), serum potassium was found to be significantly lower in sirolimus-treated patients compared to cyclosporine-treated patients at week 4, 12, 24, and 52 ($p < 0.01$). Hypokalemia occurred in 34%, and potassium supplementation was required in 27% of patients in the sirolimus-treated group.[36] Similar results were obtained in the European phase II trial where sirolimus was compared to cyclosporine in a triple therapy regimen where azathioprine was replaced by mycophenolate mofetil. Serum potassium was significantly lower in sirolimus-treated group compared to cyclosporine-treated group at week 4, 12, and 52. There was a trend for a higher incidence of hypokalemia in the sirolimus-treated group compared to cyclosporine-treated group, 20% vs. 16%, $p > 0.05$, respectively.[37]

Hypophosphatemia

Hypophosphatemia of varying degrees is frequently encountered after successful renal transplantation. The concomitant presence of hypercalcemia suggests that hypophosphatemia may result from the introduction of a well-functioning kidney allograft into a persistently hyperparathyroid milieu whereas the absence of hypercalcemia or hyperparathyroidism suggests renal phosphate wasting syndrome or even malnutrition.[48] Early after transplantation, hypophosphatemia has been attributed to a massive initial diuresis particularly following a living-donor renal transplant, defective renal phosphate reabsorption due to allograft injury, glucosuria, magnesium depletion, and corticosteroid use – the latter by inhibiting proximal tubular reabsorption of phosphate. Recent studies have suggested other less well-defined causes.[49–51] Severe hypophosphatemia may cause rhabdomyolysis, left ventricular dysfunction, respiratory muscle weakness, hemolysis, defects in erythrocyte metabolism, insulin resistance, osteomalacia, and renal tubular defects. The treatment of hypophosphatemia involves correcting the underlying conditions and phosphate replacement therapy. Mild hypophosphatemia (>2.0 mg/dl) (0.65 mmol/L) can generally be managed with a high phosphorus dietary intake while phosphate supplementation may be necessary for more pronounced hypophosphatemia. Suppression of hyperparathyroidism with cinacalcet, a calcium receptor agonist, has generally been recommended. In a small study consisting of 10 stable kidney transplant recipients with persistent hyperparathyroidism, cinacalcet effectively corrected urinary phosphate wasting, resulting in normalization of serum phosphorous levels. The phosphatemic effects of cinacalcet correlated with a marked decrease in the phosphatemic hormone PTH, rather than with a change in fibroblast growth factor 23 (FGF-23) levels or acid–base status, underscoring the importance of PTH in post-transplant hypophosphatemia.[52]

The use of calcitriol – a vitamin D analogue, has also been variably suggested to be beneficial. However, the risk of hypercalcemia or hypercalciuria associated with its use should not be overlooked.

Hypercalcemia

Hypercalcemia is common after transplantation and is generally due to persistent secondary hyperparathyroidism. The concomitant presence of severe hypophosphatemia particularly in patients with excellent graft function may exacerbate hypercalcemia through stimulation of renal proximal tubular 1α-hydroxylase. Resolution of soft tissue calcifications, high-dose corticosteroid therapy, and immobilization are potential contributing factors. In about two-third of cases, hypercalcemia resolves spontaneously within 6–12 months. However, spontaneous resolution occurs in less than half of those whose hypercalcemia existed before transplantation. Persistent hyperparathyroidism has generally been attributed to continued autonomous production of PTH from nodular hyperplastic glands, reduced density of calcitriol receptors, and decreased expression of the membrane calcium sensor receptors that render cells more resistant to physiologic concentrations of calcitriol and calcium. The risk of developing persistent hyperparathyroidism is increased with the duration of dialysis and the severity of pre-transplant hyperparathyroidism. Severe hypercalcemia or persistent hypercalcemia (≥ 12 months) requires further evaluation. Initial assessment should include an intact parathyroid hormone level. Imaging studies including neck ultrasound or parathyroid technetium 99mTc-sestamibi scan should be done at the clinicians' discretion to exclude parathyroid adenoma or parathyroid gland hyperplasia, and/or hyperplastic nodular formation of the parathyroid glands.

Cinacalcet has been shown to reduce serum calcium in renal transplant recipients with hypercalcemic hyperparathyroidism.[52,53] In an early study involving 11 renal transplant recipients with persistent hyperparathyroidism (≥ 6 months posttransplant) and normal allograft function (measured CrCl ≥ 40 ml/min/1.73 m2), Serra et al.[52] have shown that treatment with cinacalcet resulted in significant reduction in serum calcium and PTH levels (serum calcium decreased from 2.73 ± 0.05 to 2.4 ± 0.05 and 2.42 ± 0.04 mmol/L after 2 and 10 weeks of treatment, respectively, whereas plasma intact PTH levels fell by 16.1 and 21.8% at study weeks 2 and 10, respectively). The reduction in intact PTH was accompanied by an increase in serum phosphate and unchanged calcium $\times$ phosphate product. Renal function remained unchanged and no allograft rejection occurred during the study period. Similarly, Kruse et al.[54] have shown that cinacalcet treatment in renal transplant recipients with persistent hyperparathyroidism resulted in significantly decreased in serum calcium level. However, no significant changes in PTH or phosphate levels were observed while renal function slightly declined at months 2 and 3 ($p < 0.05$). Limited studies suggest that the calcium lowering effect of cinacalcet is caused in part by increased urinary calcium excretion.[53] Correction of hypercalcemia and PTH with cinacalcet has also been shown to simultaneously improve bone mineral density.[55]

Parathyroidectomy is warranted in patients with tertiary hyperparathyroidism or persistent severe hypercalcemia (>11.5 mg/dl (2.87 mmol/L)) for more than 6–12 months, symptomatic or progressive hypercalcemia, nephrolithiasis, persistent metabolic bone disease, calcium-related renal allograft dysfunction, or progressive vascular calcification and calciphylaxis.[56] Whether the advent of calcimimetics to traditional medical therapy confers better normalization of biochemical parameters and obviates the need for parathyroidectomy remains to be studied.

Hypomagnesemia

Hypomagnesemia was rarely seen in renal allograft recipients until the advent of cyclosporine. The association between the calcineurin inhibitors cyclosporine and tacrolimus and hypomagnesemia is now well established and has been shown to be due to urinary magnesium wasting.[57] Sirolimus, which has a mechanism of action distinct to that calcineurin inhibitors, has also been shown to cause urinary magnesium wasting and hypomagnesemia. Other factors that may contribute to post-transplant hypomagnesemia include loop diuretic therapy, post-ATN or post-obstructive polyuria, and/or renal tubular acidosis. In addition, the propensity toward hypomagnesemia may be more pronounced among diabetics. In the first 3 months following transplantation, a magnesium level less than 1.5 mg/dL (0.62 mmol/L) is commonly seen. Dietary magnesium intake is usually insufficient and high-dose oral magnesium supplement (i.e., 400–800 mg magnesium oxide three times a day) may be required to compensate for the ongoing magnesuria. Intravenous magnesium should be considered in severe hypomagnesemia (<1.0 mg/dl or 0.41 mmol/L) particularly in patients with a prior history of coronary artery disease or cardiac arrhythmias and in those taking digitalis. Aggressive treatment of hypomagnesemia has also been suggested to be beneficial in renal transplant recipients in terms of improvement of lipid profile (↓total cholesterol, ↓low-density lipoprotein and ↓total cholesterol/high-density lipoprotein ratio),[58] cyclosporine-induced neurotoxicity, and hypertension.

Transaminitis

Elevation of hepatic enzymes is common in the early post-transplant period and is generally due to drug-related toxicity. Potential culprits include acyclovir, ganciclovir, trimethoprim–sulfamethoxazole, cyclosporine, tacrolimus, statin therapy, and proton pump inhibitors. Cyclosporine, and less commonly, tacrolimus, may cause transient, self-limited, dose-dependent elevations of transaminase levels and mild hyperbilirubinemia secondary to defective bile secretion. Drug-related transaminitis generally improves or resolves following drug discontinuation or dose reduction.

Persistent or profound elevation in hepatic liver enzymes should prompt further evaluation to exclude infectious causes including CMV, HBV, and HCV. In high-risk candidates for primary CMV infections (recipient seronegative, donor seropositive) it may occasionally be necessary to initiate CMV therapy while awaiting laboratory results, particularly, when there is a high index of clinical suspicion (fever, fatigue, malaise, gastroenteritis, leukopenia, and/or thrombocytopenia). Evidence of post-transplant HBV reactivation should be treated with lamivudine (elevated ALT, histologic hepatitis, and serum DNA>10^5 copies/ml). Some programs routinely initiate lamivudine prophylaxis in all HbsAg+ candidates at the time of transplantation. Pre-transplant lamivudine prophylactic therapy is recommended in renal transplant candidates who have HBV DNA > 10^5 copies/ml and active liver disease defined as ALT more than two times the upper limit of normal or biopsy-proven hepatic disease.[59] There is currently no effective treatment for chronic hepatitis C in renal transplant recipients. Although treatment with interferon-α may result in clearance of HCV RNA in 25–50% of cases, rapid relapse following drug withdrawal is nearly universal.[59,60] More importantly, interferon-α treatment has been shown to precipitate acute allograft rejection and graft loss and is currently not routinely recommended for renal transplant recipients with HCV infection. Its use should be individualized at the discretion of the transplant nephrologist and hepatologist. Management of HCV infection in this patient population should probably rely on manipulation of immunosuppressive therapy. Experiences gained from liver transplantation indicate that corticosteroid therapy and antilymphocyte antibody treatment are associated with enhanced viral replication and more rapid progression to cirrhosis. Based on these observations, it is advisable to avoid antilymphocyte antibody induction therapy and minimize steroid dosage in transplant recipients with chronic HCV infection. Although early reports suggested that mycophenolate mofetil may reduce HCV replication and delay the recurrence of hepatitis C in Hep C liver transplant recipients,[61] the antiviral properties of MMF and its impact on HCV replication and hepatitis C recurrence have not been consistently demonstrated in subsequent studies.[62,63] Suggested algorithms for the management of renal transplant recipients with elevated hepatic enzymes is shown in Fig. 14.2.

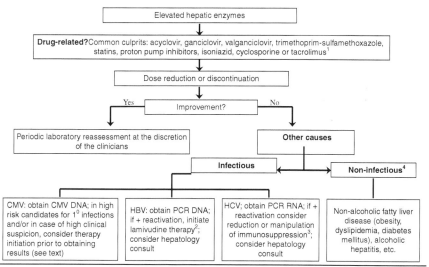

[1]Cyclosporine and less commonly tacrolimus, may cause transient, self-limited dose-dependent elevations of aminotransferase levels & mild hyperbilirubinemia secondary to defective bile secretion. [2]Some programs routinely commence lamivudine prophylactic therapy in all HBsAg positive candidates at the time of transplantation. [3]There is currently no effective treatment for chronic hepatitis C in renal transplant recipients (see text). [4]Appropriate evaluation and management similar to non-transplant settings

Fig. 14.2 Suggested algorithm for the management of elevated hepatic enzymes in renal transplant recipients

Outpatient Care

The frequency of outpatient clinic visits may vary among centers. In general, patients should be seen two to three times a week for the first 2 weeks after transplantation, twice a week for the next 2 weeks, and weekly for the next month. After the first 2 months, the frequency of outpatient visits largely depends on the complexity of the patient's early postoperative course. Most patients with stable graft function and an uneventful postoperative course can return to work or their regular daily activities 2–3 months post-transplant. Laboratory assessment during the first month after transplantation should include serum creatinine, immunosuppressive drug level, a complete blood count with platelets, urinalysis, electrolyte, and a comprehensive metabolic panel. After the first post-transplant month, pertinent laboratory evaluation should be performed at the discretion of the clinician. Most patients are referred back to their primary nephrologists for long-term care at 2–3 months post-transplant. After the first post-transplant year, annual follow-up at a transplantation center is typically recommended.

References

1. Shokes DA, Cecka JM. Effect of delayed graft function on short- and long-term kidney graft survival. In: Cecka JM and Terasaki PI (eds.), Clinical Transplants. UCLA Tissue typing Laboratory, Los Angeles, CA, 1997, pp. 297–303.
2. Lehtonen SRK, Isoniemi HM, Salmela KT et al. Long-term graft outcome is not necessarily affected by delayed onset of graft function and early acute rejection. *Transplantation* 1997;64:103–107.
3. Paff WW, Howard RJ, Patton HP et al. Delayed graft function after renal transplantation. *Transplantation* 1998;65:219–223.
4. Ojo AO, Wolfe RA, Held WP et al. Delayed graft function: risk factors and implication for renal allograft survival. *Transplantation* 1997;63:968–974.
5. Marcen R, Orofino L, Pascual J et al. Delayed graft function does not reduce the survival of renal transplant allografts. *Transplantation* 1998;66:461–466.
6. Dawidson I et al. Perioperative albumin and verapamil improve early outcome after cadaveric renal transplantation. *Transplant Proc* 1994;26:3100–3101.
7. Gritsch HA, Rosenthal JM. The transplant operation and its surgical complications. In: GM Danovitch, (ed.), Handbook of Kidney Transplantation, 3rd ed. Lippincott, Williams and Wilkins, Philadelphia, PA, 2001, pp. 146–162.
8. Gritsch HA, Rosenthal JT, Danovitch GM. Living and cadaveric kidney donation. In Danovitch GM (ed.), Handbook of Kidney Transplantation. Little, Brown, Boston, 2001, pp. 111–129.
9. Fotiadas CN, Govani MV, Heldeman JH. Renal allograft dysfunction. In Massary SG, Galssock RJ (eds.), Textbook of Nephrology. Lippincott, Williams and Wilkins, Philadelphia, 2001, pp. 1617–1635.
10. Pham PT, Pham PC, Wilkinson AH. Management of the transplant recipient in the early postoperative period. In: Davison AM, Cameron JS, Grunfeld J-P, Ponticelli C, Ritz E, Winearls C, van Ypersele C (eds), Oxford Textbook Of Clinical Nephrology, 3rd ed. Oxford University Press, Oxford/New York, 2005, pp. 2087–2101.
11. Fernandez-Najera JE, Beltran S, Aparicio M et al. Transplant renal artery stenosis: association with vascular rejection. *Transplant Proc* 2006;38(8):2404–2405.

12. Hawkins IF, Maynar M. Carbon dioxide digital subtraction angiography. In: Castadena Z (ed), Interventional Radiology, 3rd ed. Williams and Wilkins, Philadelphia, PA, 1997.

13. Kay J. Nephrogenic systemic fibrosis: a gadolinium-associated fibrosing disorder in patients with renal dysfunction. *Ann Rheum Dis* 2008;67(Suppl 3):66–69.

14. Ploeg RJ, van Bockel JH, Langendijk PT et al. for the European Multicentre Study Group: Effect of preservation solution on results of cadaveric kidney transplantation. *Lancet* 1992;340:129–137.

15. Yarlagadda SG, Klein CL, Jani A. Long-term renal outcomes after delayed graft function. *Adv Chronic Kidney Dis* 2008;15(3):248–256.

16. Shokes DA, Halloran PF. Delayed graft function in renal transplantation: etiology, management, and long-term significance. *J Urol* 1996;155:1831-1840.

17. Phillips AO, Deanne C, O'Donnell P et al. Evaluation of Doppler ultrasound in primary non-function of renal transplants. *Clin Transplant* 1994;8:83–86.

18. Pham PT, Peng A, Wilkinson AH et al. Cyclosporine and tacrolimus-associated thrombotic microangiopathy. *Am J Kidney Dis* 2000;36:844–850.

19. Barone GW, Gurley BJ, Abul-Ezz SR et al. Sirolimus-induced thrombotic microangiopathy in a renal transplant recipient. *Am J Kidney Dis* 2003;42:202–206.

20. Baid S, Pascual M, Williams WW et al. Renal thrombotic microangiopathy associated with anti-cardiolipin antibodies in hepatitis C-positive renal allograft recipients. *J Am Soc Nephrol* 1999;10:146–153.

21. Choy BY, Chan TM, Lai KN. Recurrent glomerulonephritis after kidney transplantation. *Am J Transplant* 2006;6:2535–2542.

22. Sharma M, Sharma R, Reddy SR et al. Proteinuria after injection of human focal segmental glomerulosclerosis factor. *Transplantation* 2002;73(3):366–372.

23. Watschinger B, Pascual M. Capillary C4d deposition as a marker of humoral immunity in renal allograft rejection. *J Am Soc Nephrol* 2002; 13:2420–2423.

24. Mauiyyedi S, Covin RB. Humoral rejection in kidney transplantation: new concepts in diagnosis and treatment. *Curr Opin Nephrol Hypertens* 2002;11:609–618.

25. Solez K, Colvin RB, Racusen LC et al. Banff 2007 classification of renal allograft pathology: updates and future directions. Am J Transplant 2008; 8(4): 753–760.

26. Gaber AO et al. Results of double blind, randomized, phase III clinical trial of thymoglobulin versus Atgam in the treatment of acute allograft rejection episodes after renal transplantation. *Transplantation* 1998;96:29–37.

27. Ibernon M, Gil-Vernet S, Carrera M et al. Therapy with plasmapheresis and intravenous immunoglobulin for acute humoral rejection in kidney transplantation. *Transplant Proc* 2005;37(9):743–745.

28. Jordan SC, Vo AA, Tyan D et al. Current approaches to treatment of antibody-mediated rejection. Pediatr Transplant 2005;9(3):408–415.

29. Akalin E, Ames S, Sehgal V et al. Intravenous immunoglobulin and thymoglobulin facilitate kidney transplantation in complement-dependent cytotoxicity B-cell and flow cytometry T- or B-cell crossmatch-positive patients. *Transplantation* 2003;76(10):1444–1447.

30. Berger PM, Diamond JR. Ureteral obstruction as complication of renal transplantation: a review. *J Nephrol* 1998;11:20–23.

31. Nargund VH, Cranston D. Urologic complications after renal transplantation. *Transplant Rev* 1996;10:24.

32. Mylonakis E, Goes N, Rubin RH et al. BK virus in solid organ transplant recipients: an emerging syndrome. *Transplantation* 2002;72:1587–1592.

33. Singer J, Gritsch AH, Rosenthal JT. The transplant operation and its surgical complications. In: Danovitch GM (ed.), Handbook of Kidney Transplantation. Little, Brown, Boston, 2004, pp. 193–211.

34. Jaster R, Bittorf T, Klinken SP et al. Inhibition of proliferation but not erythroid differentiation of j2E cells by rapamycin. *Biochem Pharmacol* 1996;51:1181–1185.

35. Augustine JJ, Rodriguez V, Padiyar A et al. Reduction of erythropoietin resistance after conversion from sirolimus to enteric coated mycophenolate sodium. *Transplantation* 2008;86(4):548–553.

36. Groth CG, Backman L, Morales JM et al. Sirolimus (rapamycin)-based therapy in human renal transplantation. Similar efficacy and different toxicity compared with cyclosporine. *Transplantation* 1999;67:1036–1042.

37. Kreis H, Cisterne JM, Land W et al. Sirolimus in association with mycophenolate mofetil for the prevention of acute graft rejection in renal allograft recipients. *Transplantation* 2000;69:1252-1260.

38. Luisa M et al. Thrombotic microangiopathy associated with parvovirus B19 infection after renal transplantation. *J Am Soc Nephrol* 2000;11:1132-1137.

39. Hartmann EL, Gatesman M, Roskopf-Somerville J et al. Management of leukopenia in kidney and pancreas transplant recipients. *Clin Transplant* 2008;22(6):822–888.

40. Vlahakos DV, Marathias KP, Agroyannis B et al. Posttransplant erythrocytosis. Kidney Int 2003;63(4):1187–1194.

41. Bacon BR, Rothman SA, Ricanati ES et al. Renal artery stenosis with erythrocytosis after renal transplantation. *Arch Intern Med* 1980;140:1206–.

42. Wicker CG, Norman DJ, Bennison A et al. Postrenal transplant erythrocytosis: a review of 53 patients. *Kidney Int* 1983;23:731–.

43. Brox AG et al. Erythrocytosis after renal transplantation represents an abnormality of insulin-like growth factor-I and its binding protein. *Transplantation* 1998;66:1053–1058.

44. Gupta M, Miller BA, Ahsan N et al. Expression of angiotensin II type 1 receptor on erythroid progenitors of patients with post transplant erythrocytosis. *Transplantation* 2000;70(8): 1188–1194.

45. Lezaic V et al. Erythrocytosis after kidney transplantation: the role of erythropoietin, burst promoting activity and early erythroid progenitor cells. *Eur Med Res* 2001;6:27–32.

46. Heering P, Degenhart S, Garbensee B. Tubular dysfunction following kidney transplantation. *Nephron* 1996;74:501–511.

47. Pirenne J, Lledo-Garcia E, Benedetti E et al. Colon perforation after renal transplantation a single-institution review. Clin Transplant 1997; 11(2): 88–93.

48. Ward HN, Pabico RC, McKenna BA et al. The renal handling of phosphate by renal transplant recipients: correlation with serum parathyroid hormone, cyclic $3'5'$-adenosine monophosphate urinary excretion and allograft function. Adv Exp Med Biol 1997;81:173–181.

49. Kawarazaki H, Shibagaki Y, Shimizu H et al. Persistent high level of fibroblast growth factor 23 as a cause of post-renal transplant hypophosphatemia. *Clin Exp Nephrol* 2007;11(3): 255–257.

50. Ghanekar H, Welch BJ, Moe OW et al. Post-renal transplantation hypophosphatemia: a review and novel insights. *Curr Opin Nephrol Hypertens* 2006;15(2):97–104.

51. Levi M. Post transplant hypophosphatemia. *Kidney Int* 2001; 59:2377–2387.

52. Serra AL, Wuhmann C, Wuthrich RP. Phosphatemic effect of cinacalcet in kidney transplant recipients with persistent hyperparathyroidism. *Am J Kidney Dis* 2008;52(6):1151–1157.

53. Borchhardt KA, Heinz H, Mayerwoger E et al. Cinacalcet increases calcium excretion in hypercalcemic hyperparathyroidism after kidney transplantation. *Transplantation* 2008;86(7):919–924.

54. Kruse AE, Eisenberger U, Frey FJ et al. The calcimimetic cinacalcet normalizes serum calcium in renal transplant patients with persistent hyperparathyroidism. *Nephrol Dial Transplant* 2005;20(7):1311–1314.

55. Bergua C, Torregrosa JV, Fuster D et al. Effect of cinacalcet on hypercalcemia and bone mineral density in renal transplanted patients with secondary hyperparathyroidism. *Transplantation* 2008;86(3):413–417.

56. Pham PC, Pham PT:. Parathyroidectomy. In: Nissebson AR and Fine RN, (eds.), Handbook of Dialysis Therapy. Saunders, Elsevier, London, 2008, pp. 1024–1038.

57. Barton CH. Hypomagnesemia and renal magnesium wasting in renal transplant recipients receiving cyclosporine. *Am J Med* 1987;83:693–699.

58. Gupta BK, Glicklich TVA. Magnesium repletion therapy improves lipid metabolism in hypomagnesemic renal transplant recipients. *Transplantation* 1999;67:1485-1487.

59. Gane E, Pilmore H. Management of chronic hepatitis before and after renal transplantation. *Transplantation* 2002;74:427–437.
60. Fabrizio F, Martin P. In: Danovitch GM(ed.). Handbook of Kidney Transplantation. Hepatitis in kidney Transplantation, 3rd ed. Lippincott Williams and Wilkins, Philadelphia, PA, 2001, pp. 263–271.
61. Fasola CG, Netto G, Christensen LL et al. Delay of hepatitis recurrence in liver transplant recipients treated with mycophenolate mofetil. *Transplant Proc* 2002;34:1561–1562.
62. Bahra M, Neumann UIF, Jacob D et al. MMF and calcineurin inhibitor taper in recurrent hepatitis C after liver transplantation: Impact on histological course. *Am J Transplant* 2005;5:406–411.
63. Nanmoku K, Imaizumi R, Tojimbra T et al. Effects of immunosuppressants on the progression of hepatitis C in hepatitis C virus-positive renal transplantation and the usefulness of interferon therapy. *Transplant Proc* 2008;40(7):2382–2385.
64. Amend WJ, Vincenti I, Tamlonovich SJ. The first two post-transplant months. In: Danovitch GM (ed.), Handbook of Kidney Transplantation. Little, Brown & Co, Boston, 2001, p. 167.
65. Takemoto SK, Zeevi A, Feng S, et al. National conference to assess antibody-mediated rejection in solid organ transplantation. *Am J Transplant* 2004; 4(7): 1033–1041.

Chapter 15
Post-transplant Cardiovascular Disease

Phuong-Anh T. Pham, Carmen Slavov, Phuong-Thu T. Pham,
and Alan H. Wilkinson

Introduction

Renal transplantation is the treatment modality of choice for virtually all suitable candidates with end-stage renal disease. Compared to dialysis, kidney transplantation improves both patient survival and quality of life. Studies suggest that the survival advantage of transplantation may be largely attributed to the reduction in cardiovascular disease (CVD) associated with the improvement in renal function following a successful renal transplant. In a retrospective analysis of the United States Renal Data System consisting of more than 60,000 adult primary kidney transplant recipients transplanted between 1995 and 2000 and more than 66,000 adult wait-listed patients over the same time period, Meier-Kriesche et al.[1] demonstrated a progressive decrease in cardiovascular death rates by renal transplant vintage for both diabetic and non-diabetic recipients of both living and deceased donor transplants. In contrast, the CVD death rates in wait-listed patients appeared to increase steadily by dialysis vintage. Although the CVD death rate among transplant recipients was higher in the early postoperative period compared to wait-listed patients, it fell significantly by 3 months post-transplant. On long-term follow-up, while there seemed to be a modest rise in CVD death rates in the second transplant year, the rates actually remained low even among high CVD risk groups including those with end-stage renal disease secondary to diabetes mellitus or hypertension. Nonetheless, despite the well-established survival advantage of transplantation over dialysis, CVD death has emerged as the most frequent cause of late graft loss. Although renal transplantation ameliorates CVD risk factors by restoring renal function, it introduces new cardiovascular risks including impaired glucose tolerance or diabetes mellitus, hypertension, and dyslipidemia that are derived, in part, from immunosuppressive medications such as calcineurin inhibitors (CNI),

P.-A.T. Pham (✉)
Mercy General Hospital, Heart and Vascular Institute, Cardiovascular Diseases, Sacramento, CA,
USA
e-mail: phounganh.pham@chw.edu

D.B. McKay, S.M. Steinberg (eds.), *Kidney Transplantation: A Guide to the Care
of Kidney Transplant Recipients*, DOI 10.1007/978-1-4419-1690-7_15,
© Springer Science+Business Media, LLC 2010

corticosteroids, or mammalian target of rapamycin (mTOR) inhibitors. Hence, identification and aggressive management of CVD risk factors should begin in the early post-transplant period and should remain an integral part of long-term care in renal transplant recipients. The following chapter provides an overview of the literature on conventional and unconventional CVD risk factors after renal transplantation and a discussion of an approach to their medical management.

Post-transplant Cardiovascular Disease Risk Factors

Although all the determinants of enhanced CVD risks in renal transplant recipients have not been well defined, both conventional and unconventional risk factors are thought to be contributory (Table 15.1). The former risks include age, male gender, diabetes mellitus, hypertension, dyslipidemia, obesity (measured as body mass index), cigarette smoking, and family history. The latter risks include pre-existing left ventricular hypertrophy, coronary artery vascular calcification, impaired allograft function, proteinuria, anemia, acute rejection episodes, deceased (vs. living donor), hyperhomocysteinemia, hyperuricemia, elevated C-reactive protein,

Table 15.1 CVD risk factors (adapted and modified from Pham et al.[2])

Conventional		Unconventional	
Modifiable	Non-modifiable	Modifiable (± potentially modifiable)	Non-modifiable
Hypertension	Family history	Anemia[a]	Prior acute rejection episodes
Dyslipidemia	Diabetes mellitus	Proteinuria[a]	Pre-existing CAC
Obesity	Male gender	Hyperhomocysteinemia[a]?	Deceased vs. living donor
Smoking	Age	Inflammatory cytokines[a] ↑C-reactive protein[a]	Pre-transplant splenectomy
			CMV infection[b]
			Hyperuricemia
			Impaired allograft function[c]
			Left ventricular hypertrophy[d]
			CD4 lymphopenia[e]
			Low albumin
			Steroids[a], cyclosporine > tacrolimus[a]

[a] See text for more detail.
[b] Strict adherence to CMV prophylaxis protocol/CMV surveillance in high-risk candidates.
[c] CNI minimization or withdrawal at the discretion of the clinician (variable results/difficult-to-modify risk factor).
[d] Optimize BP control; use ACE-I, angiotensin receptor AT1 blockers.
[e] Assess risks and benefits of T-cell-depleting antibody treatment. Further studies are needed.
CAC: coronary artery calcification.

low serum albumin, inflammatory cytokines, CD4 lymphopenia, pre-transplant splenectomy, and cytomegalovirus (CMV) infection among others.[2,3] Pre-transplant hypertension and CNI therapy are thought to be the most potent etiologic factors for post-transplant hypertension.[3] Selected CVD risks are discussed. New onset diabetes mellitus after transplantation (NODAT) is discussed elsewhere.

Conventional CVD Risk Factors

Post-transplant Hypertension

Hypertension is a well-known risk factor for cardiovascular disease and stroke in the general population as well as in renal transplant recipients. In addition, elevated blood pressure has also been shown to be an independent risk factor for kidney graft failure. In an analysis of the Collaborative Transplant Study (CTS) registry consisting of nearly 30,000 renal transplant recipients, increased levels of systolic and diastolic blood pressure post-transplant were found to be associated with a graded increased risk of subsequent graft failure ($P < 0.0001$).[4] Whether aggressive lowering of blood pressure retards the progression of graft failure similar to that observed in the general population with chronic kidney disease (CKD) remains to be studied. Hypertension is common after transplantation and is present in 50–90% of renal transplant recipients.[5,6] The wide range in the frequency may reflect the variable definitions of hypertension, donor source, immunosuppressive medications, time post-transplantation, and level of allograft function. Systolic BP is highest immediately after transplantation and declines during the first year.[5] In a Collaborative Transplant Study (CTS) registry analysis involving nearly 25,000 recipients of deceased donor transplants, only 8% had a systolic blood pressure less than 120 mmHg at 1 year; 33% had a BP in the pre-hypertension range; 39% had stage 1 hypertension; and 20% had stage 2 hypertension despite antihypertensive therapy.[4] Pre-existing hypertension, tacrolimus, and to a greater degree cyclosporine, corticosteroids, quality of donor organ, delayed graft function, chronic allograft nephropathy, high body mass index or excess weight gain, acute rejection episodes independent of creatinine clearance, recurrent or de novo glomerulonephritis, and transplant renal artery stenosis have all been implicated in post-transplant hypertension. In rare cases, excess renin output from the native kidneys has also been suggested to contribute to post-transplant hypertension.[5] In renal transplant recipients with severe hypertension refractory to medical therapy, bilateral native nephrectomy has been reported to ameliorate blood pressure control.[7]

The contributory role of calcineurin inhibitors (CNI) and glucocorticoids in the development of post-transplant hypertension has been well established. In a large randomized trial consisting of over 400 patients randomized to remain on sirolimus–cyclosporine–steroid or to have cyclosporine withdrawn (sirolimus–steroid) at 3 months, systolic and diastolic BP were significantly lower in the sirolimus–steroid compared to the sirolimus–cyclosporine–steroid groups at 36 months follow-up (systolic blood pressure: 131.3 vs. 140.1 mmHg, respectively; P=0.002 and diastolic BP: 76.3 vs. 81.2 mmHg, respectively; P=0.006). Moreover, this difference was observed despite significantly (P=0.001) lower use of antihypertensive medication in the sirolimus–steroid group.[8] Compared to cyclosporine, tacrolimus has been suggested to have a more favorable effect on blood pressure and lipid profile (discussed in further details under dyslipidemia). In an open, prospective, multicenter study consisting of 72 stable adult kidney transplant recipients who underwent cyclosporine to tacrolimus conversion therapy for poorly controlled hypertension, significant improvement in blood pressure was seen after 6 months of tacrolimus treatment. Paired analysis demonstrated a mean change in SBP from baseline of –15.8 ± 19.32 mmHg ($P < 0.001$) and a mean change in DBP of –5.17 ± 13.05 mmHg (P =0.0015) at week 24.[9] Similar favorable effect of tacrolimus over CsA on blood pressure was also demonstrated in a study in which CsA-treated patients were converted to tacrolimus followed by a return to CsA-based immunosuppression after 4 weeks of tacrolimus therapy. Mean daytime BP decreased from 149 ± 12/95 ± 8 mmHg to 138 ± 13/87 ± 9 mmHg ($P < 0.001$), whereas mean nighttime BP decreased from 140 ± 12/86 ± 7 mmHg to 132 ± 17/79 ± 10 mmHg ($P < 0.05$). Return to CsA caused an increase in BP to values similar to those in the first CsA phase.[10]

A 3-year observational follow-up of a European, multicenter, randomized clinical trial comparing triple therapy with tacrolimus, steroids, and mycophenolate mofetil (MMF) with withdrawal of either steroids or MMF at 3 months post renal transplantation demonstrated that, compared with other groups, steroids withdrawal was advantageous in reducing hypertension, hyperlipidemia, and diabetes mellitus.[11] Mean systolic blood pressure was lower in the steroid stop group compared to the steroid maintenance groups (steroid stop, 133.6 mmHg; triple therapy, 136.2 mmHg; MMF stop 139.8; P=0.002). Mean diastolic blood pressure was similar in all groups. Renal function was maintained in all groups, and patient and graft survival at 3 years were not compromised by the withdrawal of either steroids or MMF at 3 months from a tacrolimus-based regimen.

Management of post-transplant hypertension should include attempts to identify and treat the underlying etiology, lifestyle modifications, and treatment of associated cardiovascular risk factors. Lifestyle modifications should be similar to those used in the non-transplant population. The goal of treatment is to reduce blood pressure to < 130/80 mmHg as recommended by the K/DOQI practice guidelines. In proteinuric renal transplant recipients, the European best practice guidelines recommend a blood pressure goal of less than 125/75 mmHg.[12]

There is a paucity of controlled clinical trials to determine the superiority of one class of antihypertensive agent over the other in the transplant setting. In general, there is no absolute contraindication to the use of any antihypertensive agent in renal transplant recipients. All classes of antihypertensives have been used in various combinations with good results. In the perioperative setting, the use of perioperative beta-blockade has been shown to reduce ischemic heart disease events in high-risk candidates. In the early post-transplant period, non-dihydropyridine calcium channel blockers and diuretics are frequently used, the former for their beneficial effect on intraglomerular hemodynamics and the latter for their ability to eliminate salt and water in patients who are volume expanded postoperatively. In a single-center retrospective study to identify ischemic heart disease (IHD) risk after renal transplantation, Kasiske et al.[13] unexpectedly found an association between the use of dihydropyridine calcium channel antagonists and an increased IHD risk. In other studies, the use of dihydropyridine calcium channel blockers in proteinuric chronic kidney disease patients was also shown to be associated with increased risk of renal disease progression and death except when used in conjunction with angiotensin II blockade therapy.[1,2,14,15] The mechanism(s) for the potential adverse effects of dihydropyridine calcium channel blockers was suggested to be due, in part, to increased catecholamine levels.[16] Nonetheless, it should be noted that whether short-acting or long-acting dihydropyridine calcium channel blockers were used in previous studies that revealed adverse outcomes is not clear. Short-acting, but not long-acting dihydropyridine calcium channel blockers may cause frequent fluctuations in hemodynamics, hence undesirable cardiovascular events. In addition, the Antihypertensive and Lipid-Lowering Treatment to Prevent Heart Attack Trial (ALLHAT) showed that the long-term risk for fatal and non-fatal coronary events in patients who were treated with DHP-CCB (amlodipine) was similar to that in patients who were treated with ACE inhibitors or diuretics.[17] However, there was a 38% higher risk of heart failure among patients assigned to DHP-CCB compared with diuretics. Similar studies in the setting of renal transplantation are lacking. Until further evidence becomes available, monotherapy with dihydropyridine calcium channel antagonists should be used with caution. The beneficial effects of ACE-I or ARB on post-transplant patient and graft survival have not been consistently demonstrated. In a meta-analysis of 21 randomized controlled trials ($n=1,549$ patients) conducted to determine the effect of ACE-inhibitor or ARB use following kidney transplantation with a median follow-up of 27 months, ACE-I and ARB use was associated with clinically significant reductions in proteinuria (–0.47 g/day; 95% CI –0.86 to –0.08), hematocrit (–3.5%; 95% CI –6.1 to –0.95), and glomerular filtration rate (–5.8 ml/min; 95% CI –10.6 to –0.99). However, there were insufficient data to determine the effect of ACE-I or ARB use on patient or graft survival.[18] Of interest, in a meta-analysis of 7 trials conducted to examine the safety or efficacy of the early use of ACE inhibitors and ARBs in post-transplant patients, initiation of an ACE inhibitor within 12 weeks after transplant was suggested to be more effective than a beta-blocker in reducing left ventricular hypertrophy and proteinuria after 24 months of treatment. In addition, the use of ACE-I and ARBs in the early post-transplant period was shown to be safe in those with functioning grafts.[19] Results of a small single-center double-blind, placebo-controlled, crossover study demonstrated that compared with placebo and beta-blocker (carvedilol), the use of ARB (losartan) for a period of 8 weeks reduces proteinuria as well as the associated tubular damage and graft fibrosis – namely the expression of transforming growth factor beta-1 (TGF-beta1) and amino-terminal propeptide of type III procollagen (PIIINP).[20]

Further recommendations on the routine use of ACE-I and/or ARB await large, randomized controlled clinical trials with long-term follow-up. Nonetheless, because the antiproteinuric and cardioprotective effects of ACE-I and/or ARB have been well established, it is advisable to consider these agents as first-line therapy in transplant recipients with hypertension and compelling indications such as diabetes or heart failure. However, these drugs should be used with caution because of their potential to cause or exacerbate anemia, hyperkalemia, and renal dysfunction. A rising serum creatinine (i.e., greater than 30% above baseline) associated with their use should alert clinicians to the possibility of renal artery stenosis. Caution should be exercised when used with diuretics because ACE-I or ARB may potentiate volume depletion-induced fall in glomerular filtration. In patients with slow or delayed graft function, ACE-I and ARB are generally held until allograft function recovers. Although the use of ACE-I and ARB is not contraindicated in patients with mild to moderate renal allograft dysfunction, serum potassium and creatinine must be closely monitored. Beta-blockers should be considered in patients with known coronary artery disease or other atherosclerotic vascular disease, while alpha-2 blockers may be beneficial in patients with benign prostatic hypertrophy and neurogenic bladder. Symptomatic bradycardia and blunting of hypoglycemic awareness may limit the use of the former. Although aggressive blood pressure control is vital in reducing cardiovascular morbidities and mortalities as well as improving graft survival, this is not recommended in the early perioperative period due to the potential precipitation of acute tubular necrosis and/or graft thrombosis.

Potential advantages and disadvantages of different classes of antihypertensive agents in renal transplant recipients are shown in Table 15.2.

Post-transplant Dyslipidemia

Dyslipidemia is common following transplantation. The hyperlipemic effect of immunosuppressive agents including corticosteroids, cyclosporine, tacrolimus, and sirolimus has been well documented. While tacrolimus-based therapy has been suggested to be associated with better lipid profiles than cyclosporine-based therapy, sirolimus and everolimus have been shown to be associated with a significantly greater incidence and severity of dyslipidemia than cyclosporine-based therapy, including higher total cholesterol and triglyceride levels. The hypercholesterolemic and hypertriglyceridemic effects of sirolimus have been suggested to be dose-dependent. A dose-ranging study of sirolimus for the treatment of acute rejection in heart transplant recipients demonstrated significant dose-related increases in total cholesterol and triglyceride (TG) after 2 weeks of drug exposure. Improvement and normalization of lipid profiles were seen 4 weeks after discontinuation of the offending agent.[21] A recent systematic review of 17 randomized controlled trials revealed that kidney transplant recipients treated with mammalian target of rapamycin (mTOR) inhibitor-based immunosuppressive regimens have a higher incidence of elevated total cholesterol and TG compared to non-mTOR-treated controls.[22] Approximately 60% of mTOR inhibitor-treated patients received lipid-lowering agents (twofold higher than controls). Although only few trials (4/17) measured lipoproteins, the increases in cholesterol and TG from mTOR inhibitors

Table 15.2 Potential advantages and disadvantages of different classes of antihypertensive agents[a]

Classes of drugs	Advantages	Disadvantages
β-blockers	Perioperative use ↓ischemic heart disease	↑Risk of symptomatic bradycardia when used with non-dihydropyridine CCB Blunting of hypoglycemic awareness
CCB	↓CNI-induced renal vasoconstriction[b] ↑CNI level (may permit CNI dose reduction by up to 40%)[c]	Monotherapy with dihydropyridine CCB should be used with caution[d]
Diuretics	Beneficial in patients who are volume expanded	Hyperuricemia, gout postoperatively
ACE-I/ARB	↓Proteinuria Potential renal- and cardioprotective effects Beneficial in patients with post-transplant erythrocytosis	Potential worsening of anemia
Aldosterone receptor	May improve outcomes in heart failure	Severe hyperkalemia when used in blockers in combination with β-blockers, ACE-I/ARB or in patients with poor kidney function
β-blockers	Benign prostatic hypertrophy Neurogenic bladder	
Direct vasodilators		Tachycardia
Central alpha agonist		Depression

[a]In general there is no absolute contraindication to the use of any antihypertensive agent in renal transplant recipients.
[b]Both dihydropyridine and non-dihydropyridine CCB.
[c]Non-dihydropyridine CCB blockers.
[d]See text.
CCB: calcium channel blockers; ACE-I: angiotensin converting enzyme inhibitors; ARB: angiotensin receptor blockers.

are thought to be likely due to increases in LDL, VLDL, and non-HDL cholesterol. It is speculated that sirolimus-induced hyperlipidemia in renal transplant recipients is due to reduced catabolism of $apoB_{100}$-containing lipoproteins. In a small study consisting of five kidney transplant recipients, increases in VLDL (triglycerides) and LDL (cholesterol) after sirolimus treatment was found to coincide with higher $VLDL\text{-}apoB_{100}$ concentrations. Kinetic analysis demonstrated that sirolimus-induced increase in $VLDL\text{-}apoB_{100}$ was due to a reduction in the catabolism of $VLDL\text{-}apoB_{100}$ rather than enhanced $VLDL\text{-}apoB_{100}$ synthesis.[23]

Whether the dyslipidemic effect of mTOR inhibitors alters the risk for CVD events after kidney transplantation is currently unknown. Nonetheless, unless there is evidence to the contrary, mTOR inhibitor-induced dyslipidemia should be treated aggressively.

Other potential etiologic factors for post-transplant dyslipidemia include age, diet, rapid weight gain, hyperinsulinemia, pre-existing hypercholesterolemia, allograft dysfunction, proteinuria, and the use of β-blockers and diuretics (Table 15.3).

Table 15.3 Causative factors for post-transplant dyslipidemia (adapted and modified from Pham et al.[2])

Age
Diet
Rapid weight gain
Hyperinsulinemia
Pre-existing hypercholesterolemia
Allograft dysfunction
Proteinuria
β-blockers and diuretic therapy
Immunosuppressive agents[a]: sirolimus > corticosteroids > cyclosporine > tacrolimus

[a]See text.

Although hyperlipidemia often improves within the first 6 months after transplantation when the doses of prednisone, cyclosporine/tacrolimus or sirolimus are reduced, total and LDL cholesterol goals as defined by the National Cholesterol Education Program (NCEP) guidelines (http://www.nhlbi.nih.gov/about/ncep/index.htm) are usually not achieved and treatment is frequently still required. Management of hyperlipidemia includes therapeutic lifestyle changes and pharmacotherapy.

Statins or the HMG-CoA reductase inhibitors are the most widely used lipid-lowering agents in both the non-transplant and transplant settings. The clinical benefits of statins have been demonstrated in several large randomized controlled trials including the Heart Protection Study (HPS)[24] and the Lescol Intervention Prevention Study (LIPS).[25] Results of the Assessment of Lescol in Renal Transplantation (ALERT) study revealed that treatment of renal transplant recipients with fluvastatin over a 5- to 6-year period significantly and safely reduced LDL cholesterol levels. The incidence of major adverse cardiac events was also shown to be reduced, albeit not statistically significant. However, further analysis demonstrated a beneficial effect of early initiation of fluvastatin on outcome – the earlier the initiation of therapy, the greater the reduction in cardiac events. Patients who received statin therapy within the first 4 years post-transplant had a risk reduction of 64% compared to 19% for those who received therapy after 10 years. No statin effect on graft loss or doubling of serum creatinine was observed.[26,27] In another study, Masterson et al.[28] found better renal function at 12-month post-transplant in recipients who received statins compared to those who did not receive statin therapy (Δ creatinine clearance 6.1 ml/min, $P < 0.00$); in addition, less interstitial fibrosis was seen on protocol biopsies.

Despite the well-established efficacy and safety of the use of statins in transplant recipients, clinicians should remain vigilant to the potential drug–drug interactions in transplant patients who often require multiple medications. The use of statins in the presence of calcineurin inhibitors, particularly cyclosporine, often results in several-fold increase in statin blood level and an increased risk for myopathy and rhabdomyolysis.[29] Cyclosporine increases plasma exposure to fluvastatin by approximately 2-fold, simvastatin (20 mg/day) by 3-fold, atorvastatin by approximately 6-fold, pravastatin by 5- to 23-fold, and lovastatin by up to 20-fold. Approximate therapeutic equivalencies are achieved by 10 mg of atorvastatin, 20 mg of simvastatin, 40 mg of pravastatin, 40 mg of lovastatin, and 80 mg of fluvastatin. At these doses, the LDL cholesterol decrease is approximately 34% with very little change in HDL levels.[19] In addition to their lipid-lowering effect, statins may offer protection against CVD *via* their antiproliferative and anti-inflammatory properties and ability to reduce circulating endothelin-1, C-reactive protein levels, systolic and diastolic BP, and pulse pressure.

Other classes of lipid-lowering agents include fibric acid derivatives, nicotinic acid, bile acid sequestrants, and ezetimibe. Ezetimibe and statin combination therapy can significantly improve cholesterol control due to their complementary mechanisms of action. Ezetimibe blocks intestinal absorption of dietary cholesterol and related phytosterols whereas statin inhibits hepatic cholesterol synthesis. There has been accumulating evidence suggesting that ezetimibe used alone or as adjunctive therapy with statin is safe and effective in the treatment of dyslipidemia in renal transplant patients who are refractory to statin therapy.[30] In one single-center study consisting of 56 recipients of renal transplants, the addition of ezetimibe to statin therapy has also been shown to have a beneficial effect in preventing the decline in renal function compared to controls.[31] To date, no significant drug to drug interaction between ezetimibe and calcineurin inhibitors or sirolimus has been reported.

Drug Therapy for Hypertriglyceridemia and Non-HDL Cholesterol

Severe hypertriglyceridemia (TG >500 mg/dL) has been encountered more frequently since the introduction of sirolimus. Management includes sirolimus dose reduction, addition of a fibric acid derivative or nicotinic acid, and in refractory cases, sirolimus to MMF or tacrolimus switch. Of the major fibric acid medications (bezafibrate, ciprofibrate, fenofibrate, and gemfibrozil), the first three have been reported to cause increases in serum creatinine in cyclosporine-treated patients as well as higher plasma homocysteine levels. Although all fibrates in combinations with statins have been associated with creatinine kinase elevations with or without overt rhabdomyolysis and myopathy, gemfibrozil may have a greater risk for the development of myopathy compared to bezafibrate or fenofibrate.[19] Niacin monotherapy has not been reported to cause myopathy, but its combined use with lovastatin, pravastatin, or simvastatin may be associated with rhabdomyolysis. Bile acid sequestrants must be used with caution due to their potential interference with the absorption of other medications vital to renal transplant recipients. In addition, it should be noted that studies in the general population suggest that bile acid sequestrants may increase triglyceride levels. For a more complete list of drug to drug interaction of statins with other lipid-lowering agents, readers are referred to reference.[29]

The 2004 National Kidney Foundation Work Group suggested that statin should be the first-line therapy for the treatment of non-HDL cholesterol because of its well-established safety and efficacy in preventing CVD in randomized trials in the general population. Fibrates should be considered in those intolerant to statin despite dose reduction or despite switching to another statin.[32] Randomized controlled trials evaluating the safety and efficacy of statins and fibrates are still needed. For patients with fasting triglycerides $\geq$ 1,000 mg/dL (11.29 mmol/L), the ATP III recommends a very low fat diet (<15% total calories), medium-chain triglycerides, and fish oils to replace some long-chain triglycerides.

Suggested guidelines for pharmacological treatment of dyslipidemia are summarized in Fig. 15.1.

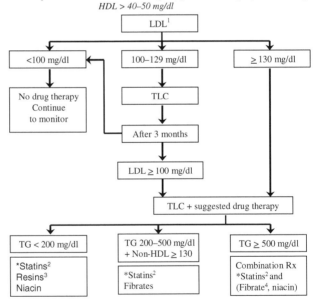

Suggested guidelines for the treatment of posttransplant dyslipidemia. *All transplant recipients should be regarded as CHD risk equivalent. Goals: LDL < 100 mg/dl (optional < 70 mg/dl), TG < 200 mg/dl, HDL > 40–50 mg/dl*

*If LDL targets not achieved with statin monotherapy consider statins + cholesterol absorption inhibitors[5] combination

[1]LDL < 70 mg/dl has been suggested for very high risk patients (NCEP, ATP III guidelines); [2]Statins are the most effective drugs and should be the agents of first choice. Start at low dose in patients on cyclosporine and tacrolimus. Monitor for myositis and transaminitis, particularly in those receiving combination therapy; [3]Bile acid sequestrans should probably not be taken at the same time as cyclosporine; [4]Extreme caution should be used with statin and fibrate combination therapy; [5]Consider cholesterol absorption inhibitors in patients intolerant to statins. TLC: therapeutic lifestyle change (see text);TG: triglyceride.

Fig. 15.1 Suggested guidelines for the treatment of post-transplant dyslipidemia

Cigarette Smoking

Similar to the general population, cigarette smoking is associated with increased CVD morbidity and mortality in renal transplant recipients. In an observational case-controlled study consisting of 780 renal transplant recipients Chuang et al.[33] demonstrated that smoking was associated with a 3.5-fold increase in acute coronary syndrome within 2 years after transplantation (OR 3.56, $P=0.034$), with the majority of cases occurring perioperatively or within the first 3 post-transplant months. Similarly, in one single-center study consisting of 1,334 renal transplant recipients in whom smoking history was available, Kasiske et al.[34] demonstrated that an 11–25 pack-year and a > 25 pack-year history of smoking at transplant resulted in a 56% and a > 100% increase in the risk for major CVD events, respectively (RR 1.56, $P=0.024$, and RR 2.14, $P < 0.001$, respectively). Compared to smoking less than 25 pack-years or no smoking, smoking more than 25 pack-years at transplant was associated with a 30% increased risk of graft failure whereas smoking cessation 5 years before transplantation reduced the relative risk of graft failure by 34% (RR 0.66, $P < 0.001$). Further analysis suggested that the adverse impact of smoking on graft survival was due to an increase in mortality (adjusted RR 1.42, $P=0.012$). Smoking cessation 5 years before transplantation reduced the risk of death by 29% (RR 0.71, $P=0.0304$). Every effort should be made to encourage patients to quit smoking. A multifaceted approach including behavioral and pharmacologic strategies appears to be most effective. To date, there have been no reports of important drug–drug interactions between currently available immunosuppressive agents and nicotine-replacement therapies.

Obesity

Obesity is a potentially detrimental condition due to its associated comorbid conditions including hyperinsulinemia and insulin resistance, diabetes mellitus, dyslipidemia, and hypertension. Obesity defined as body mass index (BMI) $\geq 30 \, \text{kg/m}^2$ has a reported prevalence of 9.5–29% at transplantation.[35] Studies in renal transplant recipients have shown that high BMI at transplant is a significant independent predictor of congestive heart failure (CHF) and atrial fibrillation. In three large historic cohort studies using the United Renal Data System Registry database, Abbott et al.[36] and Lentine et al.[35] demonstrated that a BMI ≥ 30 predicted a 43–59% relative risk increase in CHF compared to a BMI of < 30. In one registry study, a BMI > 28.3 independently predicted a 79% relative increase in the risk of hospitalized atrial fibrillation compared with a BMI of ≤ 28.3.[37] The impact of BMI on cardiac-related death has been shown to follow a U-shaped risk. In a large registry study consisting of 51,927 renal allograft recipients, the adjusted risk of cardiac death increased at both low and high BMI compared to a reference group with a BMI of 22–24 (aHR 1.3 for BMI < 20; aHR 1.2 for BMI 30–32; aHR 1.4 for BMI > 36).

In the post-transplant setting, excessive weight gain or obesity may become a problem for many patients. Patients on prednisone therapy may over-eat as they often experience constant hunger or craving for sweets. In addition, the release from pre-transplant dietary restriction and habitual physical inactivity can result in rapid post-transplant weight gain. Studies in liver transplant recipients revealed that tacrolimus immunosuppression is associated with a lower likelihood of post-transplant weight gain compared to cyclosporine (27% vs. 46%, respectively).[38] Nonetheless, cyclosporine has not consistently been found to be an independent predictor of post-transplant obesity.[2] Other suggested predictors for increased weight gain after transplantation include pre-transplant obesity, greater donor BMI, and higher cumulative doses of prednisone. It has been suggested that the steroid-sparing effect of tacrolimus may account for its lower likelihood of post-transplant weight gain compared to that of cyclosporine treatment.

Management of post-transplant obesity includes lifestyle and dietary modification. Enrollment in a diet support group and/or exercise program can be invaluable. Steroid reduction or withdrawal must be balanced against the risk of allograft rejection and graft loss. The use of pharmacologic agents for weight reduction in the post-transplant period is currently not recommended due to unknown potential drug–drug interactions. In morbidly obese patients, gastric bypass surgery has been shown to be a safe and effective means for achieving significant long-term weight loss and relief of comorbid conditions after transplantation. There is a paucity of data on the safety and efficacy of post-transplant gastric bypass surgery in ameliorating comorbid conditions such as hypertension, diabetes mellitus, or dyslipidemia. However, with the refinement in surgical techniques and advancement in postoperative care, post-transplant bariatric surgery for morbid obesity should be explored. Pre-transplant laparoscopic adjustable gastric banding has also been suggested to be an option for morbidly obese patients who would otherwise be denied for renal transplantation.[39]

Unconventional CVD Risk Factors

Hyperhomocysteinemia

Hyperhomocysteinemia occurs in about two-thirds of renal transplant recipients. In a single-center prospective study of 733 renal transplant recipients, baseline-elevated fasting plasma total homocysteine levels were independently associated with risk of death and kidney allograft loss.[40] Several randomized controlled trials of homocysteine lowering in at-risk CKD patients showed no beneficial effect on CVD risk reduction.[41,42]

Important determinants of total plasma homocysteine levels include folate, B_6 (pyridoxine), B_{12} (cyanocolabamin), and impaired renal function. The Folic Acid for Vascular Outcome Reduction in Renal Transplantation study (FAVORIT) is a multicenter double-blind randomized controlled clinical trial to evaluate whether lowering total homocysteine with either a high or low dose of folic acid (10 or 5 mg), vitamin B_6 (50 or 1.4 mg), and vitamin B_{12} (1,000 or 2 μg) reduces CVD events in stable renal transplant recipients with elevated total homocysteine levels. This is a large multicenter study consisting of more than 4,000 long-term stable renal transplant recipients with a planned follow-up of 4.5–9 years. It is expected that an extended period of follow-up may permit detection of a lag in the treatment effect, a focus not considered in most previous clinical trials.[43] Further recommendations on the use of vitamin supplement to lower CVD risks await definitive results from the FAVORIT study.

Proteinuria

Proteinuria occurs in 9–40% of kidney transplant recipients with a functioning allograft.[1] As in the non-transplant setting, post-transplantation proteinuria has been shown to be an independent risk factor for CVD. In a retrospective study consisting of over 500 Caucasian patients who received a deceased donor renal transplant and had a functioning allograft for longer than a year, Fernandez-Fresnedo et al.[44] found that compared to "no proteinuria," persistent proteinuria (defined as urine protein excretion greater than 0.5 g/day during more than 6 months; mean follow-up: 6.41 ± 3.6 years) was associated with increased mortality and graft loss (relative risk of death and graft loss; RR =1.92 and RR =4.18, respectively) and a higher incidence of CVD (RR=2.45). Similarly, Roodnat et al.[45] reported a nearly twofold risk of death in renal transplant recipients with a functioning allograft and proteinuria at 1 year compared to those without proteinuria.

  Controlled trials evaluating the beneficial effect of treating proteinuria in reducing CVD risk in the setting of renal transplantation are lacking. Nonetheless, unless contraindicated, ACE-I or ARB or both should be considered in transplant recipients with microalbuminuria or overt proteinuria due to their well-established renoprotective, antiproteinuric, and cardioprotective effects. Whether the development of proteinuria associated with sirolimus adversely affects CVD risks is currently unknown and warrants close monitoring.

Anemia

Anemia after renal transplantation has a reported prevalence of 20–80%. The wide variation in the prevalence reported is due in part to the variable definitions of anemia, immunosuppressive medications, time post-transplantation, duration of follow-up, and level of allograft function, among others. Similar to the general population and patients with chronic kidney disease, anemia adversely affects CVD in kidney transplant recipients. In a multivariate analysis of over 400 recipients of kidney alone or simultaneous kidney–pancreas transplants, Djamali et al.[46] found that diabetic transplant recipients with a hematocrit level greater than 30% were less likely to suffer from a CVD event (myocardial infarction, cardiovascular death, angina, and congestive heart failure) in the first 6 post-transplant months compared to those with a hematocrit level less than or equal to 30% (RR=0.65, P=0.22). Similarly, in a retrospective study involving consecutive de novo MMF-treated kidney recipients from the Hospital of the University of Pennsylvania between 1996 and 2002, Imoagene-Oyedeji et al.[47] revealed that the cohort with anemia at 12 months, defined as hemoglobin less than 12 g/dL, had inferior patient survival

(P=0.02, log rank) and a higher proportion of cardiovascular deaths (6.3% vs. 2.2%; P=0.017) compared to the non-anemic patients. Nonetheless, the CHOIR (Correction of Hemoglobin and Outcomes in Renal Insufficiency) study unexpectedly demonstrated increased cardiovascular events among stage 3–4 CKD patients randomized to normalization of anemia with epoetin-alpha.[48] Similarly, the CREATE (Cardiac Risk Reduction by Early Anemia Treatment with Epoetin beta) study showed a higher absolute number of cardiac events and a higher rate of dialysis event in CKD patients with hemoglobin values > 13 g/dL. Of interest, post hoc analysis of the CHOIR study suggested that toxicities related to high-dose epoetin-alpha might have contributed to worse outcomes among subjects with higher targets particularly among those who did not achieve their target hemoglobin.[49]

Studies evaluating the association between normalization of hemoglobin levels and cardiovascular disease in renal transplantation are lacking. However, until further evidence is available, the goal for anemia correction in renal transplant recipients should probably be to achieve hemoglobin levels in the 11–12 range as recommended by the K/DOQI practice guidelines. It is currently not known whether erythropoiesis-stimulating agents have a beneficial effect on CVD risk factor reduction beyond correction of post-transplant anemia alone.

Coronary Artery Calcification (CAC)

Coronary artery calcification as measured by electron beam computerized tomography (EBCT) has been studied as a non-invasive technique to diagnose coronary artery disease and as a surrogate marker of coronary plaque load. CAC as detected by EBCT has a reported sensitivity and specificity of 97 and 72%, respectively, to detect $\geq$ 50% stenosis identified angiographically.[50] Most currently available prognostic data on CAC scores were based on EBCT measurements. However, more recently CAC scoring using multidetector computed tomographic (MDCT) scanners has gained popularity in clinical practice. More importantly, Mao et al.[51] have recently demonstrated that CAC scores obtained with EBCT or newer generation 64-MDCT scanners were comparable in both Agatston score and volume score. The same group of investigators has also shown that for CAC scoring, interscan variability with newer-generation 16- and 64-MDCT scanners was similar but not superior to that with the EBCT scanner.[52]

There has been accumulating literature suggesting that CAC is a strong independent predictor of future cardiac events. However, the value of the assessment of CAC by EBCT or MDCT scanners as an independent predictor of cardiac events and a replacement for more invasive monitoring remains to be determined. Nonetheless, it should be noted that accelerated progression of CAC has been shown to be associated with higher cardiac event rates.[53] Hence, transplant recipients with CAC should be considered for aggressive risk factor reduction.

Post-transplant Screening for Cardiovascular Disease

Guidelines for cardiovascular screening of the post-transplant patients are lacking. However, early diagnosis and aggressive management of conventional CVD risk factors such as diabetes, dyslipidemia, and hypertension should be reinforced. Studies to determine the best predictive tool for identifying patients at risk for developing new onset diabetes mellitus after transplantation (NODAT) early following transplantation are scarce. Nonetheless, fasting plasma glucose should be tested at regular intervals. The utility of oral glucose tolerance test (OGTT) in the early post-transplant period as a predictor for the NODAT is currently not known and awaits studies. The routine care of patients with diabetes mellitus should include an evaluation of hemoglobin A1C level every 3 months. Fasting lipid profile should be measured annually. In transplant recipients with multiple CVD risk factors, more frequent monitoring of lipid profile should be performed at the discretion of the clinicians. Diabetes as the cause of end-stage renal disease, advanced age, and pre-transplant cardiovascular events are the most important pre-transplant predictors for post-transplant cardiovascular events. Controversies exist regarding the appropriateness of cardiac stress testing and the best screening stress test in asymptomatic renal transplant recipients. In the authors' opinion, annual or periodic screening of high-risk asymptomatic individuals is probably warranted.

Summary

Although there is no consensus on the optimal approach to the management of CVD risk in renal transplant recipients, identifying the high-risk patient and implementing primary prevention is probably the best treatment strategy. All transplant recipients should be regarded as coronary heart disease risk equivalent and, unless contraindicated, early treatment with statins, and/or beta-blockers and antiplatelets, should be considered. The beneficial effects of ACE-Is or ARBs on post-transplant patient and graft survival have not been consistently demonstrated. Further recommendations on their routine use in the post-transplant period await large, randomized controlled clinical trials. Nonetheless, unless contraindicated, ACE-I or ARB or both should be considered in transplant recipients with microalbuminuria or overt proteinuria due to their well-established renoprotective, antiproteinuric, and cardioprotective effects. Target low-density lipoprotein (LDL) concentrations should be maintained at less than 100 mg/dL (optimal < 70 mg/dL), HDL > 40 mg/dL for men and > 50 mg/dL for women. Immunosuppressive protocols should be tailored to each individual patient based on their immunological and CVD risk factor profiles. Clinicians must be familiar with the patients' immune history prior to manipulating their immunosuppressive therapy.

In addition to pharmacological treatment, emphasis should be placed on lifestyle modifications including moderation of dietary sodium and saturated fat intake, regular aerobic exercise, weight reduction, and tobacco avoidance. The management of post-transplant CVD requires a multidisciplinary approach where every potential complicating factor must be closely monitored and treated.

References

1. Meier-Kriesche HU, Schold JD, Kaplan B. Preservation of long-term renal allograft survival: a challenge for the years to come. *Am J Transplant* 2005;5:632–633.
2. Pham PT, Pham PC, Danovitch GM. Cardiovascular disease posttransplant. *Semin Nephrol* 2007;27(4):430–444.
3. Ojo AO. Cardiovascular complications after renal transplantation and their prevention. *Transplantation* 2006;82:603–611.
4. Opelz G, Wujciak T, Ritz E et al. Association of chronic kidney graft failure with recipient blood pressure. *Kidney Int* 1998;53:217–222.
5. Kasiske BL, Anjum S, Shah R et al. Hypertension after transplantation. *Am J Kidney Dis* 2004;43:1071–1081.
6. Premasathian NC, Muehrer R, Brazy PC et al. Blood pressure control in kidney transplantation. Therapeutic implications. *J Hum Hypertens* 2004;18:871–877.
7. Fricke L, Doehn C, Steinhoff J et al. Treatment of posttransplant hypertension by laparoscopic bilateral nephrectomy? *Transplantation* 1998;65(9):1182–1187.
8. Kreis H, Oberbauer R, Camoistol JM. Long-term benefits with sirolimus-based therapy after early cyclosporine withdrawal. *J Am Soc Nephrol* 2004;15:809–817.
9. Margreiter R, Pohanka E, Sparacio V et al. Open prospective multicenter study of conversion to tacrolimus therapy in renal transplant patients experiencing cyclosporine-related side effects. *Transplant Int* 2005;18(7):816–823.
10. Ligtenberg G, Hene RJ, Blankestijn PJ et al. Cardiovascular risk factors in renal transplant patients: cyclosporine A versus tacrolimus. *J Am Soc Nephrol* 2001;12(2):368–373.
11. Pascual J, Van Hooff JP, Salmela K. Three-year observational follow-up of a multicenter, randomized trial on tacrolimus-based therapy with withdrawal of steroids or mycophenolate mofetil after renal transplantation. *Transplantation* 2006;85:55–61.
12. EBPG Expert Group on Renal Transplantation. European best practice guidelines for renal transplantation. Section IV: Long-term management of the transplant recipient. IV.5.2. Cardiovascular risks. Arterial hypertension. *Nephrol Dial Transplant* 2000;17:25–26, [Abstract].
13. Kasiske BL, Chakkera H, Roel J. Explained and unexplained ischemic heart disease risk after renal transplantation. *J Am Soc Nephrol* 2001;11:1735–1743.
14. Brenner BM, Cooper ME, de Zeeuw D et al. Effects of losartan on renal and cardiovascular outcomes in patients with type 2 diabetes and nephropathy. *N Engl J Med* 2001;345:861–869.
15. Agoda LY, Appel L, Bakris GL et al. Effect of ramipril vs amlodipine on renal outcomes in hypertensive nephrosclerosis: a randomised controlled trial. *JAMA* 2001;285:2719–2728.
16. De C, Karas M, Nguyen P et al. Different effects of nifedipine and amlodipine on circulating catecholamines levels in essential hypertensive patients. *J Hypertens* 1998;16:1357–1369.
17. The ALLHAT Officers and Coordinators for the ALLHAT Collaborative Research Group. Major outcomes in high-risk hypertensive patients randomized to angiotensin-converting enzyme inhibitor or calcium channel blockers vs diuretic: The Antihypertensive and Lipid-Lowering Treatment to Prevent Heart Attack Trial (ALLHAT). *JAMA* 2002;288:2981–2997.
18. Hiremath S, Fergusson D, Doucette S et al. Renin angiotensin system blockade in kidney transplantation: a systematic review of the evidence. *Am J Transplant* 2007;7:2350–2360.
19. Jennings DL, Taber DJ. Use of rennin-angiotensin-aldosterone inhibitors within the first eight to twelve weeks after renal transplantation. *Ann Pharm Ther* 2008;42(1):116–120.
20. Tylicki L, Biedunkiewicz B, Chamienia A et al. Renal allograft protection with angiotensin II type 1 receptor antagonists. *Am J Transplant* 2007;7:243–248.

21. Miller LW. Cardiovascular toxicities of immunosuppressive agents. *Am J Transplant* 2002;2:807–818.

22. Kasiske BL, de Mattos A, Flechner SM et al. Mammalian target of rapamycin inhibitor dyslipidemia in kidney transplant recipients. *Am J Transplant* 2008;8:1384–1392.

23. Hoogeven RC, Ballantyne CM, Pownall HJ et al. Effect of sirolimus on the metabolism of apoB100-containing lipoproteins. *Transplantation* 2001;72:1244–1250.

24. Collins R, Armitage J, Parish J et al. Effects of cholesterol-lowering with simvastatin on stroke and other major vascular events in 20536 people with cerebrovascular disease or other high-risk conditions. *Lancet* 2004;363(9411):757–767.

25. Messereli AW, Aronow HD, Sprecker DL. The Lescol Intervention Prevention Study (LIPS): start all patients on statin early after PCI. *Clev Clin J Med* 2003;70:561–566.

26. Holdaas H, Fellstrom B, Jardin AG et al. Beneficial effects of early initiation of lipid-lowering therapy following renal transplantation. *Nephrol Dial Transplant* 2005;20:974–980.

27. Fellstrom B, Holdaas H, Jardine AG et al. Effects of fluvastatin end points in the Assessment of Lescol in renal transplantation (ALERT) trial. *Kidney Int* 2004;66:1549–1555.

28. Masterson R, Hweitson T, Leikis M et al. Impact of statin treatment on 1-year functional and histologic renal allograft outcome. *Transplantation* 2005;80:332–338.

29. Ballantyne CM, Corsini A, Davidson MH et al. Risk for myopathy with statin therapy in high-risk patients. *Arch Intern Med* 2003;163:553–564.

30. Chuang P, Langone AJ. Ezetimide reduces low-density lipoprotein cholesterol (LDL-C) in renal transplant patients resistant to HMG-CoA reductase inhibitors. *Am J Ther* 2007;14(5):438–441.

31. Turk TR, Voropaeva E, Kohnle M et al. Ezetimide treatment in hypercholesterolemic kidney transplant patients is safe and effective and reduces the decline of renal allograft function: a pilot study. *Nephrol Dial Transplant* 2008;23(1):369–373.

32. Kasiske BL, Cosio FG, Beto J et al. Clinical practice guidelines for managing dyslipidemias in kidney transplant patients: a report from the Managing Dyslipidemias in chronic Kidney Disease Work Group of the National Kidney Foundation Kidney Disease Outcomes Quality Initiative. *Am J Transplant* 2004;4(Suppl 7):13–53.

33. Chuang P, Gibney EM, Chan L et al. Predictors of cardiovascular events and associated mortality within two years of kidney transplantation. *Transplant Proc* 2004;36(5):1387–1391.

34. Kasiske BL, Klinger D. Cigarette smoking in renal transplant recipients. *J Am Soc Nephrol* 2000;11(4):753–759.

35. Lentine KL, Rocca-Rey LA, Bacchi G et al. Obesity and cardiac risk after kidney transplantation: Experience at one center and comprehensive literature review. *Transplantation* 2008;86(2):303–312.

36. Abbott KC, Yuan CM, Taylor AJ et al. Early renal insufficiency and hospitalized heart disease after renal transplantation in the era of modern immunosuppression. *J Am Soc Nephrol* 2003;14:2358–2365.

37. Abbott KC, Reynolds JC, Taylor AJ et al. Hospitalized atrial fibrillation after renal transplantation in the United States. *Am J Transplant* 2003;3:471–476.

38. Canzanello VJ, Schwartz L, Tater SJ et al. Evolution of cardiovascular risk after liver transplantation: a comparison of cyclosporine A and tacrolimus FK(506). *Liver Transplant Surg* 1997;3:1–9.

39. Newcombe V, Blanch A, Slater GH et al. Laparoscopic adjustable gastric banding prior to renal transplantation. *Obes Surg* 2005;15:567–570.

40. Wikelmayer WC, Kramer R, Curhan GC et al. Fasting plasma total homocysteine levels and mortality and allograft loss in kidney transplant recipients: a prospective study. *J Am Soc Nephrol* 2005;16:255–260.

41. Zoungas S, McGrath BP, Branley P et al. Cardiovascular morbidity and mortality in the Atherosclerosis and Folic acid Supplementation trial (ASFAST) in chronic renal failure: A multicenter, randomized, controlled trial. *J Am Coll Cardiol* 2006;47:1108–1116.

42. Mann JF, Sheridan P, McQueen MJ et al. Homocysteine lowering with folic acid and B vitamins in people with chronic kidney – results of the renal HOPE-2 study. *Nephrol Dial Transplant* 2008;23:645–653.
43. Bostom AG, Carpenter MA, Hunsicker L et al. Baseline characteristics of participants in the Folic Acid for Vascular Outcome Reduction in Transplantation (FAVORIT) Trial. *Am J Kidney Dis* 2009;53:121–128.
44. Fernando-Fresnedo G, Escallada R, Rodrigo E et al. The risk of cardiovascular disease associated with proteinuria in renal transplant patients. *Transplantation* 2002;73:1345–1348.
45. Roodnat JJ, Mulder PG, Rischen-Vos J et al. Proteinuria after renal transplantation affects not only graft survival but also patient survival. *Transplantation* 2001;72:438–444.
46. Djamali A, Becker YT, Simmons WD et al. Increasing hematocrit reduces early posttransplant cardiovascular risk in diabetic transplant recipients. *Transplantation* 2003;76:816–820.
47. Imoagene-Oyedeji AE, Rosas SE, Doyle AM et al. Posttransplant anemia at 12 months in kidney recipients treated with mycophenolate mofetil: risk factors and implications for mortality. *J Am Soc Nephrol* 2006;17:3240–3247.
48. Singh AK, Szczech L, Tang KL et al. Correction of anemia with epoetin alfa in chronic kidney disease. *N Engl J Med* 2006;355(20):2085–2098.
49. Szczech L, Barnhart HX, Inrig JK et al. Secondary analysis of the CHOIR trial epoetin-α dose and achieved hemoglobin outcomes. *Kidney Int* 2008;74:791–798.
50. Ishitani MB, Milliner DS, Kim DY et al. Early subclinical coronary artery calcification in young adults who were pediatric kidney transplant recipients. *Am J Transplant* 2005;5: 1689–1693.
51. Mao SS, Pal RS, McKay CR et al. Comparison of coronary artery calcium scores between electron beam computed tomography and 64-Multidetector Computed Tomographic scanner. *J Comput Assist Tomogr* 2009;33(2):175–178.
52. Budoff MJ, McClelland RI, Chung H et al. Reproducibility of coronary artery calcified plaque with cardiac 64-MDCT: The Multi-Ethnic Study of Atherosclerosis. *Am J Roentgenol* 2009;192(3):613–617.
53. Budoff MJ, Achenbach S, Blumenthal RS et al. Assessment of coronary artery disease by cardiac computed tomography: a scientific statement from the American Heart Association Committee on Cardiovascular Imaging and Intervention, and Committee on Cardiac Imaging. Council on Clinical Cardiology. *Circulation* 2006;114:1761–1791.

Chapter 16
Diabetes Mellitus and Transplantation: Risks for Post-transplant Diabetes

Phuong-Thu T. Pham, Phuong-Mai T. Pham, and Alan H. Wilkinson

Introduction

New onset diabetes mellitus after transplantation (NODAT) is a serious and frequently observed complication following solid organ transplantation. Kidney transplant recipients who develop NODAT are at increased risk of fatal and non-fatal cardiovascular events and other adverse outcomes including infection, reduced patient survival, graft rejection, and accelerated graft loss compared with those who do not develop diabetes. Identification of high-risk patients and implementation of measures to reduce the development of NODAT may improve long-term patient and graft outcome. The following chapter presents an overview of the literature on the current diagnostic criteria for NODAT, its incidence after solid organ transplantation, suggested risk factors, and potential pathogenic mechanisms. The impact of NODAT on patient and allograft outcomes and suggested guidelines for early identification and management of NODAT will also be discussed.

Definition and Diagnosis of New Onset Diabetes After Transplantation

Over the years, the precise incidence of NODAT has been difficult to determine due to the lack of a standard definition for the condition. Historically, post-transplant diabetes has been variably defined as having random glucose levels greater than 200 mg/dL or fasting glucose levels greater than 140 mg/dL, or the need for insulin therapy in the post-transplant period. In 2003, the International Expert Panel consisting of experts from both the transplant and diabetes fields set forth the International Consensus Guidelines for the diagnosis and management of NODAT.[1,2] It was recommended that the definition and diagnosis of NODAT should be based on the

P.-T.T. Pham (✉)
Division of Nephrology, Department of Medicine, Kidney and Pancreas Transplant Program, David Geffen School of Medicine at UCLA, Los Angeles, CA, USA
e-mail: ppham@mednet.ucla.edu

D.B. McKay, S.M. Steinberg (eds.), *Kidney Transplantation: A Guide to the Care of Kidney Transplant Recipients*, DOI 10.1007/978-1-4419-1690-7_16, © Springer Science+Business Media, LLC 2010

definition of diabetes mellitus and impaired glucose tolerance (IGT) described by the World Health Organization (WHO).[2] The diabetes guidelines acknowledge that both impaired fasting glucose (IFG) and IGT are important predictive factors for the progression to overt diabetes and are well-established risk factors for microvascular and cardiovascular disease.[3] The current WHO and American Diabetes Association (ADA) guidelines for the diagnosis of prediabetic states (IFG and IGT) and diabetes mellitus are provided in Table 16.1 (modified from Davidson et al.[1]).

Table 16.1 WHO and 2003 updated ADA criteria for the diagnosis of diabetes mellitus

Criteria for the diagnosis of diabetes mellitus
- Symptoms[a] of diabetes mellitus + casual[b] PG concentrations ≥ 200 mg/dL (11.1 mM)

Or
- FPG ≥ 126 mg/dL (7.0 mM). Fasting is defined as no caloric intake for at least 8 h

Or
- 2-h PG ≥ 200 mg/dL (11.1 mM) during an oral glucose tolerance test[c]

A confirmatory laboratory test based on measurements of venous PG must be done on another day in the absence of unequivocal hyperglycemia accompanied by acute metabolic decompensation

Criteria for normal FPG and IFG or IGT
FPG

WHO criteria
FPG < 110 mg/dL (6.1 mM) = normal fasting glucose
FPG ≥ 110 mg/dL (6.1 mM) and < 126 mg/dL (7.0 mM) = IFG

2003 ADA updated consensus report
FPG < 100 mg/dL (5.6 mM) = normal fasting glucose
FPG ≥ 100 mg/dL (5.6 mM) and < 126 mg/dL (7.0 mM) = IFG
or
OGTT
2-h PG < 140 mg/dL (7.8 mM) = normal glucose tolerance
2-h PG ≥ 140 mg/dL (7.8 mM) and < 200 mg/dL (11.1 nM) = IGT

WHO: World Health Organization; PG: plasma glucose; FPG: fasting plasma glucose; IFG: impaired fasting glucose; IGT: impaired glucose tolerance; OGTT: oral glucose tolerance test.
[a]Classic symptoms of diabetes include polyuria, polydipsia, and unexplained weight loss.
[b]Casual is defined as any time of day without regard to time since last meal.
[c]OGTT: the test should be performed as described by WHO, using a glucose load containing equivalent of 75 g anhydrous glucose dissolved in water.

Incidence

New onset diabetes mellitus after transplantation has been reported to occur in 4–25% of renal transplant recipients, 2.5–25% of liver transplant recipients, and 2–53% of all solid organ transplants.[1,4,5] The variation in the reported incidence may be due in part to the lack of a standard definition of the condition, the duration of follow-up, and the presence of both modifiable and non-modifiable risks factors. Over the last decade, HCV infection has increasingly been recognized as a risk factor for NODAT. In HCV-infected liver recipients, the prevalence of post-transplant diabetes ranges between 40 and 60%.[4-6] Similar to the non-transplant settings, the use of fasting plasma glucose (FPG) vs. oral glucose tolerance test (OGTT) to define diabetes mellitus also changes the prevalence of NODAT. In a prospective study designed to evaluate the use of OGTT for risk-stratifying patients for NODAT, Sharif et al.[7] demonstrated that among 122 renal transplant recipients without diabetes who had two FPG level measurements within the range of 100–125 mg/dL (5.6–6.9 mmol/L) for more than 6 months after transplantation, OGTTs revealed that 10% had overt diabetes mellitus, 9% had IGT alone, 18% had IFG alone (all defined by WHO criteria), and 14% had combined IFG and IGT.

Risk Factors for NODAT

Although risk factors for developing diabetes after transplantation may vary among studies, commonly reported predisposing factors include African American and Hispanic ethnicity, obesity defined as BMI $\geq$ 30 kg/m^2, age older than 40–45 years, family history of diabetes among first-degree relatives, impaired glucose tolerance before transplantation or presence of other components of the metabolic syndrome, recipients of deceased donor kidneys, hepatitis C infection, and immunosuppressive therapy including corticosteroids, and the calcineurin inhibitors (CNIs) tacrolimus (Tac) and, to a lesser extent, cyclosporine (CSA).[8] The antimetabolites azathioprine and mycophenolate mofetil (MMF) have not been shown to be diabetogenic. On the contrary, the concomitant use of MMF has been suggested to mitigate the diabetogenic effect of tacrolimus.[9] It is conceivable that the use of azathioprine or MMF allows clinicians to use lower doses of other diabetogenic immunosuppressive medications.

Early clinical trials suggest that sirolimus is devoid of diabetogenic effect. However, subsequent studies in animal models and in recipients of renal transplants suggest that sirolimus is associated with reduced insulin sensitivity and a defect in the compensatory β-cell response.[10,11] Studies in diabetic mice transplanted with islet cells suggest that sirolimus is associated with reduced islet engraftment and impaired β-cell function.

Other potential risk factors for the development of NODAT include the presence of certain HLA antigens such as A30, B27, and B42, increasing HLA mismatches, acute rejection history, CMV infection, male gender recipient, and male donor.[8] Polycystic kidney disease has been suggested to confer an increased risk of developing diabetes after renal transplantation in some studies but not in others.[12-15] Suggested risk factors for NODAT are summarized in Fig. 16.1. The following section provides an overview of the literature on non-modifiable and modifiable risk factors.

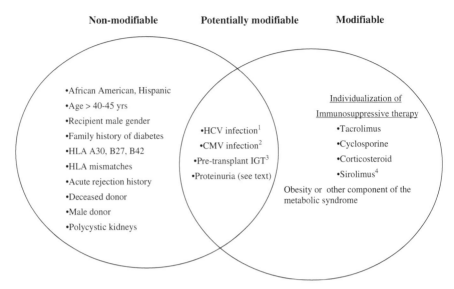

Abbreviations: HLA: human leukocyte antigen; HCV: hepatitis C virus; CMV: cytomegalovirus; IGT: impaired glucose tolerance

[1]Consider pre-tx treatment of HCV (see text). [2]Aggressive post-Tx CMV prophylaxis. [3]Counseling on life style modifications. [4]Further studies are needed.

Fig. 16.1 Risk factors for NODAT

Non-modifiable Risk Factors

Age

Older age has long been observed to be an important risk factor for the development of NODAT. In a single-center study consisting of 2,078 non-diabetic renal transplant recipients receiving cyclosporine-based immunosuppression, Cosio et al.[16] demonstrated that transplant recipients older than 45 years of age were 2.2 times more likely to develop NODAT than those who were younger than 45 at the time of transplantation ($P < 0.0001$). In their study, NODAT was defined as the need for hypoglycemic medications, starting more than 30 days after transplantation. Similarly, in an analysis of the US Renal Data System (USRDS) consisting of over 11,000 Medicare beneficiaries who received primary kidney transplants between 1996 and 2000, Kasiske et al. showed a strong association between older age and NODAT. Compared to a reference range of 18–44 years of age, transplant recipients between the age of 45 and 59 years had a relative risk for NODAT of 1.9 ($P < 0.0001$), whereas those who were ≥ 60 years of age had a relative risk of 2.09 ($P < 0.0001$).[9] The presence of NODAT was identified using data from Medicare claims.[17] Despite the heterogeneity in the diagnostic criteria used to define NODAT, the overall incidence of NODAT in this study (16% in 1 year) is in the range reported in randomized controlled trials (5–25%).

Race/Ethnicity

There has been ample literature suggesting that African Americans and Hispanics are at increased risk for developing NODAT compared to whites. In a single-center retrospective study consisting of 122 renal transplant recipients, the risk of developing NODAT as defined by the 2003 International guidelines was double in African Americans compared to whites.[18] Similarly, data from the USRDS demonstrated that NODAT was more common among African Americans (RR = 1.68, $P < 0.0001$) and Hispanics (RR = 1.35, $P < 0.0001$) compared with Caucasians. The difference in the incidence of NODAT in patients of different ethnicity has been suggested to be due in part to the differential pharmacokinetics and diabetogenic effects of immunosuppressive agents.[3] African Americans have been reported to require 37% higher dose of tacrolimus to achieve whole blood trough concentrations comparable to those observed in Caucasians.[1] In one study, the mean dose of tacrolimus was 98% higher in African Americans than the mean dose in Caucasians and Asians.[19] Tacrolimus has also been reported to have particularly potent diabetogenic effects in African Americans compared with whites.[1]

Family History of Diabetes Mellitus

Similar to type 2 diabetes in the general population, both genetic and environmental factors have been suggested to play a role in the development of NODAT. There is strong evidence suggesting that individuals with a family history of diabetes among first-degree relatives have an increased risk of developing NODAT with one study reporting a sevenfold increase in the condition.[1] The increased prevalence of NODAT associated with a family history of diabetes has been documented across all types of solid organ transplantation. In a Spanish multicenter cross-sectional study consisting of 1,410 recipients of kidney transplants, 489 liver transplants, 207 heart transplants, and 72 lung transplants, a positive family history of diabetes was associated with a 50% increase in the risk of developing NODAT (odds ratio of 1.51).[20]

Miscellaneous

Increasing HLA mismatches, DR mismatch, the presence of certain HLA antigens such as A30, B27, and B42, acute rejection history, polycystic kidney disease, male gender recipient, male donor, and deceased donor allografts have variably been reported to be associated with an increased risk of NODAT.[16,21]

Modifiable Risk Factors

Corticosteroid-Associated NODAT

The now well-established contributory role of corticosteroid on NODAT was first described by Starlz in 1964 in renal transplant recipients.[16,22] The diabetogenic effect of corticosteroids has been suggested to be dose-dependent. In a prospective study of 173 consecutive kidney transplant recipients, overt NODAT and glucose intolerance as assessed by oral glucose tolerance test developed in 18 and 31%, respectively, at 10 weeks after transplantation. A significant relationship between prednisolone dose and glucose intolerance was demonstrated by both univariate and multivariate linear regression analysis. A 0.01 mg/kg/day increase in prednisolone dose was associated with a 5% risk of developing NODAT.[23] Hjelmesaeth et al.[24] first demonstrated that oral prednisolone dose reduction to 5 mg daily significantly improves glucose tolerance during the first year after transplantation. Multiple linear regression analysis revealed that each 1-mg reduction of prednisolone dose led to an estimated decline in 2-h blood glucose of 0.12 mmol/L. In a small study involving 57 stable renal transplant recipients, Midtvedt et al.[25] found that prednisolone dose reduction from a mean of 16 mg daily (range 10–30) to 9 mg (range 5–12.5) resulted in an average increase in insulin sensitivity index of 24%. However, complete withdrawal of 5 mg/day of prednisolone did not influence insulin sensitivity significantly. Whether complete withdrawal of chronic low-dose corticosteroid therapy (prednisolone 5 mg daily) improves glucose metabolism remains to be studied. The dose-dependent diabetogenic effect of corticosteroid was also observed in recipients of non-renal organ transplants. In a retrospective review involving 88 heart transplant recipients, Depczynski et al.[26] found that patients who developed NODAT had received higher mean doses of prednisolone at 3 months compared with those who remained free of diabetes at a mean follow-up of 27 months (0.21 ± 0.03 vs. 0.19 ± 0.03 mg/kg/day, $P < 0.01$).

Experimental animal models have shown that corticosteroids affect glucose metabolism by increasing hepatic glucose production and by reducing peripheral insulin sensitivity.[27] Both insulin resistance and relative insulin deficiency have been suggested to play a role in the development of steroid-induced NODAT. Steroid-sparing or steroid withdrawal protocols in the early post-transplant period has been shown to reduce insulin resistance and improve glucose metabolism in renal transplant recipients.[28] The precise mechanism(s) of steroid-induced insulin resistance is (are) not well understood and may be multifactorial. Decreased insulin receptor number and affinity, impaired glucose uptake in skeletal muscles, impaired suppression of endogenous insulin production, activation of the glucose-free fatty acid cycle, and reduced glycogen synthesis have all been implicated.[22,29]

Calcineurin Inhibitor-Associated NODAT: Cyclosporine vs. Tacrolimus

Although clinical trials comparing the incidence of NODAT in CSA-vs. Tac-treated patients have yielded mixed results, Tac has more consistently been shown to have a greater diabetogenic effect. Data obtained from the United States Renal Data System revealed that by 1 year post-transplant the incidence of NODAT was approximately 70% greater among Tac- vs. CSA-treated patients (30% vs. 18%, respectively).[30] The incremental increase in the incidence of NODAT at 1 year were 15.4% for Tac and 9.4% for CSA. The corresponding incremental increase in the incidence of NODAT at 2 years for both groups was 17.7 and 8.4%, respectively. Recent 1-year results of the Efficacy Limiting Toxicity Elimination (ELITE)-symphony study consisting of 1,645 renal transplant recipients demonstrated a significant difference in the Kaplan–Meier estimates for NODAT at 12 months among patients receiving standard dose CSA ($n = 438$), low-dose CSA ($n = 408$), low-dose Tac ($n = 403$), or low-dose sirolimus ($n = 380$), with the highest rate occurring in the low-dose tacrolimus group (6.0% vs. 4.2% vs. 8.4% vs. 6.6%, respectively; $P = 0.02$ for all comparisons).[31] The greater diabetogenic effect of tacrolimus compared to CSA has been reported to occur across renal and non-renal transplant groups. In a meta-analysis to evaluate the reported incidence of NODAT after solid organ transplantation, Heisel et al.[32] found a higher incidence of insulin-dependent diabetes mellitus (IDDM) in Tac- vs. CSA-treated liver, heart, and lung transplant recipients. In renal transplant recipients, IDDM occurred in 9.8% of Tac- vs. 2.7% of CSA-treated patients ($P < 0.00001$). Similar trends were observed among recipients of non-renal organ transplants (11.1% vs. 6.2%, respectively, $P < 0.003$). Nonetheless, not all studies showed that Tac is more diabetogenic than cyclosporine.[33] It has been suggested that these study inconsistencies stemmed in part from the difference in the definitions of NODAT and the difference in calcineurin inhibitor dose and drug levels.[33,34] In a single-center study consisting of 139 renal transplant recipients without known pre-transplant glucose abnormalities, Maes et al.[34] have shown that high Tac trough levels, particularly levels greater than 15 ng/mL in the first month after transplant, were a significant risk factor for persistent impaired fasting glucose or diabetes mellitus beyond the first year after transplantation. In a single-center study consisting of 45 OLT recipients treated with either CSA ($n = 9$) or high- ($n = 15$) vs. low-dose ($n = 13$) Tac, the incidence of NODAT were 11, 40, and 23%, respectively.[35]

Recent retrospective single-center studies demonstrated comparable risk of NODAT and IFG in renal transplant recipients who were switched from CSA to Tac after an average of 17 months on CSA therapy.[36] Nonetheless, the results of the study should be interpreted with caution. The authors acknowledged that the mean Tac trough level within the first months following conversion was lower than the typical trough concentration when Tac is used conventionally as the de novo calcineurin inhibitor in kidney transplantation. Furthermore, patients who underwent

Tac conversion therapy were younger and had lower BMI, both of which were known risk factors for NODAT.

A potential interaction between HCV status and the use of Tac immunosuppression has also been suggested. In a retrospective study of more than 400 kidney transplant recipients with no known pre-transplant diabetes, Bloom et al.[37] have shown that among the HCV (+) cohort, NODAT occurred more often in the Tac- compared with the CSA-treated groups (57.8% vs. 7.7%, $P < 0.0001$). In contrast, among the HCV (−) cohort, the rates of NODAT were similar between the two CNI groups (Tac vs. CSA: 10% vs. 9.4%, respectively, $P = 0.521$).

Impaired insulin secretion has been suggested to contribute to the development of CNI-associated NODAT.[27] Experimental studies have shown that CNIs impair the function of cultured β-cells by impairing insulin gene expression.[27,38] In recipients of pancreas transplants, both calcineurin inhibitors CSA and Tac have been shown to cause reversible toxicity to islet cells. In a study of 26 pancreas allograft biopsies from 20 simultaneous kidney–pancreas transplant recipients, a significant correlation was seen between the presence of islet cell damage and serum levels of Tac and CSA, as well as with the Tac peak level.[39] Cytoplasmic swelling and vacuolization and marked decrease or absence of dense-core secretory granules in β-cells were demonstrated on electron microscopy. The islet cell damage was more frequent and severe in the Tac- (10/13) compared to the CSA-treated groups (5/13). Serial biopsies from two patients with hyperglycemia and evidence of islet cell damage receiving Tac immunosuppression demonstrated reversibility of the damage upon discontinuation of tacrolimus.

Effects of Sirolimus on Glucose Metabolism

Early large randomized clinical trials suggested that sirolimus is devoid of diabeto-genic effects either when used alone or in combination therapy with CNI. In recent years, these findings have been challenged by independent investigators because in these trials, NODAT was defined as the patient's requirement for insulin and OGTT was not routinely performed. Similar to type 2 diabetes in the general population, the onset of NODAT can be insidious and individuals may have a long asymptomatic pre-clinical phase, which frequently goes undetected. In one single-center study, Teutenico et al.[10] demonstrated that calcineurin inhibitors to sirolimus conversion therapy and tacrolimus withdrawal in a regimen consisting of tacrolimus and sirolimus were associated with a 30% increased incidence of impaired glucose tolerance. The authors further showed that if fasting plasma glucose alone had been used, 30% of patients with isolated IGT would have received a diagnosis of having normal glucose tolerance. Only two of four patients with 2-h blood glucose compatible with the diagnosis of NODAT had a fasting glucose level > 126 mg/dL (>7 mmol/L). In one single-center study, tacrolimus and sirolimus combination therapy was found to be associated with a higher incidence of NODAT than tacrolimus-alone immunosuppression.[18]

Suggested pathogenic mechanisms of sirolimus-induced hyperglycemia include sirolimus-associated impaired insulin-mediated suppression of hepatic glucose production, ectopic triglyceride deposition leading to insulin resistance, and direct β-cell toxicity.[27] However, studies on the effects of sirolimus on insulin action and secretion have yielded variable and conflicting results. Currently existing literature suggests that the effects of sirolimus on glucose metabolism appear to be cell-, species- and dose-dependent.[40]

Obesity

Similar to the general population, obesity has been shown to be associated with the development of NODAT in most studies.[41] Analysis of the USRDS database revealed that obesity, defined as a BMI of $\geq$ 30 kg/m^2, is one of the strongest risk factors for NODAT (relative risk of 1.73, $P < 0.0001$). Although some studies failed to demonstrate an association between obesity and the development of NODAT, obesity and its associated peripheral insulin resistance state is a known risk factor for type 2 diabetes. The mechanism whereby obesity induces insulin resistance is poorly understood. Nonetheless, the pattern of body fat distribution has been suggested to play a contributory role. Studies in healthy women showed that upper body or male-type obesity has a much greater association with insulin resistance and impaired glucose tolerance than lower body or female-type obesity.[42] Similar studies in the transplant settings is lacking. It is speculated that intra-abdominal fat or waist-to-hip ratio may be more important risk factor for NODAT than total body weight or BMI.[1]

Hypertriglyceridemia/Hypertension

The precise role of the metabolic syndrome in the development of NODAT has not been well defined. Nonetheless, the overlapping metabolic risk factors for type 2 diabetes and cardiovascular disease (e.g., obesity, hyperglycemia, dyslipidemia, hypertension) warrant early identification and aggressive management of individual risk factors. It has been suggested that the greater the number of metabolic syndrome components, the greater the risk for these outcomes.[43] The current NCEP/ATP III criteria for the metabolic syndrome require the presence of any three of the five traits including

- abdominal obesity, defined as a waist circumference in men > 102 cm (40 in.) and in women > 88 cm (35 in.);
- serum triglycerides $\geq$ 150 mg/dL (1.7 mmol/L) or drug treatment for elevated triglyceride;
- serum HDL cholesterol < 40 mg/dL (1 mmol/L) in men and < 50 mg/dL (1.3 mmol/L) in women or drug treatment for low HDL cholesterol;
- blood pressure $\geq$ 130/85 mmHg or drug treatment for elevated blood pressure; and
- fasting plasma glucose (FPG) $\geq$ 100 mg/dL (5.6 mmol/L) or drug treatment for elevated blood glucose.

Proteinuria

Early report from single-center study suggested an association between proteinuria on day 5 after transplantation and the development of NODAT.[44] However, these findings have been challenged because proteinuria on day 5 may just reflect the highly concentrated urine associated with hyperglycemia-induced osmotic diuresis from the early post-transplant use of high-dose corticosteroid or residual native kidney proteinuria. Furthermore, it has been shown that immediate post-transplant proteinuria generally resolves several weeks after transplantation.[45]

Potentially Modifiable Risk Factors

Impaired Glucose Tolerance Before Transplantation

Abnormal glucose metabolism has been reported to be a risk factor for the development of NODAT in some but not all studies. In a study consisting of 490 recipients of kidney transplants, Cosio et al.[46] demonstrated that higher pre-transplant glucose is a risk factor for NODAT at 1 year. Using patients with pre-transplant FPG levels between 90 and 100 as the reference group, patients with plasma glucose < 90 mg/dL have lower risk of NODAT (OR = 0.46, $P = 0.01$). In contrast, the risk of NODAT increases as the pre-transplant FPG levels increase (FPG = 101–110, OR = 1.5; and FPG = 110–125, OR = 7.6, $P < 0.0001$). Among patients with IFG pre-transplant, 70% had hyperglycemia at 1 year (IFG 43% and NODAT 27%).

HCV-Associated NODAT

The association between HCV infection and impaired fasting glucose or the development of frank type 2 diabetes mellitus in the non-transplant population has long been suggested. Potential mechanisms of the diabetogenic effect of HCV infection include insulin resistance, decreased hepatic glucose uptake and glucogenesis, and direct cytopathic effect of the virus on pancreatic β-cells.[47] Over the last decade, the link between hepatitis C and the development of NODAT has also been increasingly recognized in solid organ transplant recipients. The pathogenesis of HCV-associated NODAT, however, remains poorly understood. Clinical studies in orthotopic liver transplant (OLT) recipients have implicated insulin resistance associated with active HCV infection as a predominant pathogenic mechanism. Independent investigators have shown a temporal relationship between recurrent allograft hepatitis and increasing viral loads and the development of NODAT.[4,48] Furthermore, patients who responded to antiviral therapy were observed to have improvement in glycemic control.[4,48,49] In a small cohort of 17 non-diabetic HCV (+) and 33 non-diabetic HCV (–) OLT recipients, Baid et al.[4] have shown that the presence of HCV infection was independently associated with a 62% increase in insulin resistance (P=0.0005). It was suggested that the virus had a direct effect on insulin resistance as no difference in β-cell function or hepatic insulin extraction between the HCV (+) and (–) groups was observed.

In a small study consisting of 16 renal transplant candidates with sustained virologic response to interferon treatment given in the pre-transplant period, none developed NODAT at a mean follow-up of 22.5 months (range 2–88 months).[50] It is conceivable that successful pre-transplant treatment of hepatitis C could potentially reduce the incidence of NODAT after kidney transplantation.

Cytomegalovirus-Associated NODAT

The link between cytomegalovirus (CMV) infection and the development of NODAT was first reported in 1985 in a renal transplant recipient.[51] Limited studies suggested that both asymptomatic CMV infection and CMV disease are independent risk factors for the development of NODAT.[39] In a study consisting of 160 consecutive non-diabetic renal transplant recipients who were prospectively monitored for CMV infection during the first 3 months after transplantation, Hjelmesaeth et al.[52] found that asymptomatic CMV infection was associated with a fourfold increased risk of new onset diabetes (adjusted RR = 4.00; $P = 0.025$). Patients with active CMV infection had a significantly lower median insulin release compared to their CMV negative counterparts, suggesting that impaired pancreatic β-cell insulin release may be involved in the pathogenic mechanism of CMV-associated NODAT. It is speculated that CMV-induced release of proinflammatory cytokines may lead to apoptosis and functional disturbances of pancreatic β-cells.[53]

Impact of NODAT on Patient and Allograft Outcomes

Clinical studies evaluating the impact of NODAT on patient and allograft outcomes after solid organ transplantation have yielded variable results. Nonetheless, there has been ample literature suggesting that kidney transplant recipients who developed NODAT are at two- to threefold increased risk of fatal and non-fatal cardiovascular disease events as compared with non-diabetic patients.[54,55] In one single-center study, the 8-year (range 7–9 years) cumulative incidence of major cardiac events defined as cardiac death or non-fatal acute myocardial infarction was 7% in recipients without diabetes ($n = 138$) and 20% in those with NODAT ($n = 35$).[55] The development of NODAT has also been shown to be associated with an adverse impact on patient survival and an increased risk of graft rejection and graft loss, as well as an increased incidence of infectious complications. In a study consisting of 173 renal transplant recipients, 1-year patient survival in those with vs. without NODAT was 83% vs. 98%, respectively ($P < 0.01$).[56] In a single-center study consisting of 40 renal transplant recipients with NODAT and 30 non-diabetic control patients, 12-year graft survival in diabetic vs. non-diabetics was 48% vs.

70%, respectively ($P = 0.04$).[44] Data from the United Renal Data System consisting of over 11,000 Medicare beneficiaries who received primary kidney transplants between 1996 and 2000 demonstrated that compared to "no diabetes," NODAT was associated with a 63% increased risk of graft failure ($P < 0.0001$), a 46% increased risk of death-censored graft failure ($P < 0.0001$), and an 87% increased risk of mortality ($P < 0.0001$).[9]

Detection and Management of Diabetes Mellitus in Recipients of Solid Organ Transplants

Early detection and management of CVD risk factors in general and of diabetes mellitus in particular should be an integral part in the management of the transplant recipients. The following discussion focuses on the diagnosis and management of diabetes mellitus in the pre- and post-transplant period.

Pre-transplant Baseline Evaluation

The 2004 updated International Consensus Guidelines on New-onset Diabetes after Transplantation suggest that a pre-transplant baseline evaluation should include a complete medical and family history, including documentation of glucose history.[2] Fasting plasma glucose (FPG) should be tested at regular intervals and a 2-h oral glucose tolerance test (OGTT) be performed in those with normal FPG. The use of OGTT is recommended for screening purposes because it is more predictive of increased CVD risk and mortality than FPG testing, particularly in individuals with IGT. Furthermore, it has been suggested that the OGTT diagnostic criteria may be more sensitive in identifying patients with IGT than those set for FPG.[1] Patients with evidence of IGT or abnormal OGTT before transplantation should be counseled on lifestyle modifications including weight control, diet, and exercise. In a large multicenter randomized clinical trial involving more than 3,000 non-diabetic adult subjects with elevated fasting glucose and post-load plasma glucose concentrations, lifestyle intervention has been shown to be more effective than placebo or metformin in reducing the incidence of type 2 diabetes.[57] The lifestyle intervention reduced the incidence of type 2 diabetes by 58% (95% confidence interval 48–66%) and metformin by 31% (95% confidence interval 17–43%) as compared with placebo. The goals for the lifestyle modification involved achieving and maintaining a weight reduction of at least 7% of initial body weight through a healthy low-calorie, low-fat diet and at least 150 min of physical activity per week.

Pre-transplant treatment of HCV-infected renal transplant candidates should be considered. Selection of an immunosuppressive regimen should be tailored to each individual patient, weighing the risk of developing diabetes after transplantation against the risk of acute rejection. Suggested pre-transplant baseline evaluation of potential transplant candidates is shown in Fig. 16.2.

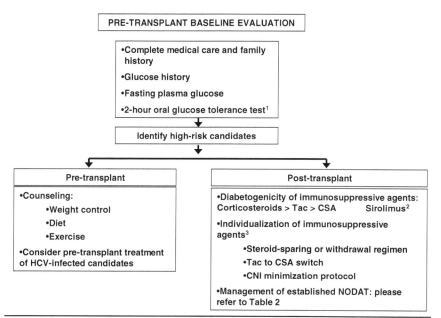

PRE-TRANSPLANT BASELINE EVALUATION

- •Complete medical care and family history
- •Glucose history
- •Fasting plasma glucose
- •2-hour oral glucose tolerance test[1]

Identify high-risk candidates

Pre-transplant	Post-transplant

•Counseling:
  •Weight control
  •Diet
  •Exercise
•Consider pre-transplant treatment of HCV-infected candidates
	•Diabetogenicity of immunosuppressive agents: Corticosteroids > Tac > CSA Sirolimus[2]
	•Individualization of immunosuppressive agents[3]
	  •Steroid-sparing or withdrawal regimen
	  •Tac to CSA switch
	  •CNI minimization protocol
	•Management of established NODAT: please refer to Table 2

[1]Please see text; [2]Further studies are needed, see text; [3]Modification of immunosuppressive regimen should be done at the discretion of the transplant physician

Abbreviations: Tac: tacrolimus, CSA: cyclosporine, CNI: calcineurin inhibitor

Fig. 16.2 Pre-transplant baseline evaluation

Early Detection of NODAT After Transplantation

Studies investigating the best predictive tool for identifying patients at risk for developing NODAT early after transplantation are currently lacking. In a single-center prospective study consisting of 359 de novo renal transplant recipients, Kuypers et al.[44] demonstrated that a normal (vs. diabetic) OGTT on day 5 was associated with a significantly reduced risk for NODAT (odds ratio 0.03, $P = 0.0002$). A similar reduction in the risk of NODAT was conferred by a normal FPG on day 5 (odds ratio 0.06; $P < 0.0001$). [NODAT was defined as the uninterrupted need for glucose-lowering therapy for at least 3 months following transplantation. The up-to-date American Diabetes Association criteria were used to define impaired glucose tolerance (IGT), impaired fasting glucose (IFG), and diabetes mellitus (DM).] Although an OGTT at 5 days after transplantation might prove to be a clinically useful predictive diagnostic tool for the eventual development of NODAT, Kuypers et al.'s study results should be interpreted with caution. The study included predominantly white patients (91.4%), negligible number of black (1.4%), and no Hispanics. The inclusions of more blacks or Hispanics or both would most probably have increased the percentage of patients destined to develop NODAT, thereby increasing the positive predictive values of both OGTT and FPG on day 5, while decreasing their negative predictive values. Furthermore, baseline evaluation of pre-existing glucose metabolism disorders was not performed. Assessment of glucose metabolic disorders and performing OGTT before transplantation might have revealed patients destined to develop type 2 DM independently of the transplantation process. Although the natural history of IFG and IGT in renal transplant recipients has not been defined, an estimated 25% of the non-transplant population with either IFG or IGT will eventually progress to overt diabetes over a period of 3–5 years. In essence, the late development of NODAT (i.e., years) may simply reflect recipients' intrinsic characteristics and is independent of the transplantation process, while DM occurring early (i.e., months) after transplantation may represent true NODAT or transplantation-induced DM. In addition, it is noteworthy that while acute rejection has been suggested to increase the risk for NODAT, it usually does not occur before day 5. Obtaining OGTT and FPG at day 5, therefore, may preclude the subset of patients with higher risk of developing NODAT. Hence, it has been suggested that performing OGTT at 10–12 weeks post-transplantation might be useful as an alternative or supplementary test to day 5 OGTT.[58] The routine recommendation of performing an OGTT early after transplantation awaits further studies.

Management of Established NODAT

The management of NODAT should follow the conventional approach for patients with type 2 diabetes mellitus as recommended by many clinical guidelines established by well-recognized organizations including the American Diabetes Association (ADA). A global guideline for the management of type 2 diabetes mellitus is available through the International Federation Global Guideline website http://www.d4pro.com/diabetesguidelines/index.htm. Similar to the non-transplant settings, a target hemoglobin A_{1C} level < 6.5% is recommended. Fasting plasma glucose should be below 100 mg/dL (6.11 mmol/L), and a 2-h postprandial plasma glucose should be below 140 mg/dL (7.77 mmol/L).[59] Nonetheless, it should be noted that recent studies demonstrated that in patients with type 2 diabetes and a median A_{1C} level of 8.1% who also had either established cardiovascular events or multiple risk factors, therapeutic strategy targeting A_{1C} levels below 6.0% increased all-cause mortality as compared with a strategy targeting levels of 7.0–7.9%.[60] At 1 year, stable median A_{1C} levels of 6.4 and 7.5% were achieved in the intensive-therapy and standard groups, respectively. The intensive-therapy group had a relative increase in mortality of 22% and an absolute increase of 1.0% during a follow-up period of 3.5 years (which is equivalent to one extra death for every 95 patients who were treated for 3.5 years). Deaths from cardiovascular causes were similar between the two treatment groups. It is also notable that hypoglycemia requiring assistance and weight gain of more than 10 kg was more frequent in the intensive-therapy group ($P < 0.001$). Similar studies in recipients of solid organ transplantation are lacking. Nonetheless, the determination of hemoglobin A_{1C} target levels for solid organ transplant recipients should be individualized based on hypoglycemia risks.

Modifiable Risk Factor Management Strategy

Diet and Physical Activity

The Diabetes Prevention Program has demonstrated that a structured diet and physical activity program that achieves and maintains modest weight loss for overweight adults with IGT can significantly reduce the development of diabetes. Emphasis should be placed on lifestyle modification including moderation of dietary sodium (< 2,400 mg sodium a day) and saturated fat intake (< 7% calories from saturated fats, 2–3% calories from trans-fatty acids), regular aerobic exercise, and weight reduction. Carbohydrate intake should be limited to 50–60% of caloric intake. The American Heart Association guidelines also suggested greater than 25 g/day of dietary fiber and 2 servings of fish per week.[61] Defining realistic goals such as a target weight loss of 5–10% of total body weight and patient-centered approach to education may be invaluable in achieving success.

Modification of Immunosuppression

Modification of immunosuppression should be considered in high-risk patients. Corticosteroid dose reduction has been shown to significantly improve glucose tolerance during the first year after transplantation.[9] However, any dose reduction should be weighed against the risk of acute rejection. Steroid-sparing regimen or steroid avoidance protocol should be tailored to each individual patient. Tac to CSA conversion therapy in patients who fail to achieve target glycemic control or in those with difficult to control diabetes has yielded variable results. Calcineurin inhibitors and steroid- minimization/avoidance/withdrawal protocols are discussed in Chapter 10.

Renin-Angiotensin Inhibition

A meta-analysis of 10 randomized controlled trials to assess the effects of rennin-angiotensin inhibition [5 with angiotensin-converting enzyme inhibitors (ACEIs) and 5 with angiotensin receptor blockers (ARBs)] on the incidence of new cases of type 2 diabetes mellitus in patients with arterial hypertension and congestive heart failure demonstrated that renin-angiotensin inhibition with either ACEIs or ARBs consistently and significantly reduced the incidence of type 2 diabetes mellitus compared with placebo, or β-blockers/diuretics or amlodipine.[62] This finding has not yet been validated in either transplant recipients or prospective trials in the general population.[63] Nonetheless, ACEI and/or ARB are commonly used due to its well-established antiproteinuric, cardioprotective, and blood pressure lowering effect.

Pharmacologic Treatment for Diabetes Mellitus

When lifestyle modification fails to achieve adequate glycemic control, medical intervention is recommended. Orally administered agents can be used either alone or in combination with other oral agents or insulin. Although oral hypoglycemic agents may be effective in many patients with corticosteroids or cyclosporine- or tacrolimus-induced NODAT, insulin therapy may ultimately be necessary in up to 40% of patients,[64] particularly in the early post-transplant period.

Oral Hypoglycemic Agents

The choice of pharmacologic therapy is based on the potential advantages and disadvantages associated with the different classes of oral agents (Table 16.2). Although metformin (*a biguanide derivative*) is the preferred agent for overweight patients, its

Table 16.2 Non-insulin drug therapy for NODAT

Agent	Adverse effects
Insulin sensitizers (Suppress hepatic glucose production, increase glucose uptake by skeletal muscle)	
Metformin, buformin, phenformin (e.g., Glucophage® and others)	Diarrhea, dyspepsia, lactic acidosis w/renal insufficiency
Insulin secretagogues (Increase insulin release from pancreatic β-cells)	Hypoglycemia (especially renal insufficiency and elderly patients)
Sulfonylureas (e.g., Glucotrol®, Diabeta®, Amaryl®)	Weight gain, edema, hypoglycemia
Meglitinides (e.g., Prandin®, Starlix®)	Weight gain, hypoglycemia (lower risk than sulfonylureas)
Others with different actions Thiazolidinedione derivatives (TZDs) (e.g., Avandia®, Actos®, Rezulin®) (Bind to PPARs[a] and stimulate insulin-sensitive genes)	May allow reduction in insulin. Side effects – weight gain, peripheral edema (especially when used with insulin), anemia, pulmonary edema, and CHF. Possible higher risk of bone fractures (especially in women)
Glucagon-like peptide-1 analogues (GLP-1) (e.g., Byetta®) (Increase insulin release from pancreas)	Either favorable or neutral effect on weight gain
Dipeptidil peptidase-4-inhibitors (DPP-4) (e.g., Januvia®) (Increase blood concentration of incretin GLP-1[b])	Either favorable or neutral effect on weight gain. Avoid vildagliptin in patients with hepatic impairment and dose of sitagliptin should be adjusted for renal insufficiency. Watch immunosuppressive drug interactions

[a]PPARs – peroxisome proliferator-activated receptors.
[b]GLP-1 – glucagon-like peptide-1 analogues

use should be avoided in patients with impaired allograft function due to the possibility of lactic acidosis. Care should also be taken when the *sulfonylurea derivatives* are prescribed to patients with impaired allograft function or to elderly patients due to the increased risk of hypoglycemia. In general, it is best to start with a low dose and titrate upward every 1–2 weeks. The "non-sulfonylureas" *meglitinides* are insulin secretagogues with a mechanism of action similar to that of the sulfonylureas. Nonetheless, they have a more rapid onset and shorter duration of action and seemingly lower risks of hypoglycemia and the amount of weight gain.[64,65] These agents are therefore best suited for patients whose food intake is erratic, elderly patients, and patients with impaired graft function. They are best taken before meals and the dose may be omitted if a meal is skipped.

The *thiazolidinedione derivatives* (TZD) are insulin sensitizers that may allow for a reduction in insulin requirement. Potential adverse effects of these agents include weight gain, peripheral edema, anemia, pulmonary edema, and congestive heart failure. The incidence of peripheral edema is increased when TZDs are used in combination with insulin.[65] More recently, during the A Diabetic Outcome Progression Trial (ADOPT) conducted to compare glycemic control in patients on rosiglitazone, metformin, or glyburide, a higher incidence of fractures on the upper arm, hand, and foot among female patients treated with rosiglitazone were noted.[66,67] Subsequently, pioglitazone was also recognized to have similar increased risks of fractures in women but not in men although further studies are needed.[67] The risk of fractures associated with the use of the TZD derivatives in the transplant settings is currently not known. Nonetheless, TZD should be used with caution particularly in female transplant recipients who are also receiving steroid immunosuppressive therapy.

The incretin mimetics *glucagon-like peptide-1 analogues* (GLP-1) and incretin enhancers *dipeptidil peptidase-4 inhibitors* (DPP-4) belong to a novel class of drugs that have been approved for use in type 2 diabetes.[68] In contrast to insulin and most other glucose-lowering agents that cause weight gain and hypoglycemia, GPL-1 inhibitors and DPP-4 inhibitors have either a favorable or neutral effect on weight reduction and a lower risk of hypoglycemia. Exenatide is an incretin mimetic that stimulates insulin biosynthesis and secretion in a glucose-dependent manner and has been shown to lower both fasting and postprandial glucose. When added to sulfonylureas, thiazolidinediones, and/or metformin, it results in additional lowering of hemoglobin A_{1c} by approximately 0.5–1%. It also promotes weight loss through its effects on satiety and delayed gastric emptying. Sitagliptin and vildagliptin are DPP-4 inhibitors that act by enhancing the sensitivity of β-cells to glucose, thereby enhancing glucose-dependent insulin secretion. It has also been shown to improve markers of β-cell function. Overall, this class of drugs has been shown to have neutral effects on weight.

Incretin-based therapy appears to provide an attractive treatment option for patients with NODAT owing to its favorable effect on weight reduction/weight neutrality. Data on its safety and efficacy in renal transplant recipients are currently lacking. Caution should be exercised when these agents are used in the transplant setting, particularly with regard to drug to drug interactions. Vildagliptin should be avoided in patients with hepatic impairment and the dose of sitagliptin should be adjusted for renal insufficiency.[68] It has been suggested that DPP-4 substrates include several immune-related molecules such as chemokines CCL-2 (MCP-1), CCL-5 (RANTES), and CCL-11 (eotaxin) and cytokines interleukin 1 and interleukin 2.[59] Whether DPP-4 inhibition may have an adverse impact on allograft function is currently unknown and awaits studies.

Drug to drug interactions should be carefully considered. The meglitinide derivatives repaglinide and, to a lesser extent, nateglinide are metabolized through the cytochrome p450 isozyme CYP 3A4, therefore glucose level should be monitored closely when the patient also receives a strong inhibitor (e.g., cyclosporine, gemfibrozil, or the azole antifungal) or inducer (e.g., rifampin, carbamazepine, phenytoin, or St John's wort) of the CYP 3A4 system.[64] The use of gemfibrozil, a CYP 3A4 inhibitor, and repaglinide combination therapy has been shown to dramatically increase the action of the latter, resulting in prolonged hypoglycemia. Co-administration of cyclosporine and repaglinide has also been shown to enhance the blood glucose-lowering effect of repaglinide and increase the risk of hypoglycemia.[69] In contrast, rifampin, a strong inducer of the CYP 3A4, considerably decreases the plasma concentration of repaglinide and also reduces its effects.[70] Although tacrolimus is also metabolized via the CYP 3A4 system and should therefore be susceptible to many drug interactions similar to those of cyclosporine, these interactions have not been similarly well documented.

Summary

The routine care of patients with post-transplant diabetes mellitus should include an evaluation of hemoglobin A_{1C} level every 3 months and regular screening for diabetic complications including microalbuminuria, retinopathy, and polyneuropathy with associated lower extremity ulcerations and infections.

It should also be noted that hemoglobin A_{1C} cannot be accurately interpreted within the first 3 months post-transplantation due to various factors including possible blood transfusions in the early post-transplant period and the presence of anemia or impaired allograft function. Blood transfusions may render the test invalid until new hemoglobin is formed and the presence of anemia and kidney impairment can directly interfere with the A_{1C} assay. More recently, an artifactual reduction in A_{1C} level has been reported in islet cell transplant recipients taking dapsone for *Pneumocystis carinii* (*P. jiroveci*) prophylaxis. The cause is yet unknown, but a reduction in red blood cell life span and/or hemolysis has been implicated.[71]

Fasting lipid profile should be measured annually. In transplant recipients with multiple CVD risk factors, more frequent monitoring of lipid profile should be performed at the discretion of the clinicians. Statins or the HMG-CoA reductase inhibitors are the most widely used lipid-lowering agents in both the non-transplant and transplant settings. Management of post-transplant dyslipidemia is discussed in Chapter 15. Table 16.3 summarizes the suggested guidelines for the management of NODAT.[72]

Table 16.3 Management of new onset diabetes mellitus after transplantation (adapted and modified from Pham et al.[72])

Dietary modification
  Dietitian referral
  For diabetic dyslipidemia: a diet low in saturated fats and cholesterol and high in complex carbohydrates and fiber is recommended
  The AHA[a] guidelines suggest limiting cholesterol (<200 mg/day for those with DM), $\leq 7\%$ calories from saturated fats, 2–3% calories from trans-fatty acids, and $\leq 2,400$ mg sodium/day. Greater than 25 g/day of dietary fiber and 2 servings of fish a week are also recommended

Lifestyle modifications
  Exercise
  Weight reduction or avoidance of excessive weight gain
  Smoking cessation

Adjustment or modification in immunosuppressive medications[b]
  Rapid steroid taper, steroid-sparing or steroid avoidance protocols
  Tacrolimus to cyclosporine conversion therapy

Pharmacologic therapy
  Acute, marked hyperglycemia (may require in-patient management):
  Intensive insulin therapy (consider insulin drip when glucose ≥ 400 mg/dL)
  Chronic hyperglycemia: treat to target $HbA_{1C} < 6.5\%$
  Oral glucose-lowering agent monotherapy or combination therapy[c] and/or insulin therapy
  Consider diabetologist referral if HbA_{1C} remains $\geq 9.0\%$

Monitoring of patients with NODAT
  Hemoglobin A_{1C} every 3 months
  Screening for microalbuminuria
  Regular ophthalmologic exam
  Regular foot care
  Annual fasting lipid profile
  Aggressive treatment of dyslipidemia and hypertension

---

[a]AHA – American Heart Association.
[b]Clinicians must be familiar with the patients' immune history prior to manipulating their immunosuppressive therapy.
[c]The choice of a particular agent should be based on the characteristics of each individual patient (see text).

References

1. Davidson J, Wilkinson AH, Dantal J et al. New-onset diabetes after transplantation: 2003 International Consensus Guidelines. *Transplantation* 2003;7:SS3–SS24.
2. Wilkinson AH, Davidson J, Dotta F et al. Guidelines for the treatment and management of new-onset diabetes after transplantation. *Clin Transplant* 2005;19:291–298.
3. Montori VM, Velosa JA, Basu A et al. Posttransplantation diabetes: A systematic review of the literature. *Diabetes Care* 2002;25:583–592.
4. Baid S, Cosimi AB, Farrell ML et al. Posttransplant diabetes mellitus in liver transplant recipients: risk factors, temporal relationship with hepatitis C virus allograft hepatitis, and impact on mortality. *Transplantation* 2001;72:1066–1072.

5. Knobbler H, Stagnaro-Green A, Wallenstein S et al. Higher incidence of diabetes in liver transplant recipients with hepatitis C. *J Clin Gastroenterol* 1998;26:30–.

6. Bigam D, Pennington J, Carpentier A et al. hepatitis-C related cirrhosis: a predictor of diabetes after orthotopic liver transplantation. *Gastroenterology* 2000;32:87.

7. Sharif A, Moore RH, Baboolal K. The use of oral glucose tolerance tests to risk stratify for new-onset diabetes after transplantation: an underdiagnosed phenomenon. *Transplantation* 2006;82:1667–1672.

8. Pham PT, Danovitch GM, Pham PC. The medical management of the renal transplant recipient. In: Johnson RJ, John F (eds.), Comprehensive Clinical Nephrology, 3rd ed. Mosby, Philadelphia, PA, 2007, 1085–1101.

9. Kasiske BL, Snyder JJ, Gilbertson D et al. Diabetes mellitus after kidney transplantation in the United States. *Am J Transplant* 2003;3:178–185.

10. Teutonico A, Schena PF, Di Paolo S. Glucose metabolism in renal transplant recipients: Effect of calcineurin inhibitor withdrawal and conversion to sirolimus. *J AM Soc Nephrol* 2005;16:3128–3135.

11. Zhang N, Su D, Qu S et al. Sirolimus is associated with reduced islet engraftment and impaired beta-cell function in transplants. *Diabetes* 2006;55:2429–2436.

12. Hamer RA, Chow CL, Ong AC et al. Polycystic kidney disease is a risk factor for new-onset diabetes after transplantation. *Transplantation* 2007;83:36–40.

13. Ducloux D, Motte G, Vautrin P et al. Polycystic kidney disease as a risk factor for post-transplant diabetes mellitus. *Nephrol Dial Transplant* 1999;14:1244–1246.

14. de Mattos AM, Olyaei AJ, Prather JC et al. Autosomal dominant polycystic kidney disease as a risk factor for diabetes mellitus following transplantation. *Kidney Int* 2005;67:714–720.

15. Hjelmesaeth J. Hartmann: insulin resistance in patients with adult polycystic kidney disease. *Nephrol Dial Transplant* 1999;14(10):2521–2522.

16. Cosio FG, Pesavento TE, Osei K et al. Post-transplant diabetes mellitus: increasing incidence in renal allograft recipients transplanted in recent years. *Kidney Int* 2001;59:732–737.

17. Hebert PL, Geiss LS, Tierney EF et al. Identifying persons with diabetes using Medicare claims data. *Am J Qual* 1999;14(6):270–277.

18. Sulanc E, Lane JT, Puumala SE et al. New-onset diabetes after kidney transplantation: an application of 2003 International Guidelines. *Transplantation* 2005;80(7):945–952.

19. Andrews PA, Sen M, Chang RW. Racial variation in dosage requirements for tacrolimus. *Lancet* 1996;348(9039):1446.

20. Martinez-Castelao A, Hernandez MD, Pascual J et al. Detection and treatment of post kidney transplant hyperglycemia: A Spanish multicenter cross-sectional study. *Transplant Proc* 2005;37(9):3813–3816.

21. Pham PT, Pham PC, Lipshutz G et al. New onset diabetes mellitus after transplantation. *Endocrinol Metab Clin North Am* 2007;36(4):873–890.

22. Jindal RM, Revanur VK, Jardine AG. Immunosuppression and diabetogenicity. In: Hakim N, Stratta R, Gray D, (eds.), Pancreas and Islet Transplantation, 1st ed. Oxford University Press, New York, 2002, 247–275.

23. Hjelmesaeth J, Hartmann A, Kofstad J et al. Tapering off prednisolone and cyclosporine the first year after renal transplantation: the effect on glucose tolerance. *Nephrol Dial Transplant* 2001;16:829–835.

24. Hjelmesaeth J, Hartmann A, Kofstad J et al. Glucose intolerance after renal transplantation depends upon prednisolone dose and recipient age. *Transplantation* 1997;64(7):979–983.

25. Midtvedt K, Hjemesaeth J, Hartmann A et al. Insulin resistance after renal transplantation: the effect of steroid dose reduction and withdrawal. *J Am Soc Nephrol* 2004;15(12): 3233–3239.

26. Depcynski B, Daly B, Campbell LV et al. Predicting occurrence of diabetes mellitus in recipients of heart transplants. *Diabetes Med* 2000;17:15–19.

27. Crutchlow MF, Bloom RD. transplant-associated hyperglycemia: a new look at an old problem. *Clin J Am Soc Nephrol* 2007;2:343–355.

28. Van Hooff JP, Christiaans MHL, van Duijhoven EM. Evaluating mechanisms of post-transplant diabetes mellitus. *Nephrol Dial Transplant* 2004;19(Suppl 6):vi18-vi12.

29. Venkatesan N, Davidson MB, Huchinson A. Possible role of the glucose-fatty acid cycle in dexamethasone-induced insulin antagonism in rats. *Metabolism* 1987;36: 883–891.
30. Woodward RS, Schnitzler MA, Baty J et al. Incidence and cost of new onset diabetes mellitus among U.S. wait-listed and transplanted renal allograft recipients. *Am J Transplant* 2003;3(5):590–598.
31. Ekberg H, Tedesco-Silva H, Demirbas A et al. Reduced exposure to calcineurin inhibitors in renal transplantation. *N Engl J Med* 2007;357:2562–2575.
32. Heisel O, Heisel R, Balshaw R et al. New onset diabetes mellitus in patients receiving calcineurin inhibitors: a systematic review and meta-analysis. *Am J Transplant* 2004;4(4):583–595.
33. Meiser BM, Uberfuhr P, Fuchs A et al. Single-center randomized trial comparing tacrolimus (FK506) and cyclosporine in the prevention of acute myocardial rejection. *J Heart Lung Transplant* 1998;17:782–788.
34. Maes BD, Kuypers D, Messiaen T et al. Posttransplant diabetes mellitus in FK-506-treated renal transplant recipients: analysis of incidence and risk factors. *Transplantation* 2001;72(10):1655–1661.
35. Cai TH, Esterl RM, Nichols F et al. Improved immunosuppression with combination tacrolimus (FK506) and mycophenolic acid in orthotopic liver transplantation. *Transplant Proc* 1998;30:1413–1414.
36. Luan FL, Zhang H, Schaubel DE et al. Comparative risk of impaired glucose metabolism associated with cyclosporine versus tacrolimus in the late posttransplant period. *Am J Transplant* 2008;8:1871–1877.
37. Bloom RD, Rao V, Weng F et al. Association of hepatitis C with posttransplant diabetes in renal transplant patients on tacrolimus. *J Am Soc Nephrol* 2002;13:1374–1380.
38. Redmon JB, Olson LK, Armstrong MB et al. Effects of tacrolimus (FK506) on human insulin gene expression, insulin mRNA levels, and insulin secretion in HIT-T15 cells. *J Clin Invest* 1996;98:2786–2793.
39. Drachenberg CB, Klassen DK, Weir MR et al. Islet cell damage associated with tacrolimus and cyclosporine: morphological features in pancreas allograft biopsies and clinical correlation. *Transplantation* 1999;68(3):396–402.
40. Subramanian S, Trence DL. Immunosuppression agents: effects on glucose and lipid metabolism. *Endocrinol Metab Clin North Am* 2007;36:891–905.
41. Bonato V, Barni R, Cataldo D et al. Analysis of posttransplant diabetes mellitus prevalence in a population of kidney transplant recipients. *Transplant Proc* 2008;40(6):1888–1890.
42. Kissebah AH, Vydelingum N, Murray R et al. Relation of body fat distribution to metabolic complications of obesity. *J Clin Endocrinol Metab* 1982;54(2):254–260.
43. Eckel RH. Mechanisms of the components of the metabolic syndrome that predispose to diabetes and atherosclerotic CVD. *Proc Nutrition Soc* 2007;66:82–95.
44. Kuypers DR, Claes K, Bammens B et al. Early clinical assessment of glucose metabolism in renal allograft recipients: diagnosis and prediction of post-transplant diabetes mellitus. *Nephrol Dial Transplant* 2008;23:2033–2042.
45. Myslak M, Amer H, Morales P et al. Interpreting post-transplant proteinuria in patients with proteinuria pre-transplant. *Am J Transplant* 2006;6:1660–1665.
46. Cosio FG, Kudva Y, van der Velde M, Larson TS et al. New onset hyperglycemia and diabetes mellitus are associated with increased cardiovascular risk after kidney transplantation. *Kidney Int* 2005;67(6):2415–2421.
47. Bloom RD, Lake JR. Emerging issues in hepatitis C virus-positive liver and kidney transplant recipients. *Am J Kidney Transplant* 2006;6:2232–2237.
48. Delgado-Borrego A, Casson D, Schoenfeld D et al. Hepatitis C virus is independently associated with increased insulin resistance after liver transplantation. *Transplantation* 2004;77:703–710.
49. Simo R, Lecube A, Genesca J et al. Sustained virological response correlates with reduction in the incidence of glucose abnormalities in patients with chronic hepatitis C virus infection. *Diabetes Care* 2006;29:2462–2466.

50. Kamar N, Toupance O, Buchler M et al. Evidence that clearance of hepatitis C virus RNA after α-interferon therapy in dialysis patients is sustained after renal transplantation. *J Am Soc Nephrol* 2003;14:2092–2098.
51. Lehr H, Jao S, Waltzer WC et al. Cytomegalovirus-induced diabetes mellitus in a renal transplant recipient. *Transplant Proc* 1985;17:2152–2154.
52. Hjelmesaeth J, Sagedal S, Hartmannn A et al. Asymptomatic cytomegalovirus infection is associated with increased risk for new-onset diabetes and impaired insulin release after renal transplantation. *Diabetologica* 2004;47(9):1550–1556.
53. Hjelmesaeth J, Muller F, Jenssen T et al. Is there a link between cytomegalovirus infection and new-onset posttransplant diabetes mellitus? Potential mechanisms of virus induced β-cell damage. *Nephrol Dial Transplant* 2005;20:2311–2315.
54. Ojo AO. Cardiovascular complications after renal transplantation and their prevention. *Transplantation* 2006;82:603–611.
55. Hjelmesaeth J, Hartmann A, Leivestad T et al. The impact of early-diagnosed new-onset post-transplantation diabetes mellitus on survival and major cardiac events. *Kidney Int* 2006;69:588–595.
56. Boudreaux JP, McHugh L, Canafax DM et al. The impact of cyclosporine and combination immunosuppression on the incidence of post transplant diabetes in renal allograft recipients. *Transplantation* 1987;44(3):376–387.
57. Knowler WC, Barrett-Connor E, Fowler SE et al. Reduction in the incidence of type 2 diabetes with lifestyle intervention or metformin. *N Engl J Med* 2002;12(Suppl 1):34–41.
58. Pham PT, Pham PC. Assessing the risk of post-transplantation diabetes mellitus with an oral glucose tolerance test. *Nat Clin Pract Nephrol* 2008;4(11):600–601.
59. Mannon RB. Therapeutic management of posttransplant diabetes mellitus. *Transplant Rev* 2008;22:116–124.
60. Gerstein HC, Miller ME, Bigger T et alFor The Action to Control cardiovascular Risk in Diabetes Study group. Effects of intensive glucose lowering in type 2 diabetes. *N Engl J Med* 2008;358(24):2545–2559.
61. Kraus RM, Eckel RH, Howard B et al. AHA dietary guidelines revision 2000: a statement for healthcare professionals from the nutrition committee of the American Heart Association. *Circulation* 2000;102:2284–2299.
62. Scheen AJ. Renin-angiotensin system inhibition prevents type 2 diabetes mellitus. Part 1. A meta-analysis of randomized clinical trials. *Diabetes Metab* 2004;30(6):487–496.
63. Bosch J, Yusuf S, Gerstein HC et al. Effect of ramipril on the incidence of diabetes. *N Engl J Med* 2006;355(15):1551–1562.
64. Jindal RM, Hjelmesaeth J. Impact and management of posttransplant diabetes mellitus. *Transplantation* 2000;70(Suppl 11):SS58–SS63.
65. Cheng AYY, Fantus IG. Oral antihyperglycemic therapy for type 2 diabetes mellitus. *CMAJ* 2005;172(2):213–226.
66. Kahn SE, Haffner SM, Heise MA. Glycemic durability of rosiglitazone, metformin or glyburide monotherapy for the ADOPT study. *NEJM* 2006;355:2427–2443.
67. Hampton T. Diabetes drugs tied to fractures in women. *JAMA* 2007;297:1645–1647.
68. Srinivasan BT, Jarvis J, Khunti K et al. Recent advances in the management of type 2 diabetes mellitus: a review. *Postgrad Med J* 2008;84(996):524–531.
69. Hatorp V, Hansen KT, Thomsen MS. Influence of drugs interacting with CYP3A4 on the pharmacokinetics, pharmacodynamics and safety of the prandial glucose regulator repaglinide. *J Clin Pharmacol* 2003;43(6):649–660.
70. Niemi M, Backman JT, Neuvonen PJ et al. Rifampin decreases the plasma concentrations and effects of repaglinide. *Clin Pharmacol Ther* 2000;68(5):495–500.
71. Tartiana F, Faradji RN, Monroy K et al. Dapsone-induced artifactual A_{1C} reduction in islet transplant recipients. *Transplantation* 2007;83(6):824.
72. Pham PT, Pham PC, Danovitch GM. Posttransplant cardiovascular disease. *Semin Nephrol* 2007;27(4):430–444.

Chapter 17
Infections in Kidney Transplant Recipients

Carlos A.Q. Santos and Daniel C. Brennan

Introduction

Infections are common in recipients of kidney transplants due primarily to immuno-suppressive medications prescribed to prevent rejection of the allograft. This chapter describes current strategies for preventing, recognizing, and treating infectious diseases in kidney transplant recipients.

Preventing Infectious Diseases in Kidney Transplant Recipients

Pre-transplant Evaluation – Detection of Infections Before Transplantation

Kidney transplant candidates are screened for occult and latent infectious diseases during the pre-transplant evaluation. Most diseases will be recognized by the routinely performed medical history, physical examination, and ancillary diagnostic tests (Table 17.1). The pre-transplant evaluation screens for serologic evidence of past exposure to cytomegalovirus, Epstein–Barr virus, varicella zoster virus, herpes simplex virus types 1 and 2, hepatitis A, B, and C, human immunodeficiency virus, and syphilis. High-risk patients are also screened for endemic fungi, coccidomycosis, *Toxoplasma gondii*, and *Strongyloides stercoralis*. Ongoing exposures to animals, habits, hobbies, and occupations that predispose to tick or arthropod-borne illness and soil fungi are also often identified.

Another important infectious disease consideration pertinent to the pre-transplant evaluation is the vaccination status of the transplant candidate. The immunosuppression that follows organ transplantation blunts the immune response to novel antigens and most vaccines should be administered before transplantation.[1] Vaccines are

C.A.Q. Santos (✉)
Division of Infectious Diseases, Department of Medicine, Washington University/Barnes-Jewish Hospital/St. Louis Children's Hospital Consortium, St. Louis, MO, USA
e-mail: csantos@im.wustl.edu

D.B. McKay, S.M. Steinberg (eds.), *Kidney Transplantation: A Guide to the Care of Kidney Transplant Recipients*, DOI 10.1007/978-1-4419-1690-7_17,
© Springer Science+Business Media, LLC 2010

Table 17.1 Pre-transplant screening

Serologies
  Herpes simplex virus 1 and 2
  Varicella zoster virus
  Cytomegalovirus
  Epstein–Barr virus
  Human herpesvirus 8
  Hepatitis A, B, and C viruses
  Human immunodeficiency virus
  Rapid plasma reagin
  Endemic fungi
  Tuberculin skin test or QuantiFERON-TB test
  Urinalysis with culture
  Pelvic or prostate exam
  Chest radiogram
  Dental evaluation

Tests to consider
  Toxoplasma serology
  Human T-cell leukemia virus
  Gallbladder ultrasound
  Stool culture
  Stool ova and parasite

more effective if given early rather than late in the course of renal disease because patients with long-standing end-stage renal disease are less likely to mount protective levels of immunity. Table 17.2 presents the vaccines that should be given to patients before renal transplantation and indicates those that are contraindicated after transplantation.

Prevention of Donor-Related Infectious Disease

Transmission of infections from the donor to the recipient can occur despite screening by the transplant center and the organ procurement organization (OPO). Prior to either live or deceased donation, the donor is inspected by serologic testing, specific enzyme immunoassays, and/or recombinant immunoblot assays for evidence of viruses, such as human immunodeficiency virus (HIV) types 1 and 2, human T-cell leukemia virus (HTLV), hepatitis A virus (HAV), hepatitis B virus (HBV), and hepatitis C virus (HCV), herpes simplex virus (HSV) 1 and 2, varicella zoster virus (VZV), cytomegalovirus (CMV), Epstein–Barr virus (EBV), human herpesvirus 8 (HHV-8), and West Nile virus. Testing is also performed to detect syphilis, *T. gondii*, urinary and blood-borne infections in deceased donors.

Viral infections transmitted from donor to recipient can lead to significant morbidity and mortality, causing disseminated diseases and virus-associated cancers such as post-transplantation lymphoproliferative disease (EBV) and Kaposi's sarcoma (HHV-8). Donor seropositivity for HSV, VZV, CMV, EBV, or HHV-8 is not

Table 17.2 Vaccine recommendations before and after transplantation

Recommended			Contraindicated
Before transplant	After transplant	Special circumstances	After transplant
Pneumovax *(Q 3–5 years)*	Pneumovax *(Q 3–5 years)*	Haemophilus influenzae type B (HiB)	BCG
Tetanus–diphtheria	Tetanus–diphtheria	Meningococcus[a]	Smallpox
Oral polio		Inactivated polio[b]	Oral polio[c]
Influenza A and B[d] (annual)	Influenza A and B[d] (annual)		Live attenuated influenza (LAIV)
Hepatitis B[e]		Hepatitis B	Yellow fever
Hepatitis A		Hepatitis A[f]	Live Japanese B encephalitis
Human papilloma vaccine (Gardasil®)[g]		Typhoid Vi[h]	Live oral typhoid
Varicella		Inactivated Japanese encephalitis	Varicella
MMR			MMR

[a] Recommended for specific high-risk groups: college-age patients, travelers to or residents of endemic areas and areas with active outbreaks, military recruits, patients with asplenia, and those with complement deficiencies.

[b] A booster may be given if more than 10 years have elapsed since the last polio vaccine dose.

[c] Causes vaccine-induced paralytic disease in immunosuppressed patients. Household contacts and medical staff should likewise only be immunized with the inactivated polio vaccine.

[d] Also vaccinate household contacts and medical staff.

[e] Doses (40 μg/dose) given at 0, 1, and 2 months are generally sufficient. Quantitative levels of hepatitis B surface antigen antibody (anti-HBs IgG) should be determined 4 months after the last dose. Patients who do not develop protective titers should have another dose administered, and titers rechecked.

[f] Two doses of the vaccine, 6–12 months apart, should be given to transplant recipients who are at least 1 year beyond transplant and being treated with only modest doses of immunosuppressive medications. If there is not enough time to provide active vaccination, intramuscular hepatitis A immunoglobulin may be given prior to travel.

[g] All females between the ages of 9 and 26 should be vaccinated.

[h] An inactive parenteral vaccine, Typhim Vi (Aventis Pasteur), should be given to transplant recipients several months prior to travel to endemic areas.

a contraindication to donation even when the recipient is seronegative.[2,3] Donor HIV-positive status is a contraindication to organ donation, even if the recipient is HIV-positive. Several OPOs employ nucleic acid testing (NAT) to increase the sensitivity of detection for HBV, HCV, HIV, and West Nile virus although this is not routinely done at all OPOs at this time.

Systemic bacterial infection in the donor is a relative contraindication to transplantation, although it can be performed in some cases if appropriate antibiotics are administered.[2] No evidence-based guidelines exist as to the duration of therapy but we recommend between 7 and 14 days of antibiotic therapy. Donor infections such as syphilis, tuberculosis, and fungal infections should be treated on a case-by-case basis.

Preventing Infectious Disease After Transplantation

Infections after transplantation can be divided into three different time frames: the first month, the second through sixth month, and beyond 6 months. Figure 17.1 shows typical infections that occur within these time periods and the recommended prophylactic medications. The time frames are guidelines; it is important to realize that the typical time course may change after treatment of rejection or the use of preemptive and prophylactic antibiotics.

1. The First Month. The typical infections that occur during the first post-transplant month are related to the surgical procedure and untreated infections in the donor. Nosocomial infections are common and can be reduced by the timely removal of endotracheal tubes, vascular access lines, drainage tubes and catheters, and the rigorous observation of institutional infection control policies.

Perioperative antibiotics have been shown to reduce nosocomial bacterial infections.[3] The prophylactic use of double-strength trimethoprim/sulfamethoxazole (TMP-SMX) while the bladder catheter remains in place has reduced the risk of bacterial urinary tract infections (UTI) to < 10% and the risk of blood stream infections by 10-fold.[4]

Viral reactivation is common during the first post-transplant month. The herpesviruses, HSV, notably, reactivate commonly. Other herpesviruses such as VZV, CMV, and EBV can also reactivate early in high-risk individuals. New or primary viral infections transmitted from the donor do not usually become symptomatic until after the first month post-transplant.

Low-dose acyclovir 200–400 mg PO twice daily is effective prophylaxis against reactivation of HSV 1 and 2.[5] Valganciclovir 450–900 mg PO daily is effective prophylaxis against CMV disease in high-risk patients (risk of CMV disease discussed below).[6] Prophylactic therapy is given for 100 days after transplantation.

The CMV risk profile is determined by the serologic status of the donor and recipient. CMV seronegative recipients who receive a kidney from a CMV seropositive donor (R–/D+) are at the highest risk for CMV disease. CMV seropositive recipients (R+/D+/ or R+/D–) are at intermediate risk for symptomatic disease. The optimal way to prevent CMV disease in these patients is not known. We recommend giving these patients valganciclovir prophylactically for 3 months. CMV seronegative recipients who receive a kidney from a CMV seronegative donor (R–/D–) have an extremely low risk of developing CMV disease, and neither prophylactic nor preemptive therapy is warranted. Valganciclovir also protects against HSV 1 and 2, VZV, EBV, and possibly HHV-6. Acyclovir should be discontinued in patients who are given valganciclovir. Doses of both acyclovir and valganciclovir need to be adjusted for renal insufficiency.

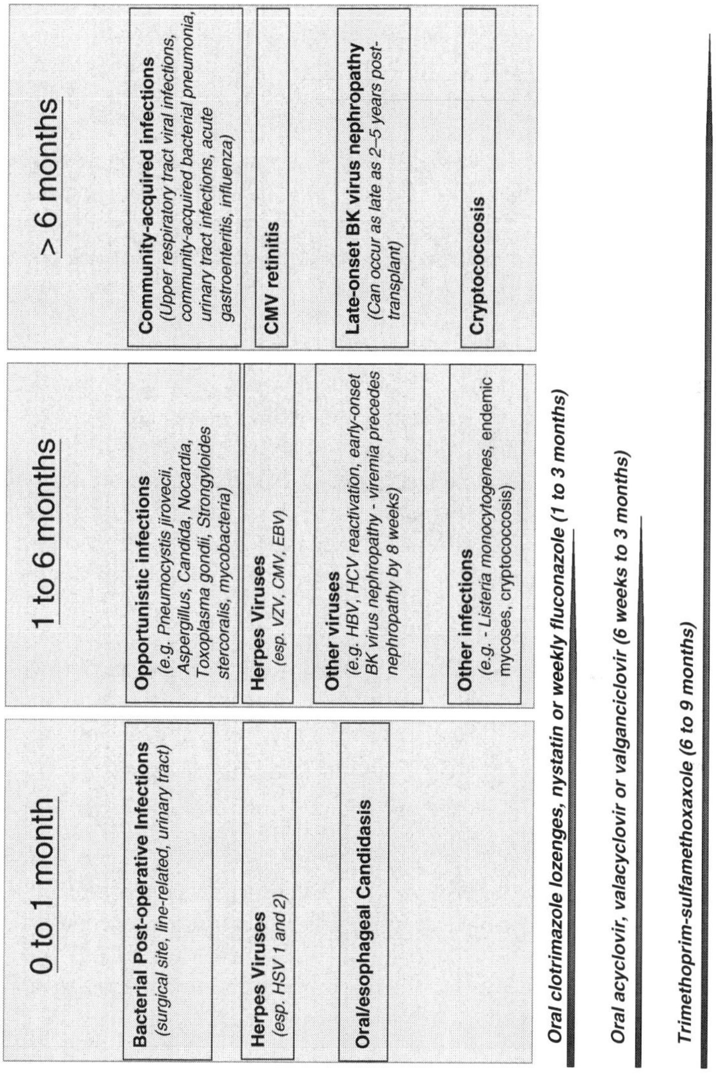

0 to 1 month	1 to 6 months	> 6 months
Bacterial Post-operative Infections *(surgical site, line-related, urinary tract)*	**Opportunistic infections** *(e.g. Pneumocystis jirovecii, Aspergillus, Candida, Nocardia, Toxoplasma gondii, Strongyloides stercoralis, mycobacteria)*	**Community-acquired infections** *(Upper respiratory tract viral infections, community-acquired bacterial pneumonia, urinary tract infections, acute gastroenteritis, influenza)*
Herpes Viruses *(esp. HSV 1 and 2)*	**Herpes Viruses** *(esp. VZV, CMV, EBV)*	**CMV retinitis**
Oral/esophageal Candidasis	**Other viruses** *(e.g. HBV, HCV reactivation, early-onset BK virus nephropathy - viremia precedes nephropathy by 8 weeks)*	**Late-onset BK virus nephropathy** *(Can occur as late as 2–5 years post-transplant)*
	Other infections *(e.g. - Listeria monocytogenes, endemic mycoses, cryptococcosis)*	**Cryptococcosis**

Oral clotrimazole lozenges, nystatin or weekly fluconazole (1 to 3 months)

Oral acyclovir, valacyclovir or valganciclovir (6 weeks to 3 months)

Trimethoprim-sulfamethoxaxole (6 to 9 months)

Fig. 17.1 Timetable indicating occurrence of various infections after kidney transplantation

2. Second to Sixth Month. The second to sixth month post-transplantation is the period when transplant-related opportunistic infections are most likely to arise. This period is characterized by intense immunosuppression. The reactivation of latent donor and recipient infections such as herpesviruses (HSV, VZV, CMV, EBV, HHV-6, HHV-7, HHV-8), HBV, HCV, BK-polyomavirus (BKV), mycobacteria, endemic mycoses, *T. gondii*, and *S. stercoralis* also occurs during this time period. Prophylactic single-strength or double-strength TMP-SMX once daily or three times per week effectively prevents infections caused by *Pneumocystis jirovecii, Nocardia, Legionella pneumophila, Listeria monocytogenes, Salmonella,* and *T. gondii.*

Patients who are allergic to TMP-SMX can be given aerosolized pentamidine 300 mg every 4 weeks, dapsone 50–100 mg once daily, or atovaquone 1,500 mg once daily. Dapsone can cause allergic reactions in patients with TMP-SMX allergies, because of the presence of sulfa moieties in its chemical structure. It should also not be used in patients with G6PD deficiency, since it causes oxidative stress and can trigger hemolysis.

3. Six Months and After. By 6 months, immunosuppressive medications have been tapered to their basal state in stable patients. After 6 months, most patients contract the same infections seen in the general population, including upper respiratory tract viral infections, community-acquired bacterial pneumonia, urinary tract infections, acute gastroenteritis, and influenza. CMV retinitis, however, tends to occur late and may occur with the reactivation of other types of herpesvirus infections including HSV, VZV, and EBV.[7] BKV nephropathy can also occur during this time period; cases presenting between 2 and 5 years post-transplant are not unusual. CMV infection or vitamin B_{12} deficiency predispose patients to the development of recurrent infections with encapsulated organisms.[8]

Transplant recipients are at risk for opportunistic infections beyond 6 months after transplantation if there is an increase in the net state of immunosuppression. Episodes of acute rejection and chronic rejection may necessitate the protracted use of prophylactic medications to prevent opportunistic infections.

Travel

Many kidney transplant recipients travel outside of North America. A high proportion of patients do not take adequate protective measures against endemic infectious diseases.[9]

We advise against traveling to developing countries within 3–6 months of kidney transplantation or for 3–6 months following treatment of acute rejection. Patients who must travel should meet with their physician to assess infection risk. The vaccines that should be given to kidney transplant recipients traveling to endemic areas are shown in Table 17.2. Yellow fever vaccine, a live attenuated vaccine, is generally contraindicated in transplant recipients, because of the risk of developing disseminated disease and death. Apart from mosquito bite prevention, there is no other way of preventing yellow fever. Patients should be advised against traveling to areas endemic for yellow fever. If travel is absolutely necessary, patients must adhere to insect bite prevention measures stringently.

The Centers for Disease Control and Prevention maintains an up-to-date traveler's health website (www.cdc.gov/travel) that could be consulted to help plan preventative measures. The pre-travel assessment must be done several months prior to the date of expected travel, since most vaccinations need to be administered several months in advance to be maximally protective.

General Measures

While traveling, kidney transplant recipients should avoid insect bites to minimize the risk of arthropod-borne diseases such as malaria, dengue fever, and yellow fever. Repellants containing DEET (*N,N*-diethyl-3-methylbenzamide), protective clothing, and bed nets should be used. Patients should not eat food sold by street vendors and should not drink tap water. Raw food should also be avoided, except for fruits and vegetables that can be peeled. We advise patients not to eat from buffets but rather the menu on cruises. These measures will decrease the risk of traveler's diarrhea.

Chemoprophylaxis

Patients who develop diarrhea for more than 1–2 days with associated fevers, chills, vomiting, or bloody stools should see a healthcare professional immediately. Treatment with ciprofloxacin 500 mg PO twice daily or levofloxacin 500 mg PO once daily for 3–7 days can be prescribed for the patient to administer while traveling. Doses for both ciprofloxacin and levofloxacin need to be adjusted for renal insufficiency. Azithromycin 500 mg PO once daily may also be used.

Chemoprophylactic agents for malaria should be given to patients who travel to endemic areas. Chloroquine is the drug of choice for travel to countries with chloroquine-sensitive malaria. Chloroquine may increase cyclosporine levels; levels should be checked prior to the patient's departure and upon their return. For areas of the world where chloroquine-resistant malaria is prevalent, atovaquone–proguanil, mefloquine, or doxycycline can be given. Like chloroquine, mefloquine and doxycycline may increase calcineurin inhibitor levels; levels must be checked prior to the patient's departure. Doses and duration of chemoprophylaxis can be found on the CDC's travel website (www.cdc.gov/travel).

Recognition and Treatment of Infectious Diseases

Evaluation of Fever in the Kidney Transplant Recipient

Fever may represent a broad range of conditions in transplant recipients, including infection and/or rejection. It is important to realize that the presenting signs and symptoms of infection may be unusual because of the use of immunosuppressive medications; therefore most patients should be evaluated and treated at the transplant center. The clinical history, environmental exposures, and physical examination help direct the investigation. Cultures of urine and blood, quantitative blood CMV polymerase chain reaction (PCR) testing, and a chest radiograph (CXR) should be obtained. Empiric syndrome-directed broad-spectrum antimicrobial therapy should be initiated early, even prior to the determination of a specific etiology. Delay in the administration of appropriate treatment may lead to excess morbidity and mortality.

Specific Conditions Causing Fever in the Transplant Recipient

Bacterial Infections

More than 50% of kidney transplant recipients will experience a bacterial infection within the first year of surgery.[10] The major sites of infection, the surgical site, urinary tract, blood stream, and the lungs, will be discussed below.

Surgical Site Infections

There has been a decline in the incidence of surgical wound infections, with rates decreasing to less than 2% in 1997 from 12% in 1988.[11,12] Intraoperative bladder irrigation, perioperative antibiotics, and improvements in surgical techniques have contributed to the decline. Gram stains and aerobic bacterial cultures of exudate from the infected site must be done to determine the causative organism. Usual causative organisms include Gram-positive skin bacteria such as *Staphylococcus aureus, S. epidermidis*, and *Streptococcus* sp. Surgical debridement may be necessary to resolve the infection.

Superficial, mild wound infections may be treated with oral TMP-SMX or clindamycin. Moderate to severe infections will require intravenous vancomycin or daptomycin. The doses for TMP-SMX, vancomycin, and daptomycin need to be adjusted for renal insufficiency. Antibiotics covering enteric Gram-negative rods should be added if there is evidence of such organisms on Gram stain or culture. The duration of therapy is dependent on response, but usually should not be more than 2 weeks.

Urinary Tract Infections

Urinary tract infections (UTIs) are the most common bacterial infections following transplantation, with an incidence ranging from 35 to 79%.[13] Treatment is important in order to avoid pyelonephritis. Typical pathogens include *Escherichia coli, Klebsiella, Proteus, Enterococcus, Enterobacter, Staphylococcus*, and *Pseudomonas*. In the case of recurrent infections, abscesses or other nidi of infection should be sought out by means of imaging with ultrasound or computed tomography.

Empiric treatment options for kidney transplant recipients who present with UTIs who are not septic include ciprofloxacin 250 mg PO twice daily, levofloxacin 500 mg PO once daily, TMP-SMX DS PO twice daily, amoxicillin 500 mg PO three times daily, and nitrofurantoin 100 mg PO twice daily for 10 days. Nitrofurantoin should not be used in patients with severe renal insufficiency. Treatment for UTIs complicated by pyelonephritis or sepsis includes anti-pseudomonal beta-lactam/beta-lactamase inhibitor combinations, such as piperacillin–tazobactam or ticarcillin–clavulanate, or carbapenems such as imipenem, meropenem, or doripenem. As part of the treatment, indwelling urinary tract catheters should be removed. Antibiotic therapy should be tailored once the offending microorganism is identified and drug susceptibilities are determined. A switch to a PO regimen is recommended once the patient has stabilized. Therapy is usually continued for 2–3 weeks.

Septicemia

The incidence of hospitalizations for septicemia among renal transplant recipients is approximately 42 times that of the general population.[14] The urinary tract is the most common source of septicemia, followed by the lungs, the surgical wound site, and the abdomen. Most cases occur within the first 6 months after transplantation.

Empiric antibiotic therapy is dictated by the suspected site of infection. If the source is unclear and the condition is life-threatening, broad-spectrum antibiotic therapy, with doses adjusted for renal insufficiency, with a carbapenem such as imipenem, meropenem, or doripenem or an anti-pseudomonal beta-lactam/beta-lactamase inhibitor such as piperacillin–tazabactam or ticarcillin–clavulanate and an anti-MRSA drug such as vancomycin, linezolid, or daptomycin is warranted.

Pneumonia

Pneumonia among kidney transplant recipients occurred with an incidence of 2.86 episodes per 100 patient-years in the United States, and a mortality rate ranging from 12.5 to 40%.[15] The infectious agent in the majority of patients is never determined. This is likely because of the low yield of blood and sputum cultures and the efficacy of antibacterial therapy. In patients who are hypoxic on presentation or do not respond to initial therapy, a bronchoscopy and bronchoalveolar lavage (BAL) is almost always warranted.

Patients should be referred if possible to a transplant center to improve the likelihood of diagnosing the etiologic agent. Common causative organisms include *Streptococcus pneumoniae*, non-typable *Haemophilus influenzae*, *Moraxella catarrhalis*, *Chlamydia pneumoniae*, *Mycoplasma pneumoniae*, and respiratory viruses such as influenza, adenovirus, and respiratory syncytial virus (RSV). Less commonly, patients may present with opportunistic organisms such as *P. jirovecii*, *L. pneumophila*, and *Mycobacterium tuberculosis*. Silver for direct fluorescent antibody (DFA) stains for *Pneumocystis* should be done on sputum or BAL specimens. A urine *Legionella* antigen test should be done on all patients on initial work-up. A delay in diagnosis and treatment of *Legionella* pneumonia is associated with increased morbidity and mortality. Outbreaks of legionellosis have been linked to drinking water, contaminated respiratory equipment, and heating and air conditioning ventilation systems. Risk assessment for tuberculosis should be done, and airborne isolation must be instituted in patients determined to be at high risk. Three sputum AFB smear and cultures should also be done.

Empiric therapy options for outpatients with suspected bacterial pneumonia include azithromycin and levofloxacin. Empiric therapy options for inpatients not needing ICU care include ceftriaxone plus azithromycin, or levofloxacin. Patients requiring ICU care need broad-spectrum combination antibiotic therapy that covers for methicillin-resistant *S. aureus* (MRSA) and resistant Gram-negative enteric rods and *Legionella*. Therapeutic options include the fourth-generation cephalosporin cefepime or a carbapenem such as imipenem, meropenem, or doripenem or an anti-pseudomonal beta-lactam/beta-lactamase inhibitor such as piperacillin–tazabactam or ticarcillin–clavulanate, combined with vancomycin or linezolid, and azithromycin. Daptomycin is inactivated by lung surfactant and should not be used to treat suspected MRSA pneumonia. Azithromycin may usually be discontinued if work-up for atypical organisms such as *Legionella* is negative. If *P. jirovecii* pneumonia is suspected, treatment doses of TMP-SMX should be administered. TMP-SMX within the first few days of administration will not reduce the diagnostic yield of a bronchoscopy for PCP. Once the causative agent of pneumonia is identified, therapy should be tailored accordingly. Duration of therapy is typically 7 days for uncomplicated bacterial pneumonia, although legionellosis is usually treated for 21 days. Care must be taken to adjust doses of antibiotics cleared by the kidney for renal insufficiency.

Viral Infections

Infections with herpes and hepatitis viruses are the most common viral infections encountered among kidney transplant recipients. Other viruses of concern include adenovirus, RSV, influenza virus, and polyomaviruses.

Herpesvirus Infections

Eight human herpesviruses (HHV) have been identified to date (Table 17.3). All are characterized by the development of a latent state and reactivation with immunosuppression.

Herpes Simplex Virus

Two types of HSV exist, HSV type 1 and HSV type 2. Type 1 is commonly associated with orolabial herpes and type 2 is associated with genital herpes. However, both types may be cultured from either location. Reactivation may occur within the first month after transplantation and most commonly presents as mild ulcer-like

Table 17.3 Human herpesviruses and associated diseases

Virus	Disease
HHV-1: herpes simplex 1 (HSV 1)	Herpes labialis
HHV-2: herpes simplex 2 (HSV 2)	Herpes genitalis
HHV-3: varicella zoster virus (VZV)	Chicken pox
	Shingles
HHV-4: Epstein–Barr virus	Mononucleosis
	Burkitt's lymphoma
	Nasopharyngeal carcinoma
	Post-transplant lymphoproliferative disorder (PTLD)
	Oral hairy leukoplakia
HHV-5: cytomegalovirus (CMV)	Cytomegalovirus disease
	Salivary gland virus disease
HHV-6: human herpes virus 6	Roseola subitum
HHV-7: human herpes virus 7	Roseola subitum
	Pityriasis rosea
HHV-8: human herpes virus 8	Kaposi's sarcoma
	Effusion lymphoma
	Multifocal Castleman's disease

mucocutaneous lesions. HSV esophagitis may cause dysphagia and mimic candidiasis. Less commonly HSV can cause pneumonitis, hepatitis, encephalitis, nephritis, and disseminated disease. Polymerase chain reaction (PCR) for detection of HSV DNA is fast becoming the diagnostic modality of choice. The standard therapy for mucocutaneous lesions is acyclovir 200 mg PO 4–5 times/day. Valacyclovir 1,000 mg PO twice daily or famciclovir 250 mg PO thrice daily are alternatives. Doses for acyclovir, valacyclovir, and famciclovir should be adjusted for renal insufficiency. More serious cases may require treatment with IV acyclovir 5–15 mg/kg every 8 h. Care must be taken to ensure adequate hydration to prevent drug-induced renal insufficiency. Patients who do not respond to treatment after 1 week or who develop new lesions while on therapy need to have the infective virus isolated and tested for antiviral drug susceptibility. Immunosuppressed patients are about 10 times more likely to have resistant HSV that requires treatment with foscarnet or cidofovir.[16] Both foscarnet and cidofovir can cause severe renal insufficiency and should be used with extreme caution in kidney transplant recipients. Uncomplicated oral or genital HSV is usually treated for 7–10 days. Chronic suppressive antiviral therapy should be considered in patients with more than 6 recurrences per year.

Varicella Zoster Virus

Over 90% of adults have evidence of prior infection with VZV. Primary VZV infection can be life-threatening in kidney transplant recipients. Reactivation of VZV in a previously exposed patient causes shingles. Dermatomal pain without zoster lesions can occur. The appearance of dermatomal vesicular lesions is usually enough to make the diagnosis but it can be confirmed with the finding of multinucleated giant cells on Tzanck smear, PCR, and DFA. Disseminated VZV infections manifesting as skin lesions, pneumonia, encephalitis, pancreatitis, hepatitis, or disseminated intravascular coagulation have a high mortality rate.

Treatment of uncomplicated herpes zoster is a 7-day course of acyclovir 800 mg PO five times daily, famciclovir 500 mg PO three times daily, or valacyclovir 1,000 mg PO three times daily. Kidney transplant recipients with primary VZV or disseminated zoster should receive acyclovir 10 mg/kg every 8 h for 7 days. These patients must be placed in negative pressure isolation until all lesions crust over to prevent spread to non-immune patients and healthcare providers. Post-herpetic neuralgia can be managed with gabapentin, tricyclic antidepressants, narcotics, pregabalin, tramadol, topical lidocaine, or topical capsaicin.[17]

The need for VZV post-exposure prophylaxis is determined by the patient's serostatus. The importance of a prophylactic intervention is underscored by the relatively high risk of complications for primary VZV in immunocompromised patients.[18] Patients who report a past history of VZV infection or who are VZV seropositive need no intervention. Patients with a negative or uncertain history of infection need to have their serostatus determined. Seronegative patients need to receive varicella immunoglobulin (VZIG or VariZIG where available) within 96 h of contact.[19] If neither VZIG or VariZIG is available, IVIG may be given. IVIG contains variable amounts of varicella immunoglobulin. The live attenuated VZV vaccine is contraindicated in patients with immunocompromise, and therefore should not be administered to renal transplant recipients. The use of prophylactic acyclovir is also not recommended. In patients who develop VZV infection despite the above measures, acyclovir should be started as soon as lesions develop to prevent the development of more serious disease.

Epstein–Barr Virus

Approximately 95% of the adult population has serologic evidence of previous infection with EBV, and the majority of seronegative recipients seroconvert within the first year after transplantation. EBV may cause a mononucleosis-like syndrome, chronic fatigue, or fever of unknown origin, but has also been associated with Burkitt's lymphoma, nasopharyngeal carcinoma, and post-transplantation lymphoproliferative disorders (PTLD). The diagnosis of PTLD is made by histology. A positive positron emission tomography (PET) test is highly suggestive. Use of EBV titers or serology is unreliable for detection of PTLD. Most PTLD cases are of B-cell origin and are associated with EBV infection. Immune-based therapies such as monoclonal anti-B-cell antibodies like rituximab, interferon-alpha, and EBV-specific donor T cells represent promising approaches for treatment of PTLD or prophylaxis in high-risk patients.[20] The use of antiviral agents such as acyclovir or ganciclovir has been explored, with mixed results.

Cytomegalovirus

CMV is a significant cause of morbidity and mortality among kidney transplant recipients. Between 60 and 90% of adults are seropositive. Symptomatic disease ranges from a relatively mild syndrome of fever, leukopenia, thrombocytopenia, and elevated liver enzymes to severe disseminated disease that involves multiple organ systems, such as the lung, liver, and gastrointestinal tract. CMV disease has been implicated as a cause of acute and chronic graft dysfunction as well as long-term graft loss. In cardiac and renal transplant recipients, CMV has been linked experimentally with arteriosclerosis of the coronary and renal arteries. CMV can also suppress the immune response which predisposes the host to infections with other viruses, bacteria, and fungi.

The incidence and severity of CMV disease has been most strongly associated with the CMV serostatus of the kidney donor and recipient. Seronegative recipients who receive a kidney from a seropositive donor (D+/R–) are at greatest risk for severe primary infection during the first 3 months post-transplant. Without antiviral prophylaxis, over 60% of patients develop active CMV infection within 100 days after transplant even without lymphocyte-depleting therapy.[21]

Rapid and accurate diagnosis of CMV is important because delayed recognition results in increased morbidity. Quantitative real-time polymerase chain reaction (RT-PCR) assays for CMV DNA and pp65 antigen detection are the most commonly used means to detect CMV viremia. The shell vial viral culture method remains a reliable way of detecting CMV in sputum.

Multiple strategies have been used to reduce the morbidity and mortality of CMV infection and its associated costs. Avoiding CMV sero-mismatching through organ allocation is not feasible or worthwhile. Universal prophylaxis refers to giving prophylactic therapy to all kidney transplant patients regardless of their CMV serostatus. Selected prophylaxis refers to giving prophylaxis to patients at high risk for CMV, namely the D+/R– category or those receiving lymphocyte-depleting therapy. The preemptive approach treats asymptomatic CMV infection in an effort to prevent CMV disease, and the deferred approach treats active CMV disease. Each approach has its advantages and disadvantages, and there is no definitive consensus on optimal preventive strategy.

Prophylactic Therapy

Prophylactic therapy is effective in preventing CMV disease in high-risk patients. Ganciclovir and valganciclovir are equally efficacious.[6] Ganciclovir 1,000 mg PO three times daily and valganciclovir 900 mg PO once daily are used. Valganciclovir is contraindicated in patients with a creatinine clearance of less than 10 ml/h. Prophylactic therapy is usually given during the first 100 days post-kidney transplant. A concern with the prophylactic strategy is that 20–30% of high-risk patients go on to develop late-onset CMV disease after the prophylaxis is stopped, and the incidence of ganciclovir resistance may be higher in those who receive prophylaxis. Since CMV infection occurs in only 66–88% of D+/R– patients, critics of the universal prophylactic approach claim that it exposes a significant proportion of patients who would never have developed disease to a prolonged course of antiviral therapy, with the attendant risks of adverse reactions and emergence of viral resistance. Moreover, it is costly and may only be delaying disease onset.

Preemptive Therapy

Preemptive therapy of CMV infection involves monitoring for CMV viremia and starting treatment before the development of signs or symptoms of disease. It has been shown to be as effective as prophylactic therapy in preventing CMV disease. Both oral ganciclovir and valganciclovir have been shown to be effective in treating viremia. Preemptive therapy has the advantage of avoiding the costs and complications of antiviral therapy in low-risk patients while at the same time initiating treatment early to avoid symptomatic disease in high-risk patients.[22,23] It has also been shown to decrease the development of late CMV disease.[24] Its major limitation is the need to perform frequent determinations of CMV viremia, and therefore may not be practical in an outpatient setting. Extreme vigilance is required to achieve successful outcomes.

Ganciclovir Resistance

Ganciclovir resistance is becoming more common among solid-organ transplant recipients. In one study, 6.2% of CMV isolates had UL97 or UL54 mutations.[25] Viral strains with mutations in the UL97 gene, which encodes for a viral protein kinase, remain susceptible to foscarnet and cidofovir. Mutations in the UL54 gene that encodes DNA polymerase can result in resistance to ganciclovir, foscarnet, and cidofovir. The emergence of ganciclovir-resistant CMV underscores the importance of optimizing preventive strategies.

Other Human Herpesviruses

HHV-6 causes self-limited febrile illnesses often followed by a rash in children. Reactivation can occur in kidney transplant recipients and is associated with active CMV infection. It has been reported to cause hepatitis, encephalitis, and hemophagocytic syndrome. Ganciclovir, foscarnet, and cidofovir are thought to be effective therapy. Ganciclovir prophylaxis is associated with a decrease in HHV-6 reactivation.[26]

HHV-7 is associated with roseola and pityriasis rosea in children. Reactivation in kidney transplant patients is common and is associated with graft rejection.[27] It is intrinsically resistant to ganciclovir; cidofovir is the treatment of choice.

HHV-8 can cause Kaposi's sarcoma (KS), multifocal Castleman's disease, and primary effusion lymphoma. The seroprevalence of HHV-8 ranges from less than 3% in the United States to over 25% in Italy and some regions of Africa.[28] The incidence of KS in transplant recipients is 0.1–5% and varies according to the regional seroprevalence of HHV-8.[29] Reduction in immunosuppression may lead to regression of the tumor. Treatment options include radiation and cytotoxic chemotherapy. The use of antiviral agents and sirolimus in the treatment of KS remains speculative.

Hepatitis Viruses

Chronic liver disease affects about 15% of kidney allograft recipients.[30] Kidney transplant recipients with chronic viral hepatitis have significantly increased mortality rates attributable to hepatic failure and sepsis.[31]

Hepatitis B Virus

HBV is a DNA virus seen in dialysis and transplant patients. Its prevalence has fallen from 7.8% in 1976 to 1.4% in 1989 because of patient monitoring for HBV infection, the use of universal precautions, the screening of blood products for HBV, widespread HBV vaccination, and the provision of separate rooms and dialysis machines for patients infected with HBV.[32] Patients infected with HBV before transplantation are at risk for reactivation of infection, worsening of liver disease and cirrhosis, and development of hepatocellular cancer. Reactivation of HBV even among HBsAg-negative transplant recipients is well documented.[33] Similarly, recipients of HBsAg-negative/HBcAb-positive donor kidneys have been shown to have seroconverted, albeit without evidence of hepatitis. The risk of progression to active infection is higher if HBsAg seropositivity is noted in the donor or recipient prior to transplantation. The effect of HBsAg seropositivity on long-term mortality in transplant recipients is controversial, but HBsAg seronegativity likely imparts a long-term survival advantage.[34] The use of HBcAb-positive donor kidneys has been evaluated and is considered safe in vaccinated patients and those with evidence of past HBV infection.[35]

Given the increased propensity for HBV latently infected patients to develop reactivation, liver disease, cirrhosis, and hepatocellular carcinoma after transplantation, efforts have been made to examine the utility of preemptive antiviral therapy. Lamivudine 100 mg PO once daily for 4 weeks prior to transplantation, and 96 weeks after, is the most well-studied regimen.[36] Its advantages include high bioavailability, a paucity of side effects, and a lack of effect on the immune system. However, it is associated with the development of resistant variants with prolonged administration and a relatively high failure rate of about 40%. Also, its dose needs to be adjusted for moderate to severe renal insufficiency. Combination therapy with adefovir 10 mg PO once daily or tenofovir 300 mg PO once daily may ameliorate the development of resistance with lamivudine monotherapy, but is associated with increases in creatinine and renal insufficiency. If either adefovir or tenofovir is added to lamivudine preemptive therapy, close attention should be given to monitoring renal function. Entecavir 0.5 mg PO once daily is emerging as a viable alternative to lamivudine-based preemptive therapy. Its barrier to resistance is higher than that of lamivudine, and it is not associated with renal toxicity. However, experience with entecavir in this setting is limited, and its dose should be adjusted in patients with a creatinine clearance of less than 50 ml/min. Experience with telbivudine 600 mg PO once daily is likewise limited, but is likely not superior to lamivudine monotherapy. Long-term high-dose hepatitis B pooled immunoglobulin is not a viable preventative option, because of high cost, limited availability, parenteral administration, and the potential to transmit unknown viruses.

Patients who develop HBV reactivation should be treated promptly to prevent the development of catastrophic fulminant hepatic failure. Tenofovir 300 mg PO once daily, either alone or in combination with lamivudine 100 mg PO once daily, or emtricitabine 200 mg PO once daily (coformulated as Truvada) is rapidly emerging as the regimen of choice because of its high potency and its ability to suppress both wild-type and lamivudine-resistant HBV. However, it has the potential to cause renal toxicity. Therefore, the renal function of kidney transplant recipients receiving tenofovir needs to be monitored very closely. Adefovir 10 mg PO once daily is less potent than tenofovir and is less able to suppress viral replication. Its use therefore has been supplanted by tenofovir. Entecavir 0.5 mg PO once daily for nucleoside-naïve adults, and 1 mg PO once daily for patients with lamivudine-resistant HBV, is also emerging as a treatment of choice. It is highly potent and has a low rate of drug resistance.[37] Moreover, it does not appear to cause renal toxicity. However, resistance has been observed in up to 50% of lamivudine-refractory patients after 5 years of treatment. It is most likely to be useful therefore in nucleoside-naïve patients. Telbivudine 600 mg PO once daily has slightly more potent antiviral effects compared to lamivudine, but it selects for the same drug-resistant mutants as lamivudine and is more expensive. Its role in primary treatment therefore is limited. Interferon-alpha is relatively contraindicated in kidney transplant recipients. It can induce acute allograft rejection by upregulating cytokine gene expression, increasing cell surface expression of HLA antigens, and enhancing the function of immune effector cells. With the availability of efficacious antiviral drug regimens, the risk of using interferon-alpha to treat HBV disease almost always outweighs its benefits. The optimal duration of antiviral therapy in these patients is unknown. Most centers provide treatment for at least 5 years; it may even be continued for the lifetime of the patient.

An algorithm to help assess the diagnosis and treatment of hepatitis B infection in ESRD patients considered for transplantation is shown in Fig. 17.2.

Hepatitis C Virus

HCV is a major cause of morbidity and mortality among kidney transplant recipients. HCV-infected patients are at higher risk for progressive hepatic disease, new-onset diabetes after transplant (NODAT), and immune complex glomerulonephritis. Tacrolimus may increase the risk of developing NODAT and should be used with caution in these patients. The prevalence of HCV ranges from 10 to 41% among kidney transplant recipients, about 10 times that of the general population.[38] The majority of anti-HCV antibody-positive patients are also HCV RNA positive, indicating persistent viral replication and chronic disease. Patients may be HCV RNA positive and anti-HCV antibody-negative in cases of humoral immune suppression both before transplant, as a result of end-stage renal disease, and after transplant as a result of iatrogenic immunomodulatory agents. Recipient seroconversion after transplantation of a HCV RNA positive donor kidney is nearly

Approach to Known HBV in Patients Awaiting Transplantation

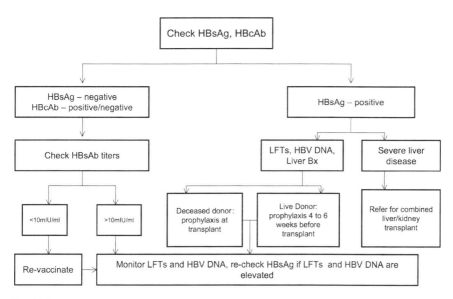

Fig. 17.2 Approach to known HBV in patients awaiting transplantation

universal. Anti-HCV antibody-positive/HCV RNA negative kidneys rarely cause infection. Because of the shortage of donor organs, these anti-HCV antibody-positive kidneys are considered for HCV RNA positive recipients. Over 60% of HCV-infected kidney transplant patients will develop chronic hepatitis.[39] The presentation may be subtle with normal liver function tests and evidence of inflammation found only on biopsy. However, long-term follow-up reveals decreased 10-year survival among HCV-positive recipients (65% vs 80% in HCV-negative recipients) and decreased graft survival (49% vs 63%). In these patients, liver function tests (LFTs) should be checked monthly for the first 6 months after transplant and every 3 months thereafter. Worsening LFTs portend progressive disease and should prompt an immediate hepatology consult for evaluation and treatment. Annual liver ultrasound and alpha-fetoprotein (AFP) should be done to screen for hepatocellular carcinoma.

Treatment of HCV in patients without renal disease consists of interferon-alpha and ribavirin. However, in patients with kidney allografts, interferon-alpha can induce acute rejection by enhancing the function of natural killer cells, cytotoxic T cells, and monocytes. We therefore do not recommend using interferon-alpha or pegylated interferon-alpha to treat HCV in kidney transplant recipients, unless the benefits of treatment clearly outweigh the risks. The use of ribavirin likewise is controversial in kidney transplant recipients. Its clearance is decreased during renal insufficiency, and its metabolites cannot be removed by hemodialysis. While it can cause proteinuria post-transplant, its ability to induce graft failure is unknown. The utility of ribavirin monotherapy in kidney transplant recipients is unstudied, and no recommendations as to its use can be given at this point.

Human Parvovirus

Parvovirus B19 is a small DNA virus that has a seroprevalence of 30–60% among adults.[40] It is the cause of fifth disease or erythema infectiosum in children, manifesting as a "slapped cheek" rash on the face, with or without erythematous exanthema of the extremities. Viral infection is efficiently aborted in immunocompetent hosts, and immunity is lifelong. However, in immunosuppressed individuals, including kidney transplant recipients, parvovirus B19 can persist as a chronic infection and manifest as red blood cell aplasia, with or without an accompanying decrease in platelets and white blood cells. Approximately one-third of patients show systemic signs of illness, including fever and malaise. Serologies for parvovirus B19 can be falsely negative in immunosuppressed patients. Bone marrow biopsies showing red cell aplasia and giant pronormoblasts are suggestive, and nucleic acid hybridization and PCR for the virus confirm the diagnosis. The treatment of choice is intravenous immunoglobulin (IVIG) 0.4–1 g/kg/day for 3–10 days. It is hypothesized that parvovirus B19 specific IgG present in IVIG helps control chronic persistent viral replication. Decreasing immunosuppression, when possible, should also be done.

Adenovirus

Adenovirus is associated with a wide range of clinical syndromes and occurs throughout the year with periodic outbreaks. Immunocompetent hosts almost always have self-limited respiratory, gastrointestinal, or conjunctival disease. Immunocompromised hosts on the other hand can present with pneumonia, colitis, hepatitis, hemorrhagic cystitis, tubulointerstitial nephritis, encephalitis, and fatal dissemination.[41] Traditional and quantitative real-time PCR techniques have been developed for diagnosis. Quantitative viral load measurements may contribute to the diagnosis of infection and act as a surrogate that correlates with clinical response to therapy.[42] Cidofovir is active against all serotypes of adenovirus in vitro and has been used with success in stem-cell transplant recipients. However, its nephrotoxicity limits its use in kidney transplant recipients. Reduction in immunosuppression aids in resolution.

Respiratory Syncytial Virus

Respiratory syncytial virus (RSV) commonly occurs in children but is seen in adult kidney transplant recipients as well. Infections typically occur between November and April and present initially as upper respiratory tract infections. However, the infection can progress to a lower respiratory tract infection with bilateral pulmonary infiltrates. It is usually diagnosed by direct fluorescent antibody staining of nasopharyngeal swab material. The treatment of upper tract RSV is supportive. In severe cases, however, ribavirin has been used successfully in kidney transplant recipients. The combination of RSV immunoglobulin and ribavirin appears effective in preventing the progression of upper tract disease to pneumonitis in bone marrow transplant patients when began early.[43] Palivizumab, a humanized monoclonal antibody against RSV, is only approved for children but appears safe and well tolerated in adult stem-cell transplant patients.[44] No studies on RSV immunoglobulin and palivizumab have been done on kidney transplant recipients.

Influenza

Influenza is a major cause of acute respiratory illness and affects immunocompromised individuals more severely than immunocompetent individuals. In addition to the typical viral prodrome of fever, headache, myalgias, and dry cough, influenza is associated with viral pneumonia, secondary bacterial pneumonia, rhabdomyolysis, and multiple neurological complications including encephalitis and hemolytic-uremic syndrome. It is recommended that transplant recipients, their family, and transplant personnel receive yearly vaccinations for influenza. Non-vaccinated patients, patients who cannot mount an immune response to the vaccine, and patients in whom the vaccine is contraindicated can receive chemoprophylaxis during the influenza season. Single therapy with adamantanes (M2 blockers) such as amantadine and rimantadine is no longer recommended for chemoprophylaxis or treatment given the high prevalence of viral resistance in the United States and Canada. There is also increasing resistance to oseltamivir. Zanamivir or combination oseltamivir–rimantadine may be therapeutic options. Up-to-date recommendations regarding chemoprophylaxis and treatment are year- and locale-specific and may be found on www.cdc.gov.

Polyomaviruses

Polyomaviruses are small DNA viruses capable of persistent infection and oncogenesis. Currently identified polyomaviruses detected in humans include JC virus, BK virus, simian virus 40 (SV-40), WU virus, KI virus, and MC virus. SV-40, WU, and KI viruses are of limited significance in kidney transplant recipients and will not be discussed.

JC/BK Virus

JC virus and BK virus are ubiquitous with seroprevalences in adults ranging from 70 to 80%.[45] The routes of acquisition and sites of primary infection are largely unknown. Both viruses can establish latent infection in the kidneys and, in the case of JC virus, in the central nervous system.

JC Virus

JC virus is the causative agent of progressive multifocal leukoencephalopathy (PML), a demyelinating disease of the brain described best among patients with advanced HIV, but also reported among other severely immunocompromised cohorts. It usually manifests with subacute neurologic deficits, including changes in mental status, motor deficits, ataxia, and visual symptoms. PML has been reported to occur in kidney transplant recipients.[46] PML should be included in the list of differentials for a transplant recipient presenting with subacute-onset patchy neurologic symptoms. Treatment consists primarily of reduction of immunosuppression. Cidofovir has been tried in patients with advanced HIV. However, nephrotoxicity limits its use in kidney transplant recipients.

BK Virus

BKV is associated with post-transplantation nephropathy, hemorrhagic cystitis, and ureteral obstruction.[47] It usually remains dormant in the urinary tract and circulating leukocytes after the primary childhood infection and becomes reactivated during immunosuppression. Adult seroprevalence rates for BKV range from 65 to 90% and BKV reactivation can come from the recipient or the donor.[48] BK viremia occurs in 13% and BK nephropathy in 8% of kidney transplant recipients.[49] Analysis of risk factors for reactivation has underscored the central role played by serologic status of the donor, immunosuppressive regimens, injury to the uroepithelial tissue, and acute rejection.[49] Distinguishing between BK infection and allograft rejection is of paramount importance, since BK infection necessitates reducing immunosuppression and allograft rejection requires the opposite.

Among kidney transplant recipients who are receiving immunosuppressive therapy, 10–60% have reactivation of BKV accompanied by shedding of urothelial cells. Shedding is inconsistently associated with allograft dysfunction. Once the virus has reactivated, an ascending infection via cell-to-cell spread occurs. The overall state of immunosuppression is the primary determinant of BKV reactivation. Viral replication begins early after transplantation and progresses through detectable stages – viruria, then viremia, then nephropathy. Viruria can be detected by PCR for BKV DNA, reverse transcription (RT)-PCR for BKV RNA, cytology for BKV inclusion bearing epithelial cells termed "decoy cells," or electron microscopy for viral particles. Viremia is a better predictor of nephropathy than viruria.[50] Although higher levels of viremia correlate with the risk of developing nephropathy, there are no established thresholds of viremia to indicate nephropathy. Therefore the gold standard for establishing BK nephropathy remains a biopsy with positive immunohistochemical or immunofluorescent staining for the SV-40 large T antigen.

Currently, no established antiviral treatment is available, and control of viral infection is tentatively obtained by means of reduction of immunosuppression. Treatment attempts have included immunoglobulins without proof of efficacy. Retinoic acid, 5-bromo-2-deoxyuridine, cidofovir, leflunomide, fluoroquinolones, and gyrase inhibitors have antiviral activity in vitro but have not been tested in patients in a systematic fashion. Cidofovir use is limited by its nephrotoxicity. Retransplantation remains an option if other therapies fail.

Most patients develop BK viruria and viremia by 3 months post-transplant. BK viruria precedes BK viremia which in turn precedes nephropathy. An effective screening strategy is to check blood for BKV DNA by PCR monthly for the first 6 months and at 9 and 12 months after transplantation, at the time of a transplant kidney biopsy, and after augmentation of immunosuppression. Because BKV nephropathy is preceded by BK viremia, asymptomatic BK viremia should prompt empiric immunosuppression reduction and continued monitoring. Blood viral levels ordinarily decline and clear within 1–6 months. However, if persistent high-level viremia, defined as greater than 10,000 copies/mL of plasma, or allograft dysfunction occurs, an allograft biopsy should be performed as soon as possible. This strategy has resulted in only one case of BKV nephropathy in more than 700 new transplants in our institution in the past 5 years, with an overall acute rejection rate of < 10% at 1 year.[51]

MC Virus

In 2008, a previously unknown polyomavirus, subsequently named MC virus, was detected in Merkel cell carcinoma (MCC) tumors.[52] MCC is a rare neuroectodermal tumor arising from mechanoreceptor Merkel cells in human skin. It is an aggressive form of skin cancer, usually presenting as flesh-colored or bluish-red nodule, and is seen most frequently among transplant recipients and patients with advanced HIV. The incidence of MCC is rising, and over 1,500 US cases per year have been reported.[53] It has a mortality of 33%, exceeding that of melanoma. Treatment options are determined by local extent and stage of disease and usually include surgery, radiation therapy, and chemotherapy. Further clinical and epidemiologic studies are needed to determine the incidence and characteristics of MCC tumors and MC virus in transplant recipients and other immunocompromised hosts.

Fungal Infections

Systemic fungal infections occur in 2–14% of kidney transplant recipients, and about two-thirds of kidney transplant recipients with fungal infections die (Table 17.4).[54] Several new antifungals have become available in the last 10 years. These include triazoles (voriconazole and posaconazole) and echinocandins (caspofungin, micafungin, and anidulafungin). Amphotericin B is still considered the drug of choice in critically ill and immunocompromised patients with fungal infections.

Voriconazole and posaconazole are broad-spectrum triazole antifungals with activity against a wide variety of yeasts, including many fluconazole-resistant *Candida* spp., and molds. The major difference in antifungal coverage between voriconazole and posaconazole is that the latter covers Zygomycetes. Both drugs

Table 17.4 Fungal infections in transplant recipients

Fungus	Common clinical syndromes	Diagnosis	Treatment options	
			Primary[a]	Secondary[a]
Aspergillus	Pneumonia/pulmonary cavity Sinusitis CNS mass Disseminated	Culture of suspected site of infection Histopathology Serum galactomannan[b]	Amphotericin[c] Voriconazole	Echinocandin[a] Itraconazole Posaconazole
Candida	Urinary tract infection Fungemia Surgical site infection	Culture of suspected site of infection	Severely ill or at risk for infection with azole-resistant strain: Amphotericin[c] Echinocandin[d] Mildly ill: Fluconazole	Itraconazole Posaconazole Voriconazole
Coccidioides	Pneumonia/pulmonary cavity Meningitis Disseminated[e]	Culture of suspected site of infection Histopathology Serology: compliment fixation	Severely ill or meningitis: Amphotericin[c] followed by fluconazole or itraconazole suppression Mild or moderately ill: Fluconazole Itraconazole	Posaconazole Voriconazole
Cryptococcus	Fungemia Meningitis Pneumonia Cellulitis	Culture of suspected site of infection Serum cryptococcal antigen CSF cryptococcal antigen Histopathology (mucicarmine stain)	*Meningitis:* Amphotericin[c] plus flucytosine followed by fluconazole suppression *No meningitis:* Amphotericin[c] followed by fluconazole suppression	Fluconazole Itraconazole Posaconazole Voriconazole

Table 17.4 (continued)

Fungus	Common clinical syndromes	Diagnosis	Treatment options	
			Primary[a]	Secondary[a]
Histoplasma	Pneumonia /pulmonary cavity Disseminated[f]	Culture of suspected site of infection (including bone marrow) Histopathology Isolator blood cultures Urine or serum histoplasma antigen Serology: compliment fixation and immunodiffusion	Severely ill: Amphotericin[c] followed by itraconazole suppression Mild or moderately ill: Itraconazole	Fluconazole Posaconazole Voriconazole
Mucormycosis	Sinusitis Pneumonia/pulmonary cavity CNS mass Disseminated	Culture of suspected site of infection Histopathology	Amphotericin[c]	Posaconazole

Abbreviations: CSF (cerebral spinal fluid), CNS (central nervous system).

[a]If more than one antifungal listed, antifungals listed alphabetically, not by order of preference.

[b]Serum galactomannan testing has a sensitivity < 50% in solid-organ transplant recipients.

[c]Amphotericin B deoxycholate, amphotericin B lipid complex, liposomal amphotericin B, or amphotericin B colloidal dispersion.

[d]Caspofungin, micafungin, and anidulafungin demonstrate similar in vitro and in vivo activity against *Candida* and *Aspergillus* species. Of note, *C. parapsilosis* has been associated with clinical failures.

[e]Disseminated coccidioides has a predilection for skin, joints, and bones.

[f]Disseminated histoplasma has a predilection for the lymphoreticular system.

increase cyclosporine and tacrolimus levels. There is currently no intravenous formulation available for posaconazole. It should be administered with food or a nutritional supplement. Alternative antifungals should be used if the patient cannot maintain an adequate caloric intake.

In contrast to the new triazoles, the antifungal activity of echinocandins is limited to *Candida* and *Aspergillus* species. These drugs are well tolerated and are rarely associated with significant adverse events. Caspofungin is hepatically metabolized; co-administration with cyclosporine will increase caspofungin levels. Caspofungin decreases cyclosporine and tacrolimus levels. Neither micafungin nor anidulafungin will interfere with the metabolism of cyclosporine or tacrolimus. Anidulafungin has the advantage of not having to be dose adjusted for either hepatic or renal insufficiency.

Candidiasis

Candidiasis is the most common fungal infection affecting kidney transplant patients. While *Candida albicans* is the usual causative yeast, the incidence of invasive disease by non-albicans species has been increasing. This includes *C. torulopsis, C. glabrata, C. parapsilosis. C. tropicalis*, and *C. krusei*. Candidal infections generally manifest as mucocutaneous overgrowth resulting in oral thrush, esophagitis, intertrigo, onychomycosis, or vaginitis. Invasive candidiasis usually occurs when the mucocutaneous barrier is breached by bladder and intravenous catheters or surgical trauma. Catheter-related sepsis may then ensue. Manifestations of disseminated candidal infections are diverse and include skin lesions, brain abscesses, endophthalmitis, arthritis, osteomyelitis, pneumonitis, and pyelonephritis. Candidal infections in kidney transplant recipients are diagnosed by performing fungal stains and cultures of appropriate specimens.

Susceptibility testing for *Candida* species is becoming more available and widely used. The incidence of *C. albicans* resistance is extremely low, with only 1.5% documented to be resistant to fluconazole in a recent surveillance study.[55] Fluconazole, therefore, remains the drug of choice for *C. albicans* infections. *C. krusei*, on the other hand, is intrinsically resistant to fluconazole. This resistance cannot be overcome with the use of higher drug doses. It also demonstrates decreased susceptibility to amphotericin B and flucytosine. *C. krusei* is susceptible to echinocandins, voriconazole, and posaconazole; these drugs therefore are the drugs of choice. Many *C. glabrata* isolates are resistant to azoles due to changes in drug efflux; this type of resistance can sometimes be overcome by using high doses of fluconazole in vivo. However, this approach may increase the risk of toxicity. Echinocandins have excellent activity against this species and are the drugs of choice. *C. parapsilosis* is very susceptible to most antifungal agents, including fluconazole. However, the MICs for *C. parapsilosis* with caspofungin are higher than for other species (2 µg/uL to > 8 µg/µL compared to 0.5 µg/µL for *C. albicans*). The clinical relevance of these observations is unclear. *C. lusitaniae* is uniquely resistant to amphotericin B. However, it is usually susceptible to azoles and echinocandins.

Treatment of candidal infections depends on the hemodynamic stability of the patient and the infecting *Candida* species. If the infecting species is unknown, the choice of agent is informed by the local prevalence of resistant *Candida* species, patient colonization history, and prior azole prophylaxis. In institutions where *C. glabrata* or *C. krusei* are commonly found, we recommend an echinocandin rather than fluconazole as first-line therapy. Hemodynamically unstable patients, and patients with neutropenia, should likewise be treated with an echinocandin. Fluconazole may be used in patients who are clinically stable and who have not received prior fluconazole prophylaxis. Oral, vaginal, and cutaneous candidasis can be treated with topical therapy with either nystatin or clotrimazole. Asymptomatic candiduria should be treated in post-transplant patients after removal of the bladder catheter because it can progress to invasive disease.[56] Invasive candidal infections require removal of foreign devices and prolonged IV antibiotic therapy.

Cryptococcosis

Pathogenic cryptococci are the most common causes of CNS fungal infection in kidney transplant patients. *Cryptococcus* sp. are saprophytes and are associated with bird guano. Infections are acquired by inhalation of basidiospores and occur in 0.3–4% of kidney transplant recipients. The most common sites of infection are the CNS (55%), skin (13%), and lungs (6%).[57] The majority of cases of cryptococcal meningitis occur 6 months after transplantation. The presentation is generally subacute or chronic. Symptoms usually include fever, headache, mental status changes, and focal neurologic deficits. Cutaneous involvement manifests as cellulitis, nodular skin lesion, or an acneiform eruption. Cryptococcal pneumonia may be indistinguishable from other community-acquired pneumonias. Amphotericin B and 5-flucytosine remain the treatments of choice for acutely ill patients. Cryptococcal pneumonia without involvement of the central nervous system can be successfully managed with fluconazole.

Aspergillosis

The most common cause of aspergillosis is *Aspergillus fumigatus*. However, other species, including *A. flavus* and *A. niger*, can cause disease. Inhalation of spores results in infections of the respiratory tract and a means of dissemination. Infection is rare except in immunocompromised hosts and occurs in up to 3% of kidney transplant recipients.[58] Characteristic presenting symptoms include fever, cough, hemoptysis, and pleuritic chest pain. Disseminated aspergillosis most often involves the CNS and manifests as meningitis, encephalitis, brain abscesses, or granulomas. Symptoms are non-specific and include headache, altered mental status, seizures, and evolving stroke.

The key to diagnosis is clinical suspicion and demonstration of *Aspergillus* in tissue biopsy or aspirate and growth in culture. Detection of *Aspergillus* in the respiratory tract (sputum, nasal swab, and bronchoalveolar lavage) is very suggestive of disease in immunocompromised patients,[59] in the presence of compatible clinical and radiologic findings.

Disseminated aspergillosis has a poor prognosis and a mortality approaching 100%. Amphotericin B has been standard therapy and often requires high-dose regimens for extended periods. Lipid-soluble formulations of amphotericin B have comparable efficacies and reduced renal side effects. Voriconazole has been shown to improve survival (70.8% vs 57.9%) at 12 weeks with fewer severe side effects compared to amphotericin B deoxycholate[60] Caspofungin has been approved as salvage therapy for invasive aspergillosis. It can be added to either voriconazole or liposomal amphotericin B in cases unimproved on monotherapy. There are no clinical data to support the use of amphotericin B–triazole combinations. In patients at high risk of zygomycosis, and in whom a diagnosis of invasive aspergillosis is not yet definite, we recommend liposomal amphotericin B rather than voriconazole, since voriconazole has no activity against Zygomycetes.

Mucormycosis

Infections with fungi of the class Zygomycetes cause mucormycosis. This class includes *Rhizopus* species, *Mucor* species, *Absidia* species, *Rhizomucor* species, and *Cunninghamella* species. These fungi are ubiquitous and are found in food, air, and soil. Invasive disease is uncommon and has a prevalence of 0–1.2%[61] in kidney transplant recipients. Its pathogenesis is similar to that of *Aspergillus*. Inhaled fungal spores develop into hyphae that then invade small vascular vessels. Secondary dissemination can then occur via the hematogenous route. Clinical manifestations include rhinocerebral, pulmonary, cutaneous, CNS, and GI mucormycosis. Signs and symptoms of infections are non-specific and can present as fever, orbital cellulitis, ophthalmoplegia, hemoptysis, cough, chest pain, headache, mental status changes, and GI bleeding. Diagnosis is made by tissue biopsy and histologic examination.

Treatment consists of aggressive surgical debridement of necrotic tissue, minimizing risk factors, and antifungal therapy. Amphotericin B remains the agent of choice. Limited clinical experience suggests that posaconazole may be efficacious as well and may be used as a step-down therapy for patients who have responded to amphotericin B. It may also be used as salvage therapy for patients who do not respond to or cannot tolerate amphotericin B. Rapid diagnosis and treatment of patients at risk are critical because of the high morbidity and mortality (80%) associated with invasive disease.

Endemic Mycoses

These infections can occur at any time following transplantation. Histoplasmosis, blastomycosis, and coccidioidomycosis are more common in transplant patients and are caused by *Histoplasma capsulatum, Blastomyces dermatitidis*, and *Coccidioides immitis*, respectively. The clinical presentation of these mycoses is varied and dissemination is common.

Histoplasmosis is endemic in the central United States. Blastomycosis is endemic to southeastern and south-central states bordering the Mississippi and Ohio River basins and the Midwestern states. Coccidioidomycosis (also called Valley Fever) is endemic in the southwestern United States, northern Mexico, and regions of Latin America. All are acquired by inhalation. Disseminated disease can occur and clinical presentation may be non-specific. They are usually diagnosed by serology, histologic examination of clinical specimens or culture. Urinary antigen detection assays exist for *Histoplasma, Blastomyces*, and *Coccidioides* and are particularly sensitive for acute disseminated infection.[62] Amphotericin B is the treatment of choice for severe disease. Milder cases may be treated with itraconazole. Fluconazole can be used for treatment of mild cases of coccidioidomycosis.

Pneumocystosis

P. jirovecii (known previously as *P. carinii*) is an extracellular organism resembling both fungi and protozoan parasites. Within the first year after transplantation, 6–20% of solid-organ transplant recipients not receiving prophylaxis develop pneumonia (PCP).[63] The clinical presentation of PCP is usually subacute with symptoms of fever, non-productive cough, dyspnea and interstitial infiltrates with or without cysts, and variable degrees of hypoxemia. Pneumocystis infection is often associated with CMV infection and may carry a high mortality rate. Diagnosis relies on identification of the organisms using silver stains or DFA staining of deep respiratory specimens. Pneumocystis infection can be prevented by using prophylaxis with TMP-SMX or alternatively with dapsone or aerosolized pentamidine for 6–12 months post-transplantation. The treatment of choice is TMP-SMX in addition to steroids in severe cases. Alternatives include primaquine plus clindamycin, dapsone or atovaquone.

Mycobacterium tuberculosis

Approximately 1–15% of kidney transplant recipients develop active *M. tuberculosis* infection (TB), with incidences varying according to geography and endemicity.[64] There is a low incidence of TB in North America in general; however, the incidence of latent TB in immigrant populations from countries with high endemicity is higher than that of the general population. Immunosuppressed patients are at increased risk for both primary infection and reactivation. Transmission of *M. tuberculosis* from the kidney allograft has been reported.

Tuberculosis can involve almost any organ system, but it most commonly presents either as pulmonary disease or as disseminated disease. Clinical manifestations include fever, weight loss, pulmonary disease with focal infiltrates (40%) or a miliary pattern (22%) on CXR.[65] The GI tract is the most common extra-pulmonary site. GI involvement occurs most commonly in the ileocecal region. Mortality in renal transplant patients is 30% overall and is greatest in disseminated TB.

Evaluation for *M. tuberculosis* infection in kidney transplant patients should begin during the pre-transplant period. Risk factors such as high-risk exposures, prior positive PPD, and prior TB treatment should be queried. A positive PPD in patients with chronic renal insufficiency is >10 mm. A PPD >5 mm is considered positive with CXR evidence of prior TB infection or close contacts of TB cases. The QuantiFERON-TB test is used to evaluate for past TB exposure at some transplant centers. Its sensitivity and specificity are similar to a PPD, but it offers the advantage of a single patient visit. Our transplant center relies on the PPD. Patients with either a positive PPD or positive QuantiFERON-TB require further evaluation for evidence of active disease.

Patients with latent disease should undergo treatment prior to transplant to prevent reactivation and medication interactions. After transplantation, a positive PPD is > 5 mm. Patients suspected of having active tuberculosis should be isolated to avoid transmission to other susceptible hosts. Three induced sputum specimens should be obtained and sent for acid-fast stain and culture. BAL and post-bronchoscopy sputum samples can also be sent for acid-fast stain and culture. Histopathologic examination of biopsy tissue (acid-fast bacilli and granulomas) may also be useful if disease is suspected and body fluid analysis is non-diagnostic. Rapid assay kits are also available and utilize nucleic acid amplification techniques to detect the organism.

Patients with latent TB require treatment with isoniazid (INH) for 9 months. Rifampin for 6 months is an alternative. Because of the high prevalence of drug-resistant *M. tuberculosis*, active TB should be treated with directly observed therapy consisting of a 2-month initial phase of INH, rifampin (RIF), pyrazinamide (PZA), and ethambutol (EMB). Alterations to this regimen are allowed if drug susceptibilities are known in advance. After 2 months, the regime can be tailored to two drugs based on the drug sensitivities, usually INH and RIF, and continued for 4–7 months. Kidney transplant recipients receiving treatment for active or latent TB should be followed closely and liver enzymes should be checked because of the high prevalence of liver disease and possible drug interactions. The adverse effects and toxicity of anti-tuberculosis agents are well described. One effect, of particular importance to patients receiving immunosuppression, is that INH and RIF induce hepatic cytochrome P450 enzymes and increase the metabolism of glucocorticoids, cyclosporine, tacrolimus, and sirolimus. This can lead to under-immunosuppression and rejection if blood levels of immunosuppressive drugs are not followed closely. Therefore it is best to treat the patient before transplantation.

Parasitic Infections

Strongyloidiasis

S. stercoralis is endemic in parts of Asia, South America, Europe, and the United States. Prevalence rates of 2.5–4% have been reported among residents of Kentucky and Tennessee.[66,67]

S. stercoralis is capable of establishing a chronic asymptomatic infection in its host through repeated low-level autoinfection. Concurrent immunosuppression may lead to accelerated autoinfection and result in hyperinfection, a syndrome characterized by disseminated invasive helminthic disease. The majority of cases of hyperinfection among solid-organ transplant recipients have occurred following kidney transplant. These cases were associated with increased corticosteroid doses in response to allograft rejection.

Multiple organ dysfunction as a result of disseminated disease leads to mortality rates that vary between 70 and 85%.[68] There are no proven parasite-specific efficacious treatments for disseminated disease. Screening at-risk individuals who are about to undergo transplantation may be life-saving. The screening modality, however, is controversial. Clinical manifestations of chronic strongyloidiasis are non-specific; moreover, many individuals are asymptomatic. Only 50–80% of patients with *S. stercoralis* infestation have eosinophilia, making a complete blood count a poor screening test. Examination of > 3 stool samples for direct identification of *S. stercoralis* larval forms has a sensitivity of only 60–70%[69] and is labor-intensive. Serologic testing is widely available and has a positive predictive value of 97% and a negative predictive value of 95% in patients residing in endemic areas[70]; however, it is costly. A reasonable approach may be to develop a standard questionnaire geared toward eliciting risk factors for strongyloidiasis, and common symptoms of strongyloidiasis, and have these incorporated into a pre-transplant evaluation. If the patient has risk factors, symptomatology consistent with strongyloidiasis or peripheral eosinophilia, serologic testing should be undertaken, and stool samples screened for confirmation.

Ivermectin (200 µg/kg/day for 2 days, repeat after 2 weeks) is the drug of choice. Its efficacy at clearing stool and improving symptoms in patients with chronic strongyloidiasis is comparable with thiabendazole (67–81%) and is much better tolerated.[71]

Summary

Infections associated with kidney transplantation are common and associated with significant morbidity, mortality, and costs. A scrupulous pre-transplant evaluation of donors and recipients can identify risks for post-transplant infection. Appropriate pre- and post-transplantation vaccination and prophylaxis reduces the impact of infection. When infection is suspected, a comprehensive evaluation with culture of urine, blood, and blood CMV-PCR and nasopharyngeal swabs and chest X-ray should be done, and broad-spectrum antibiotics and antivirals should be initiated pending results. Anti-infectives should then be tailored once a causative organism is identified. For serious fungal infections, an infectious disease consult is recommended and the patient should be referred to the transplant center. In general, stress-dose steroids are not indicated. Many antibiotics particularly macrolide antibiotics such as clarithromycin and erythromycin should not be used since they interfere with calcineurin inhibitor metabolism and lead to increased calcineurin inhibitor levels. Azithromycin, however, does not interfere with calcineurin metabolism and is safe. Antifungal "azoles" interfere with calcineurin inhibitor metabolism and lead to increased calcineurin inhibitor levels and should be used with caution; serial assessment of calcineurin inhibitor levels should be done.

References

1. Pirofski LA, Casadevall A. Use of licensed vaccines for active immunization of the immuno-compromised host. *Clin Microbiol Rev* 1998 Jan;11(1):1–26.
2. Little DM, Farrell JG, Cunningham PM, Hickey DP. Donor sepsis is not a contraindication to cadaveric organ donation. *QJM* 1997 Oct;90(10):641–642.
3. Midtvedt K, Hartmann A, Midtvedt T, Brekke IB. Routine perioperative antibiotic prophylaxis in renal transplantation. *Nephrol Dial Transplant* 1998 Jul;13(7):1637–1641.
4. Fox BC, Sollinger HW, Belzer FO, Maki DG. A prospective, randomized, double-blind study of trimethoprim-sulfamethoxazole for prophylaxis of infection in renal transplantation: clinical efficacy, absorption of trimethoprim-sulfamethoxazole, effects on the microflora, and the cost-benefit of prophylaxis. *Am J Med* 1990 Sep;89(3):255–274.
5. Seale L, Jones CJ, Kathpalia S et al. Prevention of herpesvirus infections in renal allograft recipients by low-dose oral acyclovir. *JAMA* 1985 Dec 27;254(24):3435–3438.
6. Hodson EM, Barclay PG, Craig JC et al. Antiviral medications for preventing cytomegalovirus disease in solid organ transplant recipients. *Cochrane Database Syst Rev.* 2005;(4):CD003774.
7. Lippmann BJ, Brennan DC, Wong J, Lowell JA, Singer GG, Howard TK. Are varicella zoster and herpes simplex sentinel lesions for cytomegalovirus in renal transplant recipients? *Lancet* 1995 Sep 30;346(8979):914–915.
8. Miller BW, Brennan DC, Korenblat PE, Goss JA, Flye MW. Common variable immunodeficiency in a renal transplant patient with severe recurrent bacterial infection: a case report and review of the literature. *Am J Kidney Dis* 1995 Jun;25(6):947–951.
9. Boggild AK, Sano M, Humar A, Salit I, Gilman M, Kain KC. Travel patterns and risk behavior in solid organ transplant recipients. *J Travel Med* 2004 Jan–Feb;11(1):37–43.
10. Maraha B, Bonten H, van Hooff H, Fiolet H, Buiting AG, Stobberingh EE. Infectious complications and antibiotic use in renal transplant recipients during a 1-year follow-up. *Clin Microbiol Infect* 2001 Nov;7(11):619–625.
11. Koyle MA, Ward HJ, Twomey PA, Glassock RJ, Rajfer J. Declining incidence of wound infection in cadaveric renal transplant recipient. *Urology* 1988 Feb;31(2):103–106.
12. Stephan RN, Munschauer CE, Kumar MS. Surgical wound infection in renal transplantation: outcome data in 102 consecutive patients without perioperative systemic antibiotic coverage. *Arch Surg* 1997 Dec;132(12):1315–1318;discussion 1318–1319.
13. Tolkoff-Rubin NE, Rubin RH. Urinary tract infection in the immunocompromised host. Lessons from kidney transplantation and the AIDS epidemic. *Infect Dis Clin North Am* 1997 Sep;11(3):707–717.
14. Abbott KC, Oliver JD 3rd, Hypolite I et al. Hospitalizations for bacterial septicemia after renal transplantation in the united states. *Am J Nephrol* 2001 Mar–Apr;21(2):120–127.
15. Tveit DJ, Hypolite IO, Poropatich RK et al. Hospitalizations for bacterial pneumonia after renal transplantation in the United States. *J Nephrol* 2002 May–Jun;15(3):255–262.
16. Bacon TH, Levin MJ, Leary JJ, Sarisky RT, Sutton D. Herpes simplex virus resistance to acyclovir and penciclovir after two decades of antiviral therapy. *Clin Microbiol Rev* 2003 Jan;16(1):114–128.
17. Hempenstall K, Nurmikko TJ, Johnson RW, A'Hern RP, Rice AS. Analgesic therapy in postherpetic neuralgia: a quantitative systematic review. *PLoS Med* 2005 Jul;2(7):e164.
18. Geel AL, Landman TS, Kal JA, van Doomum GJ, Weimar W. Varicella zoster virus serostatus before and after kidney transplantation, and vaccination of adult kidney transplant candidates. *Transplant Proc* 2006 Dec;38(10):3418–3419.

19. Marin M, Guris D, Chaves SS, Schmid S, Seward JF. Prevention of varicella: recommendations of the Advisory Committee on Immunization Practices (ACIP). *MMWR Recomm Rep* 2007 Jun 22;56(RR-4):1–40.
20. Taylor GS. T cell-based therapies for EBV-associated malignancies. *Expert Opin Biol Ther* 2004 Jan;4(1):11–21.
21. Sagedal S, Hartmann A, Nordal KP et al. Impact of early cytomegalovirus infection and disease on long-term recipient and kidney graft survival. *Kidney Int* 2004 Jul;66(1):329–337.
22. Jung C, Engelmann E, Borner K, Offermann G. Preemptive oral ganciclovir therapy versus prophylaxis to prevent symptomatic cytomegalovirus infection after kidney transplantation. *Transplant Proc* 2001 Nov–Dec;33(7–8):3621–3623.
23. Diaz-Pedroche C, Lumbreras C, San Juan R et al. Valganciclovir preemptive therapy for the prevention of cytomegalovirus disease in high-risk seropositive solid-organ transplant recipients. *Transplantation* 2006 Jul 15;82(1):30–35.
24. Singh N, Wannstedt C, Keyes L, Gayowski T, Wagener MM, Cacciarelli TV. Efficacy of valganciclovir administered as preemptive therapy for cytomegalovirus disease in liver transplant recipients: impact on viral load and late-onset cytomegalovirus disease. *Transplantation* 2005 Jan 15;79(1):85–90.
25. Eid AJ, Arthurs SK, Deziel PJ, Wilhelm MP, Razonable RR. Emergence of drug-resistant cytomegalovirus in the era of valganciclovir prophylaxis: therapeutic implications and outcomes. *Clin Transplant* 2008 Mar–Apr;22(2):162–170.
26. Razonable RR, Brown RA, Humar A, Covington E, Alecock E, Paya CV. Herpesvirus infections in solid organ transplant patients at high risk of primary cytomegalovirus disease. *J Infect Dis* 2005 Oct 15;192(8):1331–1339.
27. Kidd IM, Clark DA, Sabin CA et al. Prospective study of human betaherpesviruses after renal transplantation: association of human herpesvirus 7 and cytomegalovirus co-infection with cytomegalovirus disease and increased rejection. *Transplantation* 2000 Jun 15;69(11): 2400–2404.
28. Schulz TF. Epidemiology of Kaposi's sarcoma-associated herpesvirus/human herpesvirus 8. *Adv Cancer Res* 1999;76:121–160.
29. Antman K, Chang Y. Kaposi's sarcoma. *N Engl J Med* 2000 Apr 6;342(14):1027–1038.
30. Rao KV, Ma J. Chronic viral hepatitis enhances the risk of infection but not acute rejection in renal transplant recipients. *Transplantation* 1996 Dec 27;62(12):1765–1769.
31. Rao KV, Kasiske BL, Anderson WR. Variability in the morphological spectrum and clinical outcome of chronic liver disease in hepatitis B-positive and B-negative renal transplant recipients. *Transplantation* 1991 Feb;51(2):391–396.
32. Mioli VA, Balestra E, Bibiano L et al. Epidemiology of viral hepatitis in dialysis centers: a national survey. *Nephron* 1992;61(3):278–283.
33. Roberts RC, Lane C, Hatfield P et al. All anti-HBc-positive, HBsAg-negative dialysis patients on the transplant waiting list should be regarded as at risk of hepatitis B reactivation post-renal transplantation – report of three cases from a single centre. *Nephrol Dial Transplant* 2006 Nov;21(11):3316–3319.
34. Mathurin P, Mouquet C, Poynard T et al. Impact of hepatitis B and C virus on kidney transplantation outcome. *Hepatology* 1999 Jan;29(1):257–263.
35. Madayag RM, Johnson LB, Bartlett ST et al. Use of renal allografts from donors positive for hepatitis B core antibody confers minimal risk for subsequent development of clinical hepatitis B virus disease. *Transplantation* 1997 Dec 27;64(12):1781–1786.
36. Han DJ, Kim TH, Park SK et al. Results on preemptive or prophylactic treatment of lamivudine in HBsAg (+) renal allograft recipients: comparison with salvage treatment after hepatic dysfunction with HBV recurrence. *Transplantation* 2001 Feb 15;71(3):387–394.
37. Chang TT, Gish RG, de Man R et al. A comparison of entecavir and lamivudine for HBeAg-positive chronic hepatitis B. *N Engl J Med* 2006 Mar 9;354(10):1001–1010.
38. Boletis JN. Epidemiology and mode of transmission of hepatitis C virus infection after renal transplantation. *Nephrol Dial Transplant* 2000;15(Suppl 8):52–54.

39. Kallinowski B, Hergesell O, Zeier M. Clinical impact of hepatitis C virus infection in the renal transplant recipient. *Nephron* 2002 Aug;91(4):541–546.

40. Anderson LJ. Role of parvovirus B19 in human disease. *Pediatr Infect Dis J* 1987 Aug;6(8):711–718.

41. Ardehali H, Volmar K, Roberts C, Forman M, Becker LC. Fatal disseminated adenoviral infection in a renal transplant patient. *Transplantation* 2001 Apr 15;71(7):998–999.

42. Leruez-Ville M, Minard V, Lacaille F et al. Real-time blood plasma polymerase chain reaction for management of disseminated adenovirus infection. *Clin Infect Dis* 2004 Jan 1;38(1): 45–52.

43. Ghosh S, Champlin RE, Englund J et al. Respiratory syncytial virus upper respiratory tract illnesses in adult blood and marrow transplant recipients: combination therapy with aerosolized ribavirin and intravenous immunoglobulin. *Bone Marrow Transplant* 2000 Apr;25(7): 751–755.

44. Boeckh M, Berrey MM, Bowden RA, Crawford SW, Balsley J, Corey L. Phase 1 evaluation of the respiratory syncytial virus-specific monoclonal antibody palivizumab in recipients of hematopoietic stem cell transplants. *J Infect Dis* 2001 Aug 1;184(3):350–354.

45. Knowles WA. Discovery and epidemiology of the human polyomaviruses BK virus (BKV) and JC virus (JCV). *Adv Exp Med Biol* 2006;577:19–45.

46. Phillips T, Jacobs R, Ellis EN. Polyoma nephropathy and progressive multifocal leukoencephalopathy in a renal transplant recipient. *J Child Neurol* 2004 Apr;19(4):301–304.

47. van Gorder MA, Della Pelle P, Henson JW, Sachs DH, Cosimi AB, Colvin RB. Cynomolgus polyoma virus infection: a new member of the polyoma virus family causes interstitial nephritis, ureteritis, and enteritis in immunosuppressed cynomolgus monkeys. *Am J Pathol* 1999 Apr;154(4):1273–1284.

48. Bohl DL, Storch GA, Ryschkewitsch C et al. Donor origin of BK virus in renal transplantation and role of HLA C7 in susceptibility to sustained BK viremia. *Am J Transplant* 2005 Sep;5(9):2213–2221.

49. Hirsch HH, Knowles W, Dickenmann M et al. Prospective study of polyomavirus type BK replication and nephropathy in renal-transplant recipients. *N Engl J Med* 2002 Aug 15;347(7):488–496.

50. Brennan DC, Agha I, Bohl DL et al. Incidence of BK with tacrolimus versus cyclosporine and impact of preemptive immunosuppression reduction. *Am J Transplant* 2005 Mar;5(3): 582–594.

51. Bohl DL, Brennan DC. BK virus nephropathy and kidney transplantation. *Clin J Am Soc Nephrol* 2007 Jul;2(Suppl 1):S36–S46.

52. Feng H, Shuda M, Chang Y, Moore PS. Clonal integration of a polyomavirus in human Merkel cell carcinoma. *Science* 2008 Feb 22;319(5866):1096–1100.

53. Lemos B, Nghiem P. Merkel cell carcinoma: more deaths but still no pathway to blame. *J Invest Dermatol* 2007 Sep;127(9):2100–2103.

54. Tharayil John G, Shankar V, Talaulikar G et al. Epidemiology of systemic mycoses among renal-transplant recipients in India. *Transplantation* 2003 May 15;75(9):1544–1551.

55. Pfaller MA, Diekema DJ, Gibbs DL et al. Results from the ARTEMIS DISK Global Antifungal Surveillance study, 1997 to 2005: an 8.5-year analysis of susceptibilities of Candida species and other yeast species to fluconazole and voriconazole determined by CLSI standardized disk diffusion testing. *J Clin Microbiol* 2007 Jun;45(6):1735–1745.

56. Edwards JE Jr., Bodey GP, Bowden RA et al. International conference for the development of a consensus on the management and prevention of severe candidal infections. *Clin Infect Dis* 1997 Jul;25(1):43–59.

57. Husain S, Wagener MM, Singh N. Cryptococcus neoformans infection in organ transplant recipients: variables influencing clinical characteristics and outcome. *Emerg Infect Dis* 2001 May–Jun;7(3):375–381.

58. Bren A, Koselj M, Kandus A et al. Severe fungal infections in kidney graft recipients. *Transplant Proc* 2002 Nov;34(7):2999–3000.

59. Perfect JR, Cox GM, Lee JY et al. The impact of culture isolation of Aspergillus species: a hospital-based survey of aspergillosis. *Clin Infect Dis* 2001 Dec 1;33(11):1824–1833.

60. Herbrecht R, Denning DW, Patterson TF et al. Voriconazole versus amphotericin B for primary therapy of invasive aspergillosis. *N Engl J Med* 2002 Aug 8;347(6):408–415.

61. Nampoory MR, Khan ZU, Johny KV et al. Invasive fungal infections in renal transplant recipients. *J Infect* 1996 Sep;33(2):95–101.

62. Wheat LJ, Kohler RB, Tewari RP. Diagnosis of disseminated histoplasmosis by detection of Histoplasma capsulatum antigen in serum and urine specimens. *N Engl J Med* 1986 Jan 9;314(2):83–88.

63. Spieker C, Barenbrock M, Tepel M, Buchholz B, Rahn KH, Zidek W. Pentamidine inhalation as a prophylaxis against Pneumocystis carinii pneumonia after therapy of acute renal allograft rejection with orthoclone (OKT3). *Transplant Proc* 1992 Dec;24(6):2602–2603.

64. Koseoglu F, Emiroglu R, Karakayali H, Bilgin N, Haberal M. Prevalence of mycobacterial infection in solid organ transplant recipients. *Transplant Proc* 2001 Feb–Mar;33(1–2): 1782–1784.

65. Yildiz A, Sever MS, Turkmen A et al. Tuberculosis after renal transplantation: experience of one Turkish centre. *Nephrol Dial Transplant* 1998 Jul;13(7):1872–1875.

66. Simpson WG, Gerhardstein DC, Thompson JR. Disseminated Strongyloides stercoralis infection. *South Med J* 1993 Jul;86(7):821–825.

67. Berk SL, Verghese A, Alvarez S, Hall K, Smith B. Clinical and epidemiologic features of strongyloidiasis. A prospective study in rural Tennessee. *Arch Intern Med* 1987 Jul;147(7):1257–1261.

68. Lim S, Katz K, Krajden S, Fuksa M, Keystone JS, Kain KC. Complicated and fatal Strongyloides infection in Canadians: risk factors, diagnosis and management. *CMAJ* 2004 Aug 31;171(5):479–484.

69. Siddiqui AA, Berk SL. Diagnosis of Strongyloides stercoralis infection. *Clin Infect Dis* 2001 Oct 1;33(7):1040–1047.

70. Genta RM. Predictive value of an enzyme-linked immunosorbent assay (ELISA) for the serodiagnosis of strongyloidiasis. *Am J Clin Pathol* 1988 Mar;89(3):391–394.

71. Gann PH, Neva FA, Gam AA. A randomized trial of single- and two-dose ivermectin versus thiabendazole for treatment of strongyloidiasis. *J Infect Dis* 1994 May;169(5):1076–1079.

Chapter 18
Malignancies Before and After Transplantation

Mary B. Prendergast and Roslyn B. Mannon

Introduction

The success of solid organ transplantation has improved dramatically over the past decades in large part due to the potency of immunosuppressive regimens. However, these regimens, with their prolonged depression of the recipient immune response, may also enhance reactivation of latent malignancy, enhance the development of de novo malignancy and, though rare, support the inadvertent transmission of malignancy from donor to recipient. Compared to the general population, the chronic use of immunosuppressive agents increases the long-term risk of malignancy. Additionally, end-stage renal disease, in and of itself, confers an increased risk of malignancy.[1-3] When combined with immunosuppression, there is an additive effect resulting in increased cancer risk post-transplantation.[1-3] The development of cancer after transplantation is further associated with dire consequences as patients with post-transplant malignancies have higher mortality rates than their non-transplanted counterparts.[4] Cancer is also a major cause of morbidity after transplantation with one-third of recipient deaths with a functioning allograft due to cancer.[5] Thus, a fine balance must be achieved between successful prevention of allograft rejection and the potential complications of immunosuppressive therapy, particularly the risk of post-transplant malignancy. Even before transplantation, a history of previous malignancy can delay transplantation until a defined period of disease-free survival has passed. In this chapter, we will review the etiology and risk factors for malignancy, review appropriate screening strategies, and also discuss individual cancers and their management in this population.

R.B. Mannon (✉)
Division of Nephrology, Department of Medicine, University of Alabama at Birmingham, Birmingham, AL, USA
e-mail: rmannon@uab.edu

D.B. McKay, S.M. Steinberg (eds.), *Kidney Transplantation: A Guide to the Care of Kidney Transplant Recipients*, DOI 10.1007/978-1-4419-1690-7_18,
© Springer Science+Business Media, LLC 2010

Epidemiology, Etiology, and Risk Factors

The incidence of cancer after transplantation is higher than in the non-transplant population[1,2,6–9] and the relative rates are shown in Table 18.1. Of all malignancies, carcinomas of the skin (squamous cell, basal cell, Merkel cell, melanoma) and lymphoma (primarily non-Hodgkin's) are the most common post-transplant,[10] occurring at 3-fold and 20-fold greater frequencies, respectively, than in the non-transplant population. Renal cell carcinoma in patients with end-stage renal failure occurs 2.6–7.6% higher frequency than in the general population and can occur in the native kidneys of renal transplant recipients.[6,11] Genitourinary cancers such as cervical carcinoma in situ, anal cancer, testicular, and bladder are also quite common, with, for example, a 14- to 16-fold increase in the incidence of cervical carcinoma in situ in kidney transplant recipients compared with the general population. There is a twofold increase in allograft recipients of the more common solid organ malignancies, such as breast, colon, and prostate cancers, compared with the general population. Head and neck cancers (oral cavity, pharynx, larynx), and hepatocellular carcinoma, usually in context of hepatitis B or C are also seen with significant frequency in solid organ transplant recipients. However, the incidence of a second primary cancer appears to be similar to that of a first malignancy in transplant patients.

Table 18.1 Incidence of common cancers in renal transplant recipients

Increased incidence cancer type allograft recipients	Tumor type	Average time to development of post-transplant malignancy
20-Fold	Non-melanomatous skin cancer	3–8 years
	Merkel cell	7.5 years
	Kaposi's sarcoma	13–21 months
	Non-Hodgkin's lymphoma	32 months
		5 months (if donor origin)
15-Fold	Renal cell carcinoma	
5-Fold	Leukemia	142 months
	Melanoma	
	Hepatobiliary cancer	
	Cervical cancer	
	Vulvovaginal cancer	
3-Fold	Testicular cancer	
	Bladder cancer	
2-Fold	Breast, lung, colon, prostate, esophagus, stomach, pancreas, ovary	

The latency period after transplantation for a cancer diagnosis varies from 3 to 5 years with lymphoma occurring most frequently in the first post-transplant period and, in the later post-transplant period, is extremely common with the incidence of malignancy at 10 years post-transplant being 72%.[12] The average recipient age at the time of diagnosis for all cancers is 40 years and renal allograft recipients older than 55 years at the time of transplantation have a greater than 25% risk of one or more non-skin cancers after 10 years of immunosuppression. Between the ages of 35 and 45, the risk of non-skin cancers for male and female transplant recipients is 7 and 10%, respectively. In contrast, in pediatric recipients, the incidence of PTLD is higher than in adult renal transplant recipients (1.2% of adult cases versus 10.1% pediatric).[13] The disease also generally occurs sooner in children, with a higher incidence when the recipient is EBV seronegative and the allograft is from a seropositive donor (86%). Adult recipients are more likely to be EBV seropositive, which may provide some explanation for this disparity. Further discussion of this dreaded complication is covered below.

The Role of Immunosuppression

A critical risk factor for cancer development is the use of immunosuppression. Immunosuppression at the time of transplantation often includes an induction agent, either a lymphocyte-depletion antibody therapy or a non-depleting antibody therapy. Induction is then coupled to maintenance immunosuppressive therapy, which is frequently composed of a calcineurin inhibitor, such as cyclosporine or tacrolimus, an anti-metabolite agent, such as mycophenolate mofetil or azathioprine, and prednisone. It has become apparent that the overall level of immunosuppression may be a critical factor in determining risk of post-transplant malignancy as post-cardiac transplant recipients, following relatively intense immunosuppressive protocols, have higher rates of cancer than other recipients of other solid organs who receive less overall immunosuppression.[13]

Differing classes of agents have specific impacts on cancer development. Calcineurin inhibitors (CNI; cyclosporine, tacrolimus) promote malignant transformation via stimulating transforming growth factor beta (TGF-β) and increased expression of vascular endothelial growth.[14] Azathioprine is known to sensitize skin to UV damage. Sirolimus, an inhibitor of mammalian target of rapamycin (mTOR), on the other hand, has anti-proliferative properties via inhibition of p70S6K and inhibition of IL-10 and cyclins. In recipients treated with sirolimus, the incidence of cancer, particularly skin cancer, is lower and moreover regression of Kaposi lesions has been seen in transplant recipients converted to rapamycin from a calcineurin inhibitor based regimen.[15–17] Thus, some groups advocate that maintenance immunosuppression in recipients with prior cancer should include sirolimus and have also suggested converting patients to it when a cancer develops. Larger, more aggressive, and metastatic skin lesions are less likely to respond. However, there is a lack of prospective, well-controlled studies using rapamycin for prevention or management of post-transplant malignancy to support a firm conclusion about its use in patient management, though the reduced incidence of de novo post-transplant malignancies and remission and/or regression of the most lesions seems to support the use of mTORi.[18]

Finally, the anti-metabolite agent, mycophenolate mofetil (MMF), inhibits inosine monophosphate dehydrogenase resulting in impaired lymphocyte function. This enzyme is significantly elevated in many malignancies.[19,20] In some studies, MMF has been shown to be associated with lower rates of malignancy[21,22] perhaps through this mechanism.

The Role of Infection in Post-transplant Malignancy

A number of viruses have been associated with malignancy in the transplant recipient. These usually quiescent viruses, in the immunocompromised host, support malignant transformation. Post-transplant lymphoproliferative disorder (PTLD) has been strongly linked to Epstein–Barr virus infection and is one of the most common malignancies seen in solid organ transplant recipients.[10] Human herpes virus-8 has been implicated in the development of Kaposi's sarcoma after transplantation. The recently described Merkel cell polyomavirus is thought to be responsible for Merkel cell skin cancers in transplant recipients.[23] Fortunately, these tumors usually respond to a significant dose reduction in immunosuppression at the risk of rejection or a change in the maintenance immunosuppressive regimen to include sirolimus. Human papilloma virus (HPV) subtypes have been detected in benign and malignant tissue of transplant recipients and have been associated with squamous cell cancers of the skin, as well as head and neck cancers and anogenital cancers.[6] HPV DNA is detectable in up to 95% of skin cancers and some head and neck cancers in this population. Secondary squamous cell cancers are associated with warts with detectable HPV in tissue. A causative role, however, has not been established between HPV and skin cancers in organ recipients[24–31] and infection may be a surrogate for over-immunosuppression. HPV vaccine is now available, the role of vaccination in prevention in the transplant population is not known (see below).

Cancer Screening Pre-transplantation

Screening for malignancy pre-transplantation is a routine practice, and these requirements include mammography, cervical PAP smear, colonoscopy, and prostate-specific antigen as appropriate to gender and age. Each transplant program may have peculiarities specific to their screening process. Evaluation for renal cell carcinoma is often mandated for patients who have been on dialysis for a prolonged period of time, patients with polycystic kidney, or patients with unexplained hematuria or polycythemia. This includes imaging of the native kidneys for suspicious lesions and urological evaluation prior to listing for transplantation.

As prior episodes of cancer are a risk factor for post-transplant malignancy, patients with pre-existing malignancy must be carefully screened, and the disease must be deemed successfully cured. There is marked variability in the likelihood of recurrence according to tumor type that determines recommended waiting times before transplantation is considered appropriate. For each malignancy, there are specific waiting times before listing for transplantation is appropriate, as shown in Table 18.2. In general, this means a waiting time of at least 2 years for some tumors independent of staging, especially if localized disease at the time of diagnosis, and 5 years depending on tumor and more systemic disease involvement. Recurrence rates are less than 10% for localized renal cell carcinoma, testicular, cervical, thyroid cancers and lymphomas. A higher rate (11–25%) of recurrence is reported for carcinoma of breast, colon, prostate, and uterus. The highest rates of recurrence are seen in patients with a history of bladder cancer, advanced renal cell carcinoma, myeloma, and melanomatous and non-melanomatous skin cancers. No waiting time is necessary for low-grade cancers such as carcinoma in situ, basal cell carcinoma, incidental renal cell confined within capsule, or very low grade bladder cancer. Ultimately, the precise waiting period should be based, however, on an individual basis by tumor type, staging, and response to therapy, and in conjunction with information from the patient's oncologist. The Israel Penn International Transplant Tumor Registry (www.ipittr.uc.edu) is an excellent resource about malignancy and transplantation and provides a service whereby an individual physician may obtain recommendations regarding a specific patient. Ultimately, potential transplant candidates should be referred to the transplant center where this issue can be directly

Table 18.2 Recommended waiting times after primary malignancy prior to transplantation

Cancer	Recommended pre-transplant waiting time	Cancer	Recommended pre-transplant waiting time
Breast		*Kaposi's sarcoma*	
Carcinoma in situ	2 years	Limited	2 years
Cancer	5 years	Diffuse; disseminated in HIV	Not recommended
Lung Cancer	2 years	*Leukemia*	2 years
Colon cancer		*Malignant melanoma* (in situ)	5 years
Stage 1	2 years		
Stage 2 or greater	5 years		
Renal cell cancer		*Squamous cell carcinoma*	2 years
Small, low grade	2 years		
Large, high grade	5 years		
Prostate	2 years	*Basal cell carcinoma*	No waiting time
Liver	Not recommended	*Bladder*	
		Non-invasive	2 years
		Non-invasive	5 years
Multiple myeloma	Not recommended	*Cervical/uterine*	2 years
Lymphoma	2 years	*Testicular*	2 years
CNS lymphoma HIV	Not recommended		

addressed and, in some settings, patients may be wait-listed in an inactive status until deemed appropriate for transplant.

Prevention and Screening

There may be important differences between the general population, chronic kidney disease population,[32] and transplant patients in terms of preventive screening. Assay ranges, or radiologic findings, appropriate for non-transplant patients may be different from those applicable to the transplant population. Specific principles of cancer screening in the transplant population have not been clearly defined. The principles of any screening process require that early detection and recognition of a particular disease process be of value with improved health outcomes including quality and quantity of life, and that the screening procedure and societal treatment costs be economically balanced. The test itself has to be specific, sensitive, and reliable, with high positive and negative predictive values. Benefits of screening to detect early cancer must be weighed against the costs of screening and potential harm to the individual. This is even more relevant for transplant patients where an individual's life expectancy is lower than that of the general population. It is uncertain whether current screening guidelines for the general population are wholly applicable to transplant patients, not just because of expected survival differences, but because of screening test performance and interpretation, response to treatment, and the existence of comorbid factors, particularly cardiovascular disease.[33] Overdetection of disease, and its consequent treatment and attendant morbidity, by routine screening that might not otherwise have manifest in the course of the patient's lifetime is undesirable medically, psychologically, and financially.

Donor Cancer Transmission

Transmission of cancer from the donor is a relatively rare entity with living donor screening, as living donors typically have been scrutinized to be in excellent health and adequately screened for malignancy. In practical terms, it is more applicable to deceased donor organs. Given that transplant patients are immunosuppressed, microscopic disease from the donor organ could potentially proliferate in the recipient and disseminate systemically. The risk of donor having undetected cancer is of the order of 1.3% and the risk of transmission is 0.2%.[34] The rate of transmission is also dependent on tumor type. A renal cell cancer that is confined within the renal capsule, and without vascular invasion, has a very low risk of transmission. CNS tumors also carry very low risk of transmission. Melanoma and choriocarcinoma, on the other hand, have a high risk of transmission to recipient. The transmission of virus, such as Epstein–Barr virus, from donor to recipient, especially if the recipient is seronegative, may result in subsequent development of PTLD. Buell et al. reported 45% rate of malignancy in patients who received an allograft from a donor subsequently found to have a malignancy, with metastatic disease in about half of those patients.[19] The risk is very low, however, in donors with a history of past malignancy, in remission at the time of donation. In order to reduce morbidity and mortality of donor-transmitted malignancies, the United Network for Organ Sharing (UNOS) has approved accelerated re-transplantation for recipients of organs from donors found post-donation to have malignancy. Management of malignancies of donor origin, in particular, should include a reduction in immunosuppression, in addition to standard of care practices for that tumor.

Skin Cancers

Skin cancers are the most frequent malignancies after solid organ transplantation[35]; 95% of skin cancers seen are either squamous cell (SCC) or basal cell carcinomas (BCC) at a ratio 4:1 – a reversal of that seen in the general population. The incidence of rare tumors such as melanoma, Merkel cell (neuro-endocrine cancer), and Kaposi's sarcoma are also increased in this population. The incidence of non-melanoma skin cancers increase steadily with time after transplantation. In the United States and Western Europe, the 2-, 10-, and 20-year incidence is 5, 10–27, and 40–60%.[36-38] Furthermore, the greater the degree of immunosuppression the greater the incidence of skin cancer development. SCC and BCC appear principally on sun-exposed areas. Mean time to their development is 8–10 years post-transplant, but have been seen even earlier and are often associated with multiple keratotic skin lesions, whose presence denotes an increased risk of SCC or BCC. In kidney and heart transplant recipients, the presence of one SCC has been shown to be predictive of multiple subsequent SCC lesions. These cancers behave more aggressively, grow rapidly, recur locally after resection in 13.4% of patients, and metastasize in about 5–8% of patients. Interestingly, the risk of a second primary cancer is higher in transplant recipients with a history of SCCs.

Skin cancers result from a combination of a decrease in immune surveillance and from direct oncogenic properties of some immunosuppressive agents, on a background history of common sun exposure. Risk factors for skin cancer are similar to the general population and include fair skin tone, eyes, and hair and a predilection for sunburn.[14] Cumulative sun exposure is the primary responsible carcinogen, supported by the fact that most lesions appear on sun-exposed skin, and the incidence is higher in sunnier climes. Similarly, the burden of immunosuppression and type of agents used and duration of treatment are also associated with these malignancies. CD4 counts are lower in patients with these skin lesions than without. Additionally, a lower incidence of skin cancer is seen in living donor transplant recipients who require lower overall immunosuppression. Several studies have shown that patients on three-drug immunosuppressive regimens had a three-fold increased risk of non-melanomatous skin cancer compared to patients taking two-drug regimens.[1,14,39,40]

A number of studies suggest calcineurin inhibitors (cyclosporine/tacrolimus) have oncogenic properties relating to the production of cytokines that promote tumor growth, angiogenesis, and metastasis. Low-dose cyclosporine has been shown to confer a lower risk of non-melanoma skin cancer than standard dose cyclosporine.[41] On the other hand, mTOR inhibitors (sirolimus/everolimus), which inhibit angiogenesis, have been associated with a lower incidence of non-melanoma skin cancers. However, there is a lack of sufficient controlled clinical trial data to support conversion to a sirolimus-based regimen to induce tumor regression and fewer subsequent skin lesions. Finally, azathioprine has been associated with higher rates of skin cancer as it sensitizes skin cells to UVA-induced skin damage, though UVB damage seems to be of greater importance in skin cancer development.[42]

Age is another important risk factor for skin cancer. Patients who receive allograft organs after the age of 55 have a 12-fold higher risk for development of skin cancer compared to patients who received grafts before age of 34.[43] Other risk factors include male sex and polymorphisms in, for example, glutathione S-transferase and vitamin D receptor genes. Mutation of the p53 tumor suppressor gene is the most common genetic error in skin cancers. Such mutations have been detected in normal appearing skin patches of organ transplant recipients, and the frequency of these patches appears to be a risk factor for SCC. Human papilloma virus infection is also associated with an increased risk of skin cancer,[26,30] as well as head and neck cancer, and there may be a role for vaccination pre-transplant to reduce risk associated with HPV (see below).

Management of transplant-related skin cancers requires a multi-disciplinary effort and depends on the type and number of lesions. Prevention is better than cure and patient education pre- and post-transplantation in the areas of skin cancer prevention, detection, and treatment strategies is essential. Actinic keratoses are a precursor to invasive squamous cell skin cancers and should be treated aggressively to prevent progression. The development of de novo squamous cell cancer is predictive of subsequent multi-lesion development and identifies a patient as high risk for skin cancer. Strategies to reduce risk of non-melanomatous skin lesions include avoidance of sun exposure, the use of protective clothing, and the diligent application of high-factor sunscreen. Compliance in this area can be difficult, as sunscreen in this instance is not covered by insurance or Medicare. Studies have shown that the use of sunscreen in patients significantly contributes to their non-development of actinic keratoses and invasive squamous cell skin cancers compared to the untreated group over the same period of time. Complete annual dermatologic examinations are also recommended.

With suspected or proven squamous lesions, surgical excision with clear margins is standard of care. Invasive squamous cell cancers need more aggressive management since they have a higher risk of recurrence and/or metastasis. Metastatic involvement of a single regional lymph node may be curable by lymphadenectomy alone, but may require adjuvant treatment with chemotherapy or radiation. Superficial lesions may be managed with cryotherapy or electrocautery and curettage. Basal cell carcinomas generally do not metastasize and do not require care beyond the standard for an immunocompetent individual. Treatment of melanoma requires wide local excision and/or sentinel lymphadenectomy. The treatment of specific lesions, however, does not prevent recurrence or the development of new cancers. Alternative therapies that can be applied to larger treatment areas include topical imiquimod, 5-fluoruracil, photodynamic therapy, and 3% diclofenac gel. Systemic retinoids also slow down the development of new lesions, and topical retinoids reduce actinic keratoses. Regarding modification of immunosuppression, it is clear for Kaposi's sarcoma that a sirolimus-based regimen is advantageous. This is not so clear for non-melanomatous skin cancer. There are no guidelines in place that define when changes in immunosuppressive regimens should be made and whether a reduction in immunosuppression, as opposed to a change in immunosuppressive agents, is more advantageous. Reduction of immunosuppression predictably results in a lower incidence of skin cancer, but must be weighed against an increased risk of allograft rejection.

Annual examination of the skin by a dermatologist is recommended, with more frequent visits for high-risk patients. This applies to Kaposi's sarcoma also and should include examination of mucous membranes. Serologic HHV-8 positivity may warrant closer monitoring and follow-up.

Post-transplant Lymphoproliferative Disorder

The risk of post-transplant lymphoproliferative disorder (PTLD) is of the order of 1% in solid organ transplant recipients, conferring a 20- to 50-fold higher risk of lymphoma than the general population. It is a serious and potentially fatal complication of solid organ transplantation. Most PTLDs are B-cell, large non-Hodgkin's lymphomas. Few are T cell in origin, but confer a dismal prognosis. The pathogenesis appears to relate to B-cell proliferation induced by infection with Epstein–Barr virus infection in the setting of immunosuppression. Non-EBV-driven PTLD can occur, though is uncommon. Most PTLDs originate in the recipient, and donor origin tumors are less common and tend to involve the allograft. Greater than 50% of PTLD presents in extra-nodal sites and involves the gastrointestinal tract, lungs, liver, mucosal tissue, skin, and CNS. In renal allograft recipient, PTLD is more likely to develop in the renal allograft, while in heart transplant recipients, lymphoma typically presents in the heart allograft. This predilection of the transplanted organ for subsequent development of PTLD may be attributed to local immune response to foreign tissue.

The principal risk factors for PTLD are the burden of immunosuppression and EBV status of the recipient at the time of transplantation. EBV-naïve patients are at increased risk for developing PTLD post-transplantation and there is a 24-fold increased risk in PTLD among EBV-negative recipients of EBV-positive donor organs.[44] Children are at higher risk than adults, which may be reflective of a greater likelihood of EBV seronegativity at the time of transplantation. It is also recognized that allograft recipients who are managed with a lower overall immunosuppression experience PTLD less frequently. The incidence of PTLD in heart transplant recipients is higher than in renal transplant recipients, the former requiring greater immunosuppression.[45] Transplant recipients who received induction therapy have a significantly higher risk of developing subsequent PTLD than those transplanted without the use of induction agents. Interestingly, alemtuzumab ($^{®}$Campath), a profoundly immunosuppressive induction agent, has not been found to be associated with as high a rate of PTLD as other lymphocyte-depleting agents.[46] Of less importance seems to be the choice of maintenance immunosuppressive agents, though in patients transplanted without induction, the use of tacrolimus over cyclosporine is associated with a higher incidence of PTLD. Most PTLD occurs in the first post-transplant year when the burden of immunosuppression is highest or in the first year following aggressive treatment for rejection.

Evaluation and diagnosis of PTLD requires a high index of suspicion. Tissue confirmation is the gold standard. CT scan, positive emission tomography (PET) scan, quantitative EBV PCR, and increasing LDH are useful adjunctive tests. The diagnosis of CNS PTLD requires confirmation of malignant cells in CSF or from tissue biopsy. Positive MRI with gadolinium, positive CSF for EBV, and positive quantitative EBV PCR in serum are also highly suggestive of a diagnosis of PTLD.

Prevention and treatment of PTLD can be equally accomplished with minimization of immunosuppression. This has to be carefully balanced against risk of allograft loss. In terms of prevention, patients at high risk for PTLD (donor positive, recipient negative) have been treated with intravenous ganciclovir and oral acyclovir with some success, in conjunction with frequent monitoring for EBV.[47,48] The cornerstone of treatment is reduction of immunosuppression, balanced against allograft loss and patient morbidity/mortality. The degree of reduction essentially corresponds to the disease severity. For example, with extensive disease, cessation of all immunosuppressive agents except prednisone with close assessment of response for 2 or 3 weeks is appropriate. For less extensive disease, a 50% reduction in calcineurin inhibitor dose and the continuation of prednisone accompanied by a similar strategy of follow-up may be employed. There is currently no evidence to support efficacy of any anti-viral agent in the management of PTLD. Those who do not respond to this measure require more aggressive management. Rituximab, anti-CD20 antibody, is often a first step either alone or in combination with a standard lymphoma chemotherapeutic combination of cyclophosphamide, prednisone, vincristine, and doxorubicin (CHOP). Response can be determined in part with serial quantitation of EBV genome in patient's serum and serial radiologic measurements. There are other chemotherapeutic combinations available, and all require cessation of maintenance immunosuppressive agents until final chemotherapy is complete. Response rates in excess of 70% have been reported with the R-CHOP combination.[49] CNS involvement may also require field irradiation therapy.

Review of tissue by a specialist pathologist is essential to define whether the lesion is B or T cell in origin, as treatment and prognosis will differ significantly for the two tumor types. Prognosis is poor for T-cell PTLD, which is usually EBV negative and less responsive to reductions in immunosuppressive therapy. Prognosis is variable and depends on a number of factors. Increased mortality rates are seen with early diagnosis (<6 months since transplant), increasing age, multiple disease sites, performance status ≥ 2, and allograft plus other organ involvement, as opposed to allograft alone which carries a better prognosis.[50–52] Survival rates for adults, at

1 and 5 years, are reported at 93 and 86% for patient survival and 80 and 60% for allograft survival, respectively.[13] Re-transplantation can occur in these patients if graft loss does occur. There does not appear to be an increased risk of PTLD in the context of subsequent grafts, though a period of 2 years should be allowed to elapse before proceeding to re-transplant. In one large cohort, overall patient and allograft survival was 86 and 74% following re-transplant.[53]

Renal Cell and Hepatobiliary Carcinomas

The incidence of renal cell carcinoma is about 100 times greater in end-stage renal disease and transplant patients than the general population.[54–56] Most cancers arise in the native kidneys rather than the renal allograft. This is of even greater concern in renal patients with adult polycystic kidney disease (APKD), who may require more intensive screening. In general, annual surveillance of the native kidneys by ultrasound or CT scan is recommended, though there are no firm guidelines regarding frequency. In general, patients with or without APKD who have Bosniak I (simple benign cysts) or II cysts (one or two septations, fine wall calcifications, non-enhancing hyperdense cysts) should undergo renal ultrasonography twice yearly, followed by CT or MRI for suspicious lesions. Bosniak IIF patients should have ultrasound every 3 months and annual CT or MRI. Nephrectomy is indicated for progressive lesions or Bosniak III or IV lesions.[57] Routine screening is not recommended and there are no prospective data to determine if such screening strategies are cost-effective in this population.

The presence of unexplained hematuria should prompt evaluation to exclude renal or bladder lesions. There is an increased risk of developing neoplasms of the native urinary tract especially in patients with a history of analgesic nephropathy, prolonged exposure to cyclophosphamide, and with a history of Chinese Herb exposure.[58] Urine cytology is not a reliable diagnostic tool. As well as the radiologic imaging recommended above, serum BK PCR and PSA are recommended. Patients with non-glomerular hematuria should also undergo cystoscopy.

For hepatocellular carcinoma, serum AFP (high specificity) and ultrasonography (high sensitivity) should be performed annually in patients with hepatitis B or C related cirrhosis. Suspicious lesions should be evaluated with contrast CT or MRI.

Other Solid Organ Tumors

As already discussed, there is a twofold increased risk of colon, lung, prostate, breast, stomach, esophagus, pancreas, and ovarian cancers in the transplant population. In general, adherence to the routine screening guidelines already established for the general non-transplant population is appropriate for transplant patients. There are some caveats. There are also differences between how some screening tests perform in the general population compared with the transplant population.

Randomized controlled trials to support or refute the efficacy of a screening test have not been performed in the transplant population. In the case of mammography, end-stage renal failure patients and transplant patients have a higher frequency of breast calcification than women with normal renal function resulting in higher rates of referral for diagnostic biopsy. Calcineurin inhibitors, especially cyclosporine, result in increased breast density and a higher incidence of benign adenomas than in non-transplant counterparts. Current cancer screening guidelines advocate screening for prostate cancer, even though a survival advantage has not been demonstrated, with a probable overdiagnosis of inconsequential disease. Free PSA is eliminated by the kidney, and rate of excretion is determined by glomerular filtration rate (GFR). Reduced GFR will result in higher PSA levels making their interpretation more difficult, especially baseline determinations, and rendering the current normal range not readily applicable for transplant recipients. Greater prevalence of cancer amongst transplant recipients may not justify an increased and aggressive approach to early detection. Allograft function in many cases will not equal that of the patient, and renal transplant recipients have a disease process that will shorten their expected survival time in any case.

Anal and Genitourinary Cancers

Because of the increased incidence of anal cancer, screening for anal intraepithelial neoplasia should be considered for all transplant recipients.[59] Gynecologic examinations should also be performed annually as there are increased risks of cervical carcinoma in situ, vulvar cancers, and uterine malignancies. The role of HPV vaccine is controversial. Vaccination post-transplantation may be ineffective for HPV-naïve patients as antibody response may be delayed, with lower seroconversion rates and a more rapid decline in antibody levels compared to the general population.[6] Recipients may already be infected with HPV rendering vaccination futile.[60]

Summary Recommendations

Modifiable cancer risk factors for the general population also apply to cancer patients. These include healthy diet, regular exercise, smoking cessation, and the use of skin care precautions with regard to sun exposure. Education is an important component of the transplantation process and randomized controlled trials have shown that education can change people's behavior. Annual evaluation by dermatology, gynecology, etc., as well as routine screening as prescribed for the general population is strongly recommended. Special consideration for the increased risk of renal cell cancer in end-stage dialysis patients, as well as transplant recipients, should be given.

In terms of treatment of malignancy in the transplant population, a reduction in immunosuppression, in general, is not required, unless a tumor is driven by Epstein–Barr virus, is donor in origin, or in the case of multiple site invasive carcinomas of the skin, when immunosuppression modification and/or minimization should be employed. Reduction or cessation of immunosuppression may result in tumor regression in lymphoma, skin cancers, Kaposi's sarcoma, and donor-derived malignancies. When serious malignancy is diagnosed post-transplantation, a reasonable first approach is discontinuation of the anti-metabolite (mycophenolate mofetil, azathioprine), with continuation of the calcineurin inhibitor (tacrolimus, cyclosporine) and prednisone, a strategy that carries less risk of allograft rejection. For recipients of a zero-mismatched allografts, continuation of the anti-metabolite and prednisone in favor of the calcineurin inhibitor may be considered. More aggressive revision with cessation of all immunosuppression may be necessary if response is suboptimal. Loss of the renal allograft, whilst undesirable, is not a terminal event, when patient survival is of paramount importance. Close collaboration with the appropriate specialist, whether oncologic, hematologic, gynecologic, or urologic, is mandatory, as further additional therapies may be warranted in addition to modification of immunosuppression. Post-transplant malignancy detection requires a high index of suspicion, and management involves a multi-disciplinary team and participation. Prevention of tumors should be the primary goal of those managing transplant recipients.

References

1. Vajdic CM, McDonald SP, McCredie MR et al. Cancer incidence before and after kidney transplantation. *JAMA* 2006;296:2823–2831.
2. Webster AC, Craig JC, Simpson JM, Jones MP, Chapman JR. Identifying high risk groups and quantifying absolute risk of cancer after kidney transplantation: a cohort study of 15,183 recipients. *Am J Transplant* 2007;7:2140–2151.
3. Maisonneuve P, Agodoa L, Gellert R et al. Cancer in patients on dialysis for end-stage renal disease: an international collaborative study. *Lancet* 1999;354:93–99.
4. Webster AC, Hayen A, Kelly PJ, Chapman JR, Craig JC. Impact of kidney transplantation and cancer co-morbidity compared with cancer alone on expected survival: a registry analysis from Australia and New Zealand. *Transplantation* 2008;86:102–103.
5. Kauffman HM, Cherikh WS, McBride MA, Cheng Y, Hanto DW. Post-transplant de novo malignancies in renal transplant recipients: the past and present. *Transpl Int* 2006;19:607–620.
6. Webster AC, Wong G, Craig JC, Chapman JR. Managing cancer risk and decision making after kidney transplantation. *Am J Transplant* 2008;8:2185–2191.
7. Adami J, Gabel H, Lindelof B et al. Cancer risk following organ transplantation: a nationwide cohort study in Sweden. *Br J Cancer* 2003;89:1221–1227.
8. Chapman JR, Webster AC. Cancer after renal transplantation: the next challenge. *Am J Transplant* 2004;4:841–842.
9. Mihalov ML, Gattuso P, Abraham K, Holmes EW, Reddy V. Incidence of post-transplant malignancy among 674 solid-organ-transplant recipients at a single center. *Clin Transplant* 1996;10:248–255.
10. Bustami RT, Ojo AO, Wolfe RA et al. Immunosuppression and the risk of post-transplant malignancy among cadaveric first kidney transplant recipients. *Am J Transplant* 2004;4:87–93.

11. Buell JFBT, Woodle ES. Management of Posttransplant Malignancies. Online CME/CE Activity. 2004; http://www.medscape.com/viewprogram/3282_pnt.
12. Webster AC, Byrne B, McDonald S, Craig JC, Chapman JR. Incidence, risk and prediction of cancer after renal transplantation; an analysis of ANZDATA, the Australian and New Zealand Dialysis & Transplant Registry. *Transplantation* 2004;78:35.
13. Shapiro R, Nalesnik M, McCauley J et al. Posttransplant lymphoproliferative disorders in adult and pediatric renal transplant patients receiving tacrolimus-based immunosuppression. *Transplantation* 1999;68:1851–1854.
14. Ulrich C, Kanitakis J, Stockfleth E, Euvrard S. Skin cancer in organ transplant recipients – where do we stand today? *Am J Transplant* 2008;8:2192–2198.
15. Lebbe C, Euvrard S, Barrou B et al. Sirolimus conversion for patients with posttransplant Kaposi's sarcoma. *Am J Transplant* 2006;6:2164–2168.
16. Tessmer CS, Magalhaes LV, Keitel E et al. Conversion to sirolimus in renal transplant recipients with skin cancer. *Transplantation* 2006;82:1792–1793.
17. Fernandez A, Marcen R, Pascual J et al. Conversion from calcineurin inhibitors to everolimus in kidney transplant recipients with malignant neoplasia. *Transplant Proc* 2006;38: 2453–2455.
18. Monaco AP. The role of mTOR inhibitors in the management of posttransplant malignancy. *Transplantation* 2009;87:157–163.
19. Buell JF, Gross TG, Woodle ES. Malignancy after transplantation. *Transplantation* 2005;80:S254–S264.
20. Engl T, Makarevic J, Relja B et al. Mycophenolate mofetil modulates adhesion receptors of the beta1 integrin family on tumor cells: impact on tumor recurrence and malignancy. *BMC Cancer* 2005;5:4.
21. Robson R, Cecka JM, Opelz G, Budde M, Sacks S. Prospective registry-based observational cohort study of the long-term risk of malignancies in renal transplant patients treated with mycophenolate mofetil. *Am J Transplant* 2005;5:2954–2960.
22. O'Neill JO, Edwards LB, Taylor DO. Mycophenolate mofetil and risk of developing malignancy after orthotopic heart transplantation: analysis of the transplant registry of the International Society for Heart and Lung Transplantation. *J Heart Lung Transplant* 2006;25:1186–1191.
23. Feng H, Shuda M, Chang Y, Moore PS. Clonal integration of a polyomavirus in human Merkel cell carcinoma. *Science* 2008;319:1096–1100.
24. Boxman IL, Berkhout RJ, Mulder LH et al. Detection of human papillomavirus DNA in plucked hairs from renal transplant recipients and healthy volunteers. *J Invest Dermatol* 1997;108:712–715.
25. Berkhout RJ, Bouwes Bavinck JN, ter Schegget J. Persistence of human papillomavirus DNA in benign and (pre)malignant skin lesions from renal transplant recipients. *J Clin Microbiol* 2000;38:2087–2096.
26. Harwood CA, Surentheran T, McGregor JM et al. Human papillomavirus infection and non-melanoma skin cancer in immunosuppressed and immunocompetent individuals. *J Med Virol* 2000;61:289–297.
27. Arends MJ, Benton EC, McLaren KM, Stark LA, Hunter JA, Bird CC. Renal allograft recipients with high susceptibility to cutaneous malignancy have an increased prevalence of human papillomavirus DNA in skin tumours and a greater risk of anogenital malignancy. *Br J Cancer* 1997;75:722–728.
28. Meyer T, Arndt R, Nindl I, Ulrich C, Christophers E, Stockfleth E. Association of human papillomavirus infections with cutaneous tumors in immunosuppressed patients. *Transpl Int* 2003;16:146–153.
29. Euvrard S, Chardonnet Y, Pouteil-Noble C et al. Association of skin malignancies with various and multiple carcinogenic and noncarcinogenic human papillomaviruses in renal transplant recipients. *Cancer* 1993;72:2198–2206.

30. Euvrard S, Chardonnet Y, Pouteil-Noble CP, Kanitakis J, Thivolet J, Touraine JL. Skin malignancies and human papillomaviruses in renal transplant recipients. *Transplant Proc* 1993;25:1392–1393.

31. de Jong-Tieben LM, Berkhout RJ, ter Schegget J et al. The prevalence of human papillomavirus DNA in benign keratotic skin lesions of renal transplant recipients with and without a history of skin cancer is equally high: a clinical study to assess risk factors for keratotic skin lesions and skin cancer. *Transplantation* 2000;69:44–49.

32. Wong G, Webster AC, Chapman JR, Craig JC. Reported cancer screening practices of nephrologists: results from a national survey. *Nephrol Dial Transplant* 2009;24(7): 2136–2143.

33. Wong G, Chapman JR, Craig JC. Cancer screening in renal transplant recipients: what is the evidence? *Clin J Am Soc Nephrol* 2008;3(Suppl 2):S87–S100.

34. Birkeland SA, Storm HH. Risk for tumor and other disease transmission by transplantation: a population-based study of unrecognized malignancies and other diseases in organ donors. *Transplantation* 2002;74:1409–1413.

35. Euvrard S, Kanitakis J, Claudy A. Skin cancers after organ transplantation. *N Engl J Med* 2003;348:1681–1691.

36. Kasiske BL, Snyder JJ, Gilbertson DT, Wang C. Cancer after kidney transplantation in the United States. *Am J Transplant* 2004;4:905–913.

37. Ramsay HM, Reece SM, Fryer AA, Smith AG, Harden PN. Seven-year prospective study of nonmelanoma skin cancer incidence in U.K. renal transplant recipients. *Transplantation* 2007;84:437–439.

38. Bordea C, Wojnarowska F, Millard PR, Doll H, Welsh K, Morris PJ. Skin cancers in renal-transplant recipients occur more frequently than previously recognized in a temperate climate. *Transplantation* 2004;77:574–579.

39. Campistol JM, Eris J, Oberbauer R et al. Sirolimus therapy after early cyclosporine withdrawal reduces the risk for cancer in adult renal transplantation. *J Am Soc Nephrol* 2006;17:581–589.

40. Otley CC, Maragh SL. Reduction of immunosuppression for transplant-associated skin cancer: rationale and evidence of efficacy. *Dermatol Surg* 2005;31:163–168.

41. Dantal J, Hourmant M, Cantarovich D et al. Effect of long-term immunosuppression in kidney-graft recipients on cancer incidence: randomised comparison of two cyclosporin regimens. *Lancet* 1998;351:623–628.

42. O'Donovan P, Perrett CM, Zhang X et al. Azathioprine and UVA light generate mutagenic oxidative DNA damage. *Science* 2005;309:1871–1874.

43. Otley CC, Cherikh WS, Salasche SJ, McBride MA, Christenson LJ, Kauffman HM. Skin cancer in organ transplant recipients: effect of pretransplant end-organ disease. *J Am Acad Dermatol* 2005;53:783–790.

44. Walker RC. Pretransplant assessment of the risk for posttransplant lymphoproliferative disorder. *Transplant Proc* 1995;27:41.

45. Opelz G, Henderson R. Incidence of non-Hodgkin lymphoma in kidney and heart transplant recipients. *Lancet* 1993;342:1514–1516.

46. Kirk AD, Cherikh WS, Ring M et al. Dissociation of depletional induction and posttransplant lymphoproliferative disease in kidney recipients treated with alemtuzumab. *Am J Transplant* 2007;7:2619–2625.

47. Humar A, Hebert D, Davies HD, Stephens D, O'Doherty B, Allen U. A randomized trial of ganciclovir versus ganciclovir plus immune globulin for prophylaxis against Epstein-Barr virus related posttransplant lymphoproliferative disorder. *Transplantation* 2006;81:856–861.

48. Funch DP, Walker AM, Schneider G, Ziyadeh NJ, Pescovitz MD. Ganciclovir and acyclovir reduce the risk of post-transplant lymphoproliferative disorder in renal transplant recipients. *Am J Transplant* 2005;5:2894–2900.

49. Trappe R, Riess H, Babel N et al. Salvage chemotherapy for refractory and relapsed post-transplant lymphoproliferative disorders (PTLD) after treatment with single-agent rituximab. *Transplantation* 2007;83:912–918.

50. Leblond V, Dhedin N, Mamzer Bruneel MF et al. Identification of prognostic factors in 61 patients with posttransplantation lymphoproliferative disorders. *J Clin Oncol* 2001;19: 772–778.
51. Trofe J, Buell JF, Beebe TM et al. Analysis of factors that influence survival with post-transplant lymphoproliferative disorder in renal transplant recipients: the Israel Penn International Transplant Tumor Registry experience. *Am J Transplant* 2005;5:775–780.
52. Ghobrial IM, Habermann TM, Maurer MJ et al. Prognostic analysis for survival in adult solid organ transplant recipients with post-transplantation lymphoproliferative disorders. *J Clin Oncol* 2005;23:7574–7582.
53. Johnson SR, Cherikh WS, Kauffman HM, Pavlakis M, Hanto DW. Retransplantation after post-transplant lymphoproliferative disorders: an OPTN/UNOS database analysis. *Am J Transplant* 2006;6:2743–2749.
54. Doublet JD, Peraldi MN, Gattegno B, Thibault P, Sraer JD. Renal cell carcinoma of native kidneys: prospective study of 129 renal transplant patients. *J Urol* 1997;158:42–44.
55. Denton MD, Magee CC, Ovuworie C et al. Prevalence of renal cell carcinoma in patients with ESRD pre-transplantation: a pathologic analysis. *Kidney Int* 2002;61:2201–2209.
56. Brennan JF, Stilmant MM, Babayan RK, Siroky MB. Acquired renal cystic disease: implications for the urologist. *Br J Urol* 1991;67:342–348.
57. Israel GM, Bosniak MA. An update of the Bosniak renal cyst classification system. *Urology* 2005;66:484–488.
58. Morath C, Mueller M, Goldschmidt H, Schwenger V, Opelz G, Zeier M. Malignancy in renal transplantation. *J Am Soc Nephrol* 2004;15:1582–1588.
59. Koutsky LA, Holmes KK, Critchlow CW et al. A cohort study of the risk of cervical intraepithelial neoplasia grade 2 or 3 in relation to papillomavirus infection. *N Engl J Med* 1992;327:1272–1278.
60. The Future II Study Group. Quadrivalent vaccine against human papillomavirus to prevent high-grade cervical lesions. *N Engl J Med* 2007;356:1915–1927.

Chapter 19
Bone Disease in Renal Transplantation

Bradford Lee West, Stuart M. Sprague, and Michelle A. Josephson

Transplant Patients Are at Increased Risk for Fracture

The risk of suffering a bone fracture increases following kidney transplantation. This elevated risk continues for the life of the transplant,[1] only increasing with time.[2] By 5 years post-transplant up to 50% of patients experience at least one fracture. Reported fracture incidences in transplant recipients range anywhere from 5% to greater than 60%.[1,2] This wide range of reported fracture rates is a consequence of the varied methodology used in obtaining these data. Whether determining fracture rates by questionnaire or patient encounter notes or looking for radiographic evidence dramatically affects the result. As well, the relative risk of fracture depends on the populations being used as comparisons. Male kidney transplant recipients have an overall fivefold increased fracture risk compared to the general population. Female kidney transplant recipients aged 25–44 have a relative risk of 18, and the 45- to 64-year-old female cohort has a 34-fold increased risk.[3] Dialysis patients have an increased incidence of both hip and spinal fractures relative to the general population but a decreased incidence compared with transplant recipients.[4] Using kidney failure patients as the comparison group for transplant patients will dampen the magnitude of relative risk of fracture, although the difference remains noteworthy. Studies using USRDS data from over 100,000 patients reveal a 34% increased risk of hip fracture in transplant recipients compared to those with kidney failure.[5]

In the general population fractures result in significant medical costs and morbidity.[5,6] Conservative cost estimates for hip fracture are in excess of $81,300 (2001 estimate). Life expectancy can be reduced by 25% and over 300 remaining days of life can be spent in skilled nursing facilities.[6] Although these factors have not been specifically examined in the transplant population, extrapolating from the general population there is no doubt that the high fracture incidence results in significant morbidity and mortality in transplant recipients. A study of transplant patients hospitalized for fracture showed that renal transplant recipients had an adjusted risk

B.L. West (✉)
Department of Nephrology, University of Chicago Medical Center, Chicago, IL, USA
e-mail: bradfordw9@hotmail.com

D.B. McKay, S.M. Steinberg (eds.), *Kidney Transplantation: A Guide to the Care of Kidney Transplant Recipients*, DOI 10.1007/978-1-4419-1690-7_19, © Springer Science+Business Media, LLC 2010

of fracture of 4.59 (95% CI of 3.59–6.31) compared to the general population and an increased risk of mortality of 1.6 (95% CI 1.13–2.26).[7] With the aging transplant population and with the acceptance of transplanting older individuals, this problem is poised to become even larger.

Fractures result from a decrease in bone mass and quality which results in decreased bone strength.[8] In addition conditions such as peripheral neuropathy and an increased likelihood of falls contribute to fracture risk. Bone strength is determined by impaired bone quality and bone quantity. Bone quality is a function of its turnover and level of mineralization. Bone quantity is difficult to assess in patients with kidney failure, particularly those on dialysis. In the general public, bone density serves as a surrogate for bone quantity; however, it cannot assess bone quality. It is unlikely that it is as robust a surrogate in patients with kidney disease or in the transplant population.

When evaluated by bone mineral density, osteoporosis is very common in kidney transplant patients, affecting anywhere from 27 to 57%.[9,10] This decrease in bone density can be associated with an increased fracture risk in transplant patients,[11] though the risk of diminished BMDs is better characterized in non-renal patients.[12] Most studies have not found BMDs to have the same predictive value for fracture as noted in the general population. Nevertheless many physicians obtain BMD studies in transplant recipients. How BMD findings should be used to direct therapy remains to be determined.

Bone biopsies reveal an array of qualitative abnormalities both early and late after transplant including, but not limited to, low bone turnover, osteomalacia, and high-turnover disease. Low-turnover or adynamic bone disease is characterized by decreased osteoblast and osteoclast function resulting in decreased deposition of new mineralized bone and decreased removal of old and possibly microfractured bone. Osteomalacia or defective mineralization can also be found. Adynamic bone disease and osteomalacia may occur simultaneously. High-turnover bone disease is a consequence of overactive osteoblasts and osteoclasts. New osteoid and mineralized bone is laid down rapidly and old bone is quickly removed. Similarly, both high turnover and osteomalacia may occur simultaneously. When the osteoclast activity outpaces the osteoblast activity, decreased bone mass ensues. High-turnover bone disease is frequently but not universally associated with hyperparathyroidism. It is difficult to accurately estimate the prevalence of different bone lesions as a limited number of studies have included post-transplant bone biopsies. As well, the relative contribution of the different bone pathologies changes with modifications in CKD-MBD management. To that end, adynamic bone disease may be more common now than in the past.[13]

Although documenting the type or cause of bone disease in a transplant recipient may sound academic it can be clinically useful. Aside from providing a practical guide for treatment decisions it may help predict which bones are most at risk for fracture. As an example, steroids tend to affect the cancellous bone and cause adynamic bone disease whereas hyperparathyroidism primarily affects cortical bone.[10] Cancellous bone involvement affects the spine. Although spinal compression fractures can be asymptomatic they may also result in profound back pain, decreased mobility, respiratory compromise, and a decreased quality of life.[14] Cortical bone is found predominantly in long bones of the appendicular skeleton. Several studies have found a propensity for fractures in the appendicular skeleton, especially the feet, in kidney transplant recipients.[3] Evaluating 432 kidney transplant recipients Ramsey-Goldman et al. observed 33 fractures of which 28 were appendicular and 5 were axial.[3] Hip fractures are also debilitating cortical fractures and their occurrence is increased in both dialysis and transplant patients.[5,15]

CKD: Setting the Stage for Post-transplant Bone Disorders

Almost all kidney transplant recipients suffer from disturbances in mineral metabolism universally associated with chronic kidney disease, referred to as chronic kidney disease-mineral bone disease (CKD-MBD)[16] prior to transplant. Pathologically the bone disease may manifest as either low-turnover disease or high-turnover disease with or without mineralization defects.

Chronic hyperparathyroidism plays a major role in bone loss both before and after transplant.[17] Hyperparathyroidism is very common post-transplant. Some studies demonstrate that greater than 50% of transplant patients have elevated PTH levels even after 2 years.[18] Elevations in PTH are invariably a consequence of the patient's pre-transplant physiology. The longer a patient is on dialysis, the higher their PTH level. Higher PTH values pre-transplant predict higher post-transplant PTH values.[19] PTH acts on multiple sites of the body including bone and kidney via a G-coupled receptor. With prolonged or chronic hyperparathyroidism down-regulation of the osteoblast PTH receptor ensues.[20] Chronic hyperparathyroidism seen in patients with severe kidney dysfunction can be due to increased gland mass from nodular or monoclonal hyperplasia. The hyperplasia results in secondary and tertiary hyperparathyroidism. Parathyroid cells have a prolonged half-life of 20 years.[21] Consequently the pre-transplant parathyroid gland mass is predictive of the post-transplant gland mass and hormone levels. In the setting of parathyroid hyperplasia, it may take months to years after the establishment of better kidney function for the parathyroid glands to involute and produce less hormone.[22] Despite this time lag, the PTH level is consistently below pre-transplant values by 6 months post-transplant.[18] After 6 months, investigators have found a median decrease of 54% in PTH.[18] PTH decreases to variable degrees with time after transplantation.[18] PTH concentrations may remain elevated for many years.[18] In addition to the degree to which kidney function is restored, falling PTH levels are affected by low vitamin D concentrations,[23] phosphorus abnormalities, and hypocalcemia caused by hyper-calciuria and/or poor intestinal absorption secondary to steroids and/or vitamin D deficiency.

Disorders of vitamin D metabolism play a major role in bone and mineral disorders in CKD prior to transplantation which may continue into the post-transplant period. Cholecalciferol or vitamin D_3 is acquired from dietary intake or conversion from ultraviolet light, UVB. Cholecalciferol is converted by the liver to calcidiol (25-hydroxyvitamin D_3), which is a prohormone and the storage form of the active hormone, calcitriol (1,25-hydroxyvitamin D_3). Calcitriol is produced primarily by the kidneys for its systemic effect on mineral metabolism, but is also produced by numerous other tissues, where it has a local regulatory effect. Calcidiol is utilized to monitor body stores of vitamin D. Normal vitamin D levels range from 30 to 80 ng/mL. Vitamin D deficiency is essentially endemic in CKD patients,[24] which persists post-transplantation with mean vitamin D levels being reported as low as 10.9 ng/mL (95% CI 8.2–14.3).[25]

Metabolic acidosis also contributes to bone loss following transplantation. Transplant patients may have metabolic acidosis from persistent CKD, medication-induced diarrhea, and renal tubular acidosis. Hydrogen ions bind to carbonate releasing bone calcium,[26]and hydrogen ions also stimulate osteoclasts.[27] The association of metabolic acidosis with bone loss has been demonstrated in the general population. Whether extrapolating these findings to the transplant population is appropriate is unknown. Research on this topic is more limited in kidney transplant patients and some studies have been unable to demonstrate an association of bone loss and acidosis in transplant patients.[28]

Hormonal dysregulation is common in patients with advanced CKD and ESRD. Some of these abnormalities such as low testosterone and low estradiol concentrations may persist following transplant. Low sex hormone levels have been associated with bone loss in the general population; however, direct evidence for this association is sparse for transplant patients.

In addition to factors associated with ESRD and dialysis predisposing to bone loss, other patient characteristics may influence the post-transplant bone state. For example, diabetic patients have a much higher risk of fracture compared to non-diabetics. Nearly half of diabetic patients experience a fracture within 5 years of transplant. This risk is much higher than found in their non-diabetic counterparts.[5] There is also a range of relative risk for fracture within patients who have diabetes mellitus, depending on their specific characteristics. For example, patients with insulin-dependent diabetes mellitus have a higher risk for osteoporosis compared to those with type 2 diabetes. This may be at least in part attributed to their lower BMI.[29] Patients getting a simultaneous kidney pancreas transplant (SPK) have an annual fracture rate of 11% compared to about 3.9% per year for patients getting a kidney alone, although 40% of the kidney transplant patients also had diabetes.[3] A group of 31 patients with SPK were studied and 23% & 58% respectively were found to have trabecular osteoporosis and cortical osteoporosis . Vertebral fractures were found in 45% an average of 40 months (± 23) after transplantation.[30] Other studies have also shown a predominant effect on cortical bone, underscoring the idea that in diabetics, bone loss is a consequence of more than just post-transplant steroids exposure.[31]

Non-immunosuppressive Post-transplant Factors

Following transplantation numerous factors other than immunosuppression may contribute to diminished bone strength. Commonly used medications such as loop diuretics, heparin, and anti-epileptics may impact bone quality. In addition, post-operative immobilization leading to muscle weakness and bone loss, malnutrition, vitamin D deficiency, hypogonadism, and hypophosphatemia (discussed below) also contribute to post-transplant fractures. Comorbid conditions such as diabetes mellitus may further increase the risk. Diabetes mellitus is independently associated with low-turnover bone disease as well as peripheral neuropathy and decreased vision that can increase the fall risk.

Ethnicity is another factor that may independently influence bone loss after transplant. Caucasians, especially woman, tend to have a higher fracture rate than African Americans.[32] Whether or not this is due to genetic differences is unclear. It is possible that the differences may be related to the environmental effects of different diets or even differences in BMI.[33] The vitamin D receptor has different genotypes BB, Bb, or bb and the BB genotype is much more prevalent in Caucasians than in African Americans.[34]

Hypophosphatemia is a common problem following successful kidney transplantation. Hypophosphatemia can be exacerbated by immunosuppressant medications, diuretics, persistent hyperparathyroidism, and tubular dysfunction.[35] The role of phosphatonins, such as FGF-23, in perpetuating hypophosphatemia following kidney transplantation is of particular interest.[36] The majority of patients have moderate to severe hyperphosphatemia at the time of transplantation and phosphorus concentrations tend to decrease dramatically immediately after transplantation; however, this decrease can be transient.[18] For some patients hypophosphatemia persists. About 2–40% of patients can have hypophosphatemia at 6 months after transplant.[37–39] It appears that the degree of hypophosphatemia is not associated with the GFR.[40] Treatment for hypophosphatemia is phosphorus supplementation, either through foods or by oral supplements. If the phosphorous is low enough to cause muscle weakness, intravenous phosphorous supplementation may be indicated. The net effect of low phosphorus levels on bone density, strength, and risk for fracture is not well known; however, prolonged and severe hypophosphatemia could lead to osteomalacia.

Kidney transplantation improves kidney function but does not fully restore it. Transplant recipients often have some degree of impaired kidney function and CKD. If advanced enough, transplant recipients can also be afflicted by CKD-MBD.

Immunosuppression

During the initial 6 months following transplant most patients experience a rapid decline in bone mineral density. During the early perioperative period, medications, inflammation, and immobilization can contribute to bone loss. Inflammatory cytokines contribute to bone loss by affecting RANKL and osteoprotegerin influencing osteoclastogenesis.[41] Immobilization from the surgery, steroid-associated myopathy, or other causes also contribute to bone loss. Fall risk also is increased from coexisting medical conditions such as diabetic neuropathy (RR of fracture of

2.6).[1] The largest influence on early post-transplant bone loss appears to be the use of corticosteroids.

Steroids can induce bone loss in multiple different ways such as impairing bone formation, accelerating breakdown, and causing a negative calcium balance. Steroids promote a negative calcium balance by decreasing gastrointestinal absorption and increasing urinary excretion. Steroids also impair gonadal hormone production. Steroids can induce apoptosis of osteoblasts and osteocytes and inhibit osteoblast replication and differentiation resulting in an imbalance of osteoclast and osteoblast number and function causing bone loss.[42] Long-term steroid use tends to produce a low-turnover state which may play a critical role in subsequent fracture development. During the induction phase of immunosuppression high doses of steroids are used, and the dose of steroids correlates with the amount of bone loss.[43] Even small doses of steroids can result in significant bone loss.[44] Due to the deleterious effects of steroids, some centers have tried steroid withdrawal or avoidance protocols. Most, though not all, studies with variable methods ranging in size from 20 to 120 patients have shown a higher BMD in the steroid withdrawal or avoidance group compared to standard steroid immunosuppression protocols. These differences are most marked at the lumbar spine (difference in BMD of 1.4–20%).

Another potential serious adverse effect of steroids is avascular necrosis (AVN). The mechanism of AVN is not entirely clear but may be due to steroid's effect on the endothelial cells and smooth muscle cells, damaging veins resulting in venous stasis and poor drainage. AVN can affect anywhere from 3 to 41% of patients.[45] AVN tends to occur early after transplantation, usually within the first 12 months.[46] For unknown reasons, there is a higher risk of AVN in patients under 40.[46] High-dose steroids (over 4 g) given via intravenous route are associated with an increased risk of AVN.[47] The incidence of bilateral AVN has decreased from 79% in Kopecky's 1991 report to 14% in Marston's 2002 report correlating with decreased steroids usage throughout those years.[46,48] Despite decreased dependence on high doses of steroids in modern immunosuppressant protocols, AVN still occurs. This is possibly because there are no proven preventative measures. Although screening with MRI can find early-stage AVN, the implications for clinical outcomes after joint saving interventions for early AVN and cost effectiveness are not well defined.[46] While there are no proven effective means to salvage an affected joint, steroid minimization may help to limit disease progression and prevent disease in the contralateral hip.

Calcineurin inhibitors such as cyclosporine and tacrolimus affect bone as well. Studies by Epstein suggest that cyclosporine may increase high-turnover-associated bone loss in male Sprague–Dawley rats.[49] Cyclosporine is thought to affect bone metabolism by increasing osteoclast number and bone turnover as evidenced by increased osteocalcin. Although not as well studied it appears that tacrolimus has a similar effect on bone.[50] By contrast, in vitro studies have suggested that calcineurin inhibitors actually inhibit osteoclastic bone resorption.[51] Clinical observations have been unable to clarify calcineurin inhibitor's effect on bone. Some studies suggest a minimal effect on bone metabolism.[52] Others suggest that cyclosporine inhibits osteoclast differentiation.[53]

Josephson et al. found that cyclosporine resulted in bone loss, as measured by serial BMDs, independent of steroid exposure.[54] One French study did not find a difference between tacrolimus and cyclosporine other than lower estradiol levels in the tacrolimus group.[55] In contrast other studies have found cyclosporine to be more toxic to bones than tacrolimus.[56] Studies comparing tacrolimus and cyclosporine are confounded by the use of lower doses of steroids in the tacrolimus arm.[57] The physiological effect of calcineurin inhibitors is thought to be opposite to that of steroids, and consequently hypothetically they should offset each other. It has also been suggested that calcineurin inhibitors actually cause an uncoupling of bone processes and though their direct effect on bone cells is to inhibit bone resorption, they actually stimulate circulating bone-resulting in net bone loss.[58] Although there are limited available data regarding MMF, sirolimus, and azathioprine an effect on bone has not been identified.

Measuring Bone Health

Disorders of bone in transplant patients are a consequence of alterations that occur after transplant superimposed on the bone disorders that existed prior to transplant. Consequently kidney transplant osteodystrophy encompasses all of the disorders that can occur with CKD and can be characterized by the degree of mineralization, bone volume, and bone turnover.[16] Because the bone pathology of the transplant patient is complex, measuring bone loss and/or the risk for fracture can be difficult. And in considering these patients it is useful to understand not only the bone density (or quantity) but also the turnover and architecture (or quality).

Bone Mineral Density

Bone mineral density (BMD), a surrogate marker for bone volume, is strongly associated with risk of fracture in the post-menopausal Caucasian population.[59] However, this association is less clear-cut in the CKD population. In this group there is an undefined utility for hip and spine BMD.[60] BMD estimates the amount of mineralized bone, but does not reflect the degree of bone turnover. BMD cannot reveal subperiosteal resorption in patients with severe osteitis fibrosa or looser zones in those with severe osteomalacia. And so it is not surprising that BMD has not been proven to provide good fracture risk prediction in kidney transplant patients. Newer imaging modalities such as Micro-CT may help to assess bone quality in the future.[61] Further work is needed to clarify the utility of these newer techniques.

Biomarkers

Biomarkers provide a non-invasive approach to assess bone pathology. Osteoblasts synthesize type 1 collagen, alkaline phosphatase, osteocalcin, and these proteins can be used as a surrogate marker of osteoblastic bone formation and bone turnover. Osteoblasts synthesize alpha-1 and alpha-2 chains of collagen. Subsequently the proline and lysine residues in the collagen chains are hydroxylated to hydroxyproline and hydroxylysine. Hydroxyproline can also be excreted from dietary intake and non-bone collagen breakdown. Two alpha-1 and one alpha-2 chains combine to form a helical structure called tropocollagen, which has a non-helical C-telopeptide and N-peptide region. These can cross-link via N-telopeptide, C-telopeptide, and deoxypyridinoline crosslinks. Osteoclasts have a tartrate-resistant acid phosphatase on the cell membrane that is used in combination with hydrolytic enzymes to break down the collagen bone matrix. As a result, the breakdown products of the collagen matrix can be measured in both the serum and urine. The most commonly measured products are the urinary free pyridinoline and deoxypyridinoline residues. Osteocalcin which is produced by osteoblasts is generally considered a marker for bone formation (or osteoblast activity) and the collagen crosslinks are considered a marker for bone breakdown (or osteoclast activity).

The utility of bone biomarkers in transplant recipients is questionable. Although changes in biomarkers provide a sense of underlying changes in bone formation and dissolution, the values may not be discriminating enough to diagnose the underlying pathology for any given patient. Cruz et al. performed kidney biopsies at the time of transplant and 6 months later. Biomarkers normalized before the pathology did, indicating that there may be a time lag between improvements in markers and underlying bone pathology.[62] Biomarker levels change after transplant. Generally osteocalcin and parathyroid hormone change in parallel and decrease with time post-transplantation. Urinary collagen crosslinks remain stable or decrease post-transplantation, while alkaline phosphatase tends to have a more unpredictable course.[2]

Bone Biopsy

Bone biopsy is the gold standard for diagnosis of renal osteodystrophy. Intuitively it would seem that bone biopsies for transplant patients with worsening BMD or with multiple fractures would be useful. However, few centers perform bone biopsies on transplant patients. This is likely because performing a bone biopsy is costly, it may be uncomfortable for the patient, and there are few centers with the expertise to appropriately interpret the pathology. Consequently whether or not the increased use of bone biopsies would aid clinicians in providing more appropriate treatment and lead to better outcomes for patients with reduction in post-transplant fractures is unknown. Furthermore, a quantitative analysis and definition of bone histology and clinical consequences following transplantation has not been performed. Clearly a detailed study of bone histology following transplantation is required.

Treatment

How to approach or treat patients once a diagnosis is made can be even more problematic than making an appropriate diagnosis because of the limited number of studies addressing treatment of bone disorders in transplant patients. Several treatment regimens have been utilized including vitamin D, bisphosphonates, cinacalcet, teriparatide, and parathyroidectomy. For most of these treatments improvement in bone mineral density has been noted.[63] However, the studies have not been powered to demonstrate a reduction in fracture risk.[63]

Vitamin D

Both CKD and transplant patients have a high incidence of vitamin D deficiency. Studies using 1,25-OH vitamin D have shown that treatment is associated with improved BMD compared with no treatment.[54,64] and studies using 25-OH vitamin D also showed increased BMD.[65] Careful monitoring must be used when giving 1,25-OH vitamin D, as it has been associated with hypercalcemia.[54]

Bisphosphonates

Bisphosphonates act via inhibition of osteoclasts, thereby inhibiting bone resorption. A meta-analysis of bisphosphonate use in transplant recipients has demonstrated an increase in BMD, particularly at the lumbar spine.[66] However, in the only study in which bone biopsies were obtained prior to and following 6 months of therapy, the use of pamidronate was associated with low-turnover bone disorders.[67] Consequently, uniform use is not recommended and, when used, limiting treatment duration may be indicated. In addition, the patient's GFR must be taken into account when considering bisphosphonate use as it is not indicated if the GFR is less than 30 mg/dL.

PTH-Cinacalcet and Parathyroidectomy

Parathyroidectomy (either medical or surgical) may be indicated in the setting of persistent hyperparathyroidism and hypercalcemia. Cinacalcet can provide a medical parathyroidectomy by increasing the sensitivity of the calcium-sensing receptor to calcium and thus decreasing the secretion of parathyroid hormone. Cinacalcet has been studied post-transplant and found to have efficacy in ameliorating hypercalcemia post-transplantation.[68] Furthermore, case reports have suggested an improved BMD with the use of cinacalcet.[69] Surgical parathyroidectomy has also been shown to increase bone mass after renal transplantation.[70] One retrospective study of 14 patients demonstrated that parathyroidectomy post-transplantation resulted in a 10% increase in bone mass after a median follow-up of 26 months. The gain in bone density was greatest for those with osteoporosis and osteopenia; however, this study is difficult to interpret by the inclusion of 9 patients on steroid-free regimens (64%).[71] When considering cinacalcet or parathyroidectomy, it is important to understand that optimal target ranges for post-transplant PTH levels have not been established.

Using ranges of PTH established for the CKD population matching for level of kidney function, though never tested, may be a reasonable approach.

Teriparatide

Teriparatide is an amino-terminal parathyroid hormone with full physiological activity that has been shown to increase BMD and decrease fracture risk in large cohorts of post-menopausal women.[72] Teriparatide increased BMD more than bisphosphonates in a cohort of 428 men and women on steroid therapy over a 3-month period.[73] Only one study is currently available in transplant recipients. In this small randomized control trial of 26 patients treated with 20 μg of teriparatide, a benefit was not demonstrated.[74] Future studies are needed in the renal transplant population.

Summary

A recent meta-analysis found that studies examining prophylactic post-transplant bone treatment were not powered to detect a decrease in fractures.[63] Thus, while bisphosphonates and vitamin D may improve BMD, they have not been shown to lower fracture risk. Nevertheless, given the early post-transplant bone loss a prophylactic approach in the first year (with vitamin D or bisphosphonates) may be reasonable for some individuals. Data for treatment after the first year of transplantation are limited. Given the risk and differing profiles of individual patients, one should individualize the approach to post-transplant bone disease. However, how to individualize treatment remains to be determined.

Although data supporting the use of BMD are not available, BMD may be helpful to identify high-risk patients for whom additional evaluation should be performed. Patients with osteoporosis, defined as a BMD less than 2.5 standard deviations below the mean, should be considered for additional evaluation. Also patients with a history of fracture, long length of time on dialysis, with an SPK, elderly women, or history of diabetes may be considered for further evaluation. Further evaluation should include markers of bone turnover, vitamin D levels, and thyroid and parathyroid function.

In our opinion, parathyroid hormone should be measured and monitored following transplantation for at least 6 months. The ideal parathyroid hormone for a given transplant patient should depend on the time on dialysis, current GFR, and current calcium–phosphorus balance.

In selected patients a bone biopsy may be necessary to guide therapy. It is reasonable to consider performing biopsies on individuals with inconsistencies among biochemical parameters of bone turnover, unexplained fractures, repeated low-impact fractures, unexplained bone pain, unexplained hypercalcemia, and suspicion of overload of metals such as aluminum. Patients with decreasing bone density despite conservative therapy should also be considered for biopsy to help guide therapy. Bone biopsy should be considered after treatment in order to re-establish the degree of bone turnover as it can change with therapy.

Patients that are thought to have high- or low-turnover bone disease should be carefully considered for treatment. Some patients with low-turnover bone disease can be considered for teriparatide. The dose of teriparatide used in the failed study was 20 µg.[74] Whether or not higher doses of teriparatide may be beneficial requires study. In addition, cessation of therapies that lower parathyroid hormone should be considered. There are several options for treatment of high-turnover bone disease. Bisphosphonates and PTH-lowering drugs such as cinacalcet, 1,25-OH vitamin D analogues, and parathyroidectomy all can help to ameliorate high-turnover bone disease. There are no data to support one therapy over another. Treatment of high-turnover bone disease should be individualized. Further studies are needed to help illustrate the benefit of these therapies. In addition, phosphorus should be maintained within normal range. Vitamin D_3 is recommended, although studies have not been done to support or refute this recommendation. Serum levels should be monitored and supplemental vitamin D given if serum concentrations are less than 30 pg/mL.

Bone disorders such as osteonecrosis, low bone density, and fracture are very common in the renal transplant population. There are many physiological reasons for bone disease and many forms of bone disease. There are several different potential treatment and prophylactic approaches; however, none are proven. Management should be based on the individual patient's type of bone disease. The types of bone pathology can be estimated using parathyroid hormone and markers for bone turnover; however, a labeled bone biopsy remains the gold standard. Bone disease in post-transplant patients is a complex and diverse field that requires further investigation.

References

1. Vautour LM, Melton LJ 3rd, Clarke BL, Achenbach SJ, Oberg AL, McCarthy JT. Long-term fracture risk following renal transplantation: a population-based study. *Osteoporos Int* 2004 Feb;15(2):160–167.
2. Sprague SM, Josephson MA. Bone disease after kidney transplantation. *Semin Nephrol* 2004 Jan;24(1):82–90.
3. Ramsey-Goldman R, Dunn JE, Dunlop DD, Stuart FP, Abecassis MM, Kaufman DB et al. Increased risk of fracture in patients receiving solid organ transplants. *J Bone Miner Res* 1999 Mar;14(3):456–463.
4. Stehman-Breen CO, Sherrard DJ, Alem AM, Gillen DL, Heckbert SR, Wong CS et al. Risk factors for hip fracture among patients with end-stage renal disease. *Kidney Int* 2000 Nov;58(5):2200–2205.
5. Ball AM, Gillen DL, Sherrard D, Weiss NS, Emerson SS, Seliger SL et al. Risk of hip fracture among dialysis and renal transplant recipients. *JAMA* 2002 Dec 18;288(23):3014–3018.
6. Braithwaite RS, Col NF, Wong JB. Estimating hip fracture morbidity, mortality and costs. *J Am Geriatr Soc* 2003 Mar;51(3):364–370.
7. Abbott KC, Oglesby RJ, Hypolite IO, Kirk AD, Ko CW, Welch PG et al. Hospitalizations for fractures after renal transplantation in the United States. *Annals of Epidemiol* 2001 Oct;11(7):450–457.

8. Borah B, Gross GJ, Dufresne TE, Smith TS, Cockman MD, Chmielewski PA et al. Three-dimensional microimaging (MRmicroI and microCT), finite element modeling, and rapid prototyping provide unique insights into bone architecture in osteoporosis. *Anat Rec* 2001 Apr;265(2):101–110.

9. Marcen R, Caballero C, Uriol O, Fernandez A, Villafruela JJ, Pascual J et al. Prevalence of osteoporosis, osteopenia, and vertebral fractures in long-term renal transplant recipients. *Transplant Proc* 2007 Sep;39(7):2256–2258.

10. Parker CR, Freemont AJ, Blackwell PJ, Grainge MJ, Hosking DJ. Cross-sectional analysis of renal transplantation osteoporosis. *J Bone Miner Res* 1999 Nov;14(11):1943–1951.

11. Durieux S, Mercadal L, Orcel P, Dao H, Rioux C, Bernard M et al. Bone mineral density and fracture prevalence in long-term kidney graft recipients. *Transplantation* 2002 Aug 27;74(4):496–500.

12. Marshall D, Johnell O, Wedel H. Meta-analysis of how well measures of bone mineral density predict occurrence of osteoporotic fractures. *BMJ* (Clinical research ed.) 1996 May 18;312(7041):1254–1259.

13. Monier-Faugere MC, Mawad H, Qi Q, Friedler RM, Malluche HH. High prevalence of low bone turnover and occurrence of osteomalacia after kidney transplantation. *J Am Soc Nephrol* 2000 Jun;11(6):1093–1099.

14. Cockerill W, Lunt M, Silman AJ, Cooper C, Lips P, Bhalla AK et al. Health-related quality of life and radiographic vertebral fracture. *Osteoporos Int* 2004 Feb;15(2):113–119.

15. Dooley AC, Weiss NS, Kestenbaum B. Increased risk of hip fracture among men with CKD. *Am J Kidney Dis* 2008 Jan;51(1):38–44.

16. Moe S, Drueke T, Cunningham J, Goodman W, Martin K, Olgaard K et al. Definition, evaluation, and classification of renal osteodystrophy: a position statement from Kidney Disease: Improving Global Outcomes (KDIGO). *Kidney Int* 2006 Jun;69(11):1945–1953.

17. Cruz DN, Wysolmerski JJ, Brickel HM, Gundberg CG, Simpson CA, Mitnick MA et al. Parameters of high bone-turnover predict bone loss in renal transplant patients: a longitudinal study. *Transplantation* 2001 Jul 15;72(1):83–88.

18. Sprague SM, Belozeroff V, Danese MD, Martin LP, Olgaard K. Abnormal bone and mineral metabolism in kidney transplant patients – a review. *Am J Nephrol* 2008;28(2): 246–253.

19. Messa P, Sindici C, Cannella G, Miotti V, Risaliti A, Gropuzzo M et al. Persistent secondary hyperparathyroidism after renal transplantation. *Kidney Int* 1998 Nov;54(5):1704–1713.

20. Edwards RM, Contino LC, Gellai M, Brooks DP. Parathyroid hormone-1 receptor down-regulation in kidneys from rats with chronic renal failure. *Pharmacology* 2001 May;62(4):243–247.

21. Parfitt AM. The hyperparathyroidism of chronic renal failure: a disorder of growth. *Kidney Int* 1997 Jul;52(1):3–9.

22. Bonarek H, Merville P, Bonarek M, Moreau K, Morel D, Aparicio M et al. Reduced parathyroid functional mass after successful kidney transplantation. *Kidney Int* 1999 Aug;56(2): 642–649.

23. Reinhardt W, Bartelworth H, Jockenhovel F, Schmidt-Gayk H, Witzke O, Wagner K et al. Sequential changes of biochemical bone parameters after kidney transplantation. *Nephrol Dial Transplant* 1998 Feb;13(2):436–442.

24. LaClair RE, Hellman RN, Karp SL, Kraus M, Ofner S, Li Q et al. Prevalence of calcidiol deficiency in CKD: a cross-sectional study across latitudes in the United States. *Am J Kidney Dis* 2005 Jun;45(6):1026–1033.

25. Querings K, Girndt M, Geisel J, Georg T, Tilgen W, Reichrath J. 25-hydroxyvitamin D deficiency in renal transplant recipients. *J Clin Endocrinol Metab* 2006 Feb;91(2):526–529.

26. Bushinsky DA. The contribution of acidosis to renal osteodystrophy. *Kidney Int* 1995 Jun;47(6):1816–1832.

27. Krieger NS, Frick KK, Bushinsky DA. Mechanism of acid-induced bone resorption. *Curr Opin Nephrol Hypertens* 2004 Jul;13(4):423–436.

28. Welch AA, Bingham SA, Reeve J, Khaw KT. More acidic dietary acid-base load is associated with reduced calcaneal broadband ultrasound attenuation in women but not in men: results from the EPIC-Norfolk cohort study. *Am J Clin Nutr* 2007 Apr;85(4):1134–1141.

29. Tuominen JT, Impivaara O, Puukka P, Ronnemaa T. Bone mineral density in patients with type 1 and type 2 diabetes. *Diabetes Care* 1999 Jul;22(7):1196–1200.

30. Smets YF, van der Pijl JW, de Fijter JW, Ringers J, Lemkes HH, Hamdy NA. Low bone mass and high incidence of fractures after successful simultaneous pancreas-kidney transplantation. *Nephrol Dial Transplant* 1998 May;13(5):1250–1255.

31. Bruce DS, Newell KA, Josephson MA, Woodle ES, Piper JB, Millis JM et al. Long-term outcome of kidney-pancreas transplant recipients with good graft function at one year. *Transplantation* 1996 Aug 27;62(4):451–456.

32. Hochberg MC. Racial differences in bone strength. *Trans Am Clin Climatol Assoc* 2007;118:305–315.

33. Mullin BH, Prince RL, Dick IM, Hart DJ, Spector TD, Dudbridge F et al. Identification of a role for the ARHGEF3 gene in postmenopausal osteoporosis. *Am J Hum Genet* 2008 Jun;82(6):1262–1269.

34. Nelson DA, Vande Vord PJ, Wooley PH. Polymorphism in the vitamin D receptor gene and bone mass in African-American and white mothers and children: a preliminary report. *Ann Rheum Dis* 2000 Aug;59(8):626–630.

35. Ghanekar H, Welch BJ, Moe OW, Sakhaee K. Post-renal transplantation hypophosphatemia: a review and novel insights. *Curr Opin Nephrol Hypertens* 2006 Mar;15(2):97–104.

36. Pande S, Ritter CS, Rothstein M, Wiesen K, Vassiliadis J, Kumar R et al. . FGF-23 and sFRP-4 in chronic kidney disease and post-renal transplantation. *Nephron Physiol* 2006;104(1):23–32.

37. Saha HH, Salmela KT, Ahonen PJ, Pietila KO, Morsky PJ, Mustonen JT et al. Sequential changes in vitamin D and calcium metabolism after successful renal transplantation. *Scand J Urol Nephrol* 1994 Mar;28(1):21–27.

38. Cayco AV, Wysolmerski J, Simpson C, Mitnick MA, Gundberg C, Kliger A et al. Posttransplant bone disease: evidence for a high bone resorption state. *Transplantation* 2000 Dec 27;70(12):1722–1728.

39. de Sevaux RG, Hoitsma AJ, van Hoof HJ, Corstens FJ, Wetzels JF. Abnormal vitamin D metabolism and loss of bone mass after renal transplantation. *Nephron Clin Pract* 2003 Jan;93(1):C21–C28.

40. Ozdemir FN, Afsar B, Akgul A, Usluogullari C, Akcay A, Haberal M. Persistent hyper-calcemia is a significant risk factor for graft dysfunction in renal transplantation recipients. *Transplant Proc* 2006 Mar;38(2):480–482.

41. Cunningham J. Pathogenesis and prevention of bone loss in patients who have kidney disease and receive long-term immunosuppression. *J Am Soc Nephrol* 2007 Jan;18(1):223–234.

42. Weinstein RS, Jilka RL, Parfitt AM, Manolagas SC. Inhibition of osteoblastogenesis and pro-motion of apoptosis of osteoblasts and osteocytes by glucocorticoids. Potential mechanisms of their deleterious effects on bone. *J Clin Invest* 1998 Jul 15;102(2):274–282.

43. Mikuls TR, Julian BA, Bartolucci A, Saag KG. Bone mineral density changes within six months of renal transplantation. *Transplantation* 2003 Jan 15;75(1):49–54.

44. Van Staa TP, Leufkens HG, Abenhaim L, Zhang B, Cooper C. Use of oral corticosteroids and risk of fractures. *J Bone Miner Res* 2000 Jun;15(6):993–1000.

45. Meakin CJ, Hopson CN, First MR. Avascular (aseptic) necrosis of bone following renal transplantation. *Int J Artif Organs* 1985 Jan;8(1):19–20.

46. Marston SB, Gillingham K, Bailey RF, Cheng EY. Osteonecrosis of the femoral head after solid organ transplantation: a prospective study. *J Bone Joint Surg* 2002 Dec;84–A(12):2145–2151.

47. Kubo T, Fujioka M, Yamazoe S, Yoshimura N, Oka T, Ushijima Y et al. Relationship between steroid dosage and osteonecrosis of the femoral head after renal transplantation as measured by magnetic resonance imaging. *Transplant Proc* 1998 Nov;30(7):3039–3040.

340 B.L. West et al.

48. Kopecky KK, Braunstein EM, Brandt KD, Filo RS, Leapman SB, Capello WN et al. Apparent avascular necrosis of the hip: appearance and spontaneous resolution of MR findings in renal allograft recipients. *Radiology* 1991 May;179(2):523–527.
49. Epstein S, Dissanayake IR, Goodman GR, Bowman AR, Zhou H, Ma Y et al. Effect of the interaction of parathyroid hormone and cyclosporine a on bone mineral metabolism in the rat. *Calcif Tissue Int* 2001 Apr;68(4):240–247.
50. El Haggan W, Barthe N, Vendrely B, Chauveau P, Berger F, Aparicio M et al. One year evolution of bone mineral density in kidney transplant recipients receiving tacrolimus versus cyclosporine. *Transplant Proc* 2002 Aug;34(5):1817–1818.
51. Stern PH. The calcineurin-NFAT pathway and bone: intriguing new findings. *Mol Interv* 2006 Aug;6(4):193–196.
52. Brandenburg VM, Westenfeld R, Ketteler M. The fate of bone after renal transplantation. *J Nephrol* 2004 Mar–Apr;17(2):190–204.
53. Orcel P, Denne MA, de Vernejoul MC. Cyclosporin-A in vitro decreases bone resorption, osteoclast formation, and the fusion of cells of the monocyte-macrophage lineage. *Endocrinology* 1991 Mar;128(3):1638–1646.
54. Josephson MA, Schumm LP, Chiu MY, Marshall C, Thistlethwaite JR, Sprague SM. Calcium and calcitriol prophylaxis attenuates posttransplant bone loss. *Transplantation* 2004 Oct 27;78(8):1233–1236.
55. Albano L, Casez JP, Bekri S, Gigante M, Champenois I, Cassuto-Viguier E et al. Effects of tacrolimus vs cyclosporin-A on bone metabolism after kidney transplantation: a cross-sectional study in 28 patients. *Nephrol Ther* 2005 May;1(2):115–120.
56. Monegal A, Navasa M, Guanabens N, Peris P, Pons F, Martinez de Osaba MJ et al. Bone mass and mineral metabolism in liver transplant patients treated with FK506 or cyclosporine A. *Calcif Tissue Int* 2001 Feb;68(2):83–86.
57. Goffin E, Devogelaer JP, Lalaoui A, Depresseux G, De Naeyer P, Squifflet JP et al. Tacrolimus and low-dose steroid immunosuppression preserves bone mass after renal transplantation. *Transpl Int* Mar 2002;15(2–3):73–80.
58. Gal-Moscovici A, Popovtzer MM. New worldwide trends in presentation of renal osteodystrophy and its relationship to parathyroid hormone levels. *Clin Nephrol* 2005 Apr;63(4):284–289.
59. Melton LJ 3rd, Atkinson EJ, O'Fallon WM, Wahner HW, Riggs BL. Long-term fracture prediction by bone mineral assessed at different skeletal sites. *J Bone Miner Res* 1993 Oct;8(10):1227–1233.
60. Jamal SA, Hayden JA, Beyene J. Low bone mineral density and fractures in long-term hemodialysis patients: a meta-analysis. *Am J Kidney Dis* 2007 May;49(5):674–681.
61. Nickolas TL, Leonard MB, Shane E. Chronic kidney disease and bone fracture: a growing concern. *Kidney Int* 2008 Sep;74(6):721–731.
62. Cruz EA, Lugon JR, Jorgetti V, Draibe SA, Carvalho AB. Histologic evolution of bone disease 6 months after successful kidney transplantation. *Am J Kidney Dis* 2004 Oct;44(4):747–756.
63. Palmer SC, Strippoli GF, McGregor DO. Interventions for preventing bone disease in kidney transplant recipients: a systematic review of randomized controlled trials. *Am J Kidney Dis* 2005 Apr;45(4):638–649.
64. Cueto-Manzano AM, Konel S, Freemont AJ, Adams JE, Mawer B, Gokal R et al. Effect of 1,25-dihydroxyvitamin D3 and calcium carbonate on bone loss associated with long-term renal transplantation. *Am J Kidney Dis* 2000 Feb;35(2):227–236.
65. El-Agroudy AE, El-Husseini AA, El-Sayed M, Ghoneim MA. Preventing bone loss in renal transplant recipients with vitamin D. *J Am Soc Nephrol* 2003 Nov;14(11):2975–2979.
66. Mitterbauer C, Schwarz C, Haas M, Oberbauer R. Effects of bisphosphonates on bone loss in the first year after renal transplantation – a meta-analysis of randomized controlled trials. *Nephrol Dial Transplant* 2006 Aug;21(8):2275–2281.
67. Coco M, Glicklich D, Faugere MC, Burris L, Bognar I, Durkin P et al. Prevention of bone loss in renal transplant recipients: a prospective, randomized trial of intravenous pamidronate. *J Am Soc Nephrol* 2003 Oct;14(10):2669–2676.

68. Szwarc I, Argiles A, Garrigue V, Delmas S, Chong G, Deleuze S et al. Cinacalcet chloride is efficient and safe in renal transplant recipients with posttransplant hyperparathyroidism. *Transplantation* 2006 Sep 15 ;82(5):675–680.
69. Decleire PY, Devogelaer JP, Goffin E. Cinacalcet improves bone mineral density in a renal transplant recipient with persistent hyperparathyroidism. *Clin Nephrol* 2008 Mar;69(3): 231–232.
70. Chou FF, Hsieh KC, Chen YT, Lee CT. Parathyroidectomy followed by kidney transplantation can improve bone mineral density in patients with secondary hyperparathyroidism. *Transplantation* 2008 Aug 27;86(4):554–557.
71. Collaud S, Staub-Zahner T, Trombetti A, Clerici T, Marangon N, Binet I et al. Increase in bone mineral density after successful parathyroidectomy for tertiary hyperparathyroidism after renal transplantation. *World J Surg* 2008 Aug;32(8):1795–1801.
72. Neer RM, Arnaud CD, Zanchetta JR, Prince R, Gaich GA, Reginster JY et al. Effect of parathyroid hormone (1–34) on fractures and bone mineral density in postmenopausal women with osteoporosis. *New Engl J Med* 2001 May 10;344(19):1434–1441.
73. Saag KG, Shane E, Boonen S, Marin F, Donley DW, Taylor KA et al. Teriparatide or alendronate in glucocorticoid-induced osteoporosis. *New Engl J Med* 2007 Nov 15;357(20): 2028–2039.
74. Cejka D, Benesch T, Krestan C, Roschger P, Klaushofer K, Pietschmann P et al. Effect of teriparatide on early bone loss after kidney transplantation. *Am J Transplant* 2008 Sep;8(9):1864–1870.

Chapter 20
Sexuality and Pregnancy Before and After Kidney Transplantation

Martha Pavlakis and Dianne B. McKay

One of the many successes provided by solid organ transplantation is restoration of sexual and reproductive function. These are two areas often given limited discussion, yet they are important elements of a normal life. This chapter will review published literature on sexuality and reproduction and provide guidelines for the counseling and management of patients before and after pregnancy.

Sexuality

Significant improvements have occurred in the quality of life of patients with chronic kidney disease, end-stage renal disease (ESRD), and transplantation. However, problems with sexual function remain an important quality-of-life parameter that is often not fully addressed in clinical practice and may continue to plague patients with kidney disease. Despite the importance of sexuality in overall quality of life, clinicians are often unprepared to openly discuss sexuality with their patients.

Male and female patients with end-stage renal disease (ESRD) commonly experience sexual dysfunction and infertility. The potential etiologies include endocrine aberrations, vasomotor dysfunction, prescribed medications, and psychological factors.[1,2] While there is some improvement following transplantation,[3] many patients remain sexually dysfunctional 3 years after transplantation.[4] As a quality-of-life issue, this is often under-studied and under-reported to clinicians. Thus, the clinician caring for patients with end-stage renal disease (ESRD) should assume a high prevalence of sexual dysfunction in their patient population and integrate methods into routine practice that capture and address the problem.

There are many interventions possible for patients experiencing sexual dysfunction, depending on the etiology. Simple statements such as "many patients with chronic kidney disease have difficulties or concerns about their sexual function"

M. Pavlakis (✉)
Kidney and Pancreas Transplantation, Beth Israel Deaconess Medical Center, Transplant, Boston, MA, USA
e-mail: mpavlaki@bidmc.harvard.edu

D.B. McKay, S.M. Steinberg (eds.), *Kidney Transplantation: A Guide to the Care of Kidney Transplant Recipients*, DOI 10.1007/978-1-4419-1690-7_20,
© Springer Science+Business Media, LLC 2010

can serve as an introduction to patient questions and allay anxieties about perceived or real barriers against addressing these problems. Clinicians should explain the possible causes in lay terms to the patient with kidney disease (for example, hormone imbalances, blood vessel problems, medication or psychological factors such as stress and depression) in order to facilitate an environment conducive to addressing potential problems. Often, referral to a sub-specialist, such as a urologist, or adjustment in medications can lead to an improvement in sexual function.

Fertility

Fertility is affected by ESRD and transplantation in both women and men. Female infertility in ESRD results from altered hypothalamic function, due in part to high FSH, LH, and prolactin levels.[1] The hormone aberrations usually resolve after transplantation, and normal ovulatory cycles and regular menstruation often resume quickly.[5,6] Many women with chronic kidney disease experience premature menopause, on an average of 4.5 years earlier than the general population,[7] and therefore older women may not experience resolution of infertility. Since pregnancy immediately after kidney transplantation carries a high risk, all women of childbearing age (who have not had surgical sterilization) should be counseled about adequate contraception in the peritransplant period. A woman's age, the desire for genetic offspring, and risk of early menopause should be considered in the optimal timing of pregnancy following transplantation (see "Timing of Pregnancy").

Male infertility is common with ESRD, due in part to low testosterone, high LH, FSH, and prolactin levels, high estrogen levels, impotence, and spermatogenic abnormalities.[1,8] The true incidence and prevalence of male infertility after transplantation is difficult to determine and has not been quantified. Testes of men with ESRD have shown germinal aplasia and seminiferous tubule destruction, suggesting that men might experience more infertility than is generally assumed. The extent of histologic damage in ESRD determines the reversibility of male fertility following transplantation.[1] Even though transplantation restores the hormone imbalance of ESRD and sperm motility is improved, sperm counts and irregular morphology can persist indefinitely.[9] Calcineurin inhibitors and azathioprine do not appear to alter male fertility, while sirolimus has been associated with low free testosterone levels and significantly elevated levels of LH and FSH.[10,11] Several reports have suggested that sirolimus should not be prescribed to male transplant recipients interested in fathering a child.[10,12,13]

Contraception

Contraception counseling is best performed in the pre-transplant time period, due to rapid return of fertility after transplantation. Guazzelli et al. questioned 198 women who had received a transplant at a single center in Brazil and found that although most female kidney transplant recipients were sexually active before and after transplantation, many were not counseled about the need for contraception and did not use any form of birth control.[14] Of 14 post-transplant pregnancies in this population, 13 were unplanned.

Since preexisting kidney disease is an independent risk factor for preeclampsia, prematurity, low birth weight, and neonatal death,[15] it is ideal for the pregnancy to coincide with excellent allograft function (e.g., not too soon and not too late after transplantation). The immediate post-transplant period (first 3–4 months) is not the optimal time for pregnancy because the female transplant recipient is usually ingesting fetotoxic and/or teratogenic medications. In addition, this is the most important time for optimization of immunosuppression to avoid acute rejection. The advice for contraception in this population has historically been barrier methods. However, due to potential for contraception failure, the American Society of Transplantation (AST) Consensus Conference report states that transplant recipients should be advised that barrier methods and IUDs may not be the best forms of contraception.[16] Progestin-only oral contraceptives as well as estrogen/progestin are probably acceptable for use in this patient population as long as hypertension is well controlled and there is no history of thromboembolic disease.[17] Advice for the best contraceptive agent depends upon patient-specific preferences and considerations of the risks and benefits of each contraceptive method. For example, barrier methods should be advocated for any patient who is entering a new sexual relationship and as an adjunct to other methods.[18]

Timing of Pregnancy

At this time there are no specific recommendations for male transplant recipients regarding the optimal time to father a child after transplantation. The optimal timing of pregnancy for women who have undergone kidney transplantation was previously recommended to be 2 years following successful transplantation.[19] This recommendation has been replaced by the American Society of Transplantation Consensus Opinion as follows: a transplant recipient can proceed with pregnancy as long as graft function is optimal (defined as a serum creatinine <1.5 mg/dl, with less than 500 mg/24 h urinary protein excretion) and there are no concurrent fetotoxic or teratogenic medications or infections, and that immunosuppressive dosing is stable at maintenance levels.[16] This would likely be achieved by 1 year after transplantation. However, given the increasing age of the transplant population, these recommendations may apply to a waiting period of only 6 months post-transplant in specific situations.[17]

Pregnancy

While pregnancies in patients with end-stage disease are still relatively uncommon,[20] increasing numbers of pregnancies have been reported in patients with transplanted kidneys, livers, hearts, lungs, small bowels, and even in those with multiple organ transplants. In an attempt to estimate numbers of pregnancies that have occurred in transplant recipients, Davidson tabulated all pregnancies reported within the worldwide literature up to the year 2001. Reports of 14,000 pregnancies were acquired through review of case, center, and registry reports.[21] This number is of course an underestimate, as reporting of pregnancies in transplant recipients is not a widespread practice.

Data about the outcomes of pregnancy come from voluntary registries, as well as from case and center reports. Several voluntary pregnancy registries have published information on maternal, paternal, and infant outcomes. The NTPR registry in the United States has reported approximately 1,600 outcomes in female and 1,000 outcomes in male transplant recipients.[22] While registries (in the United States and in other countries) provide essential information, the registries have captured only a minority of the pregnancies that have actually occurred in transplant recipients.[21] In addition, registry data are limited by unavoidable reporting bias. It is important to realize these limitations because the registry data provide the primary source of data that currently guide patient management. Thus, there is limited published information and an absence of prospective studies that would lead to evidence-based care of the pregnant transplant recipient. Much of our preconception counseling in the transplant patient is therefore based on incomplete knowledge.

Risks of Pregnancy to the Mother and the Fetus

Several risks should be discussed with the maternal transplant recipient and her partner, ideally before the patient becomes pregnant. The risks to discuss are those specific to the transplant recipient (worsened hypertension, preeclampsia, graft rejection, graft loss) and risks specific to the fetus (malformations, immunologic and neurologic deficits). In order to minimize risks the pregnant transplant recipient should be jointly managed by her transplant nephrologists and high-risk obstetrician, preferably an obstetrician with experience in maternal–fetal medicine.

Maternal Risks

Hypertension

Hypertension is common in pregnant transplant recipients (occurring in 73% of patients reported to the NTPR), due either to preexisting chronic hypertension or to the development of hypertension during gestation.[23,24] During normal pregnancy, blood pressure is lowest in the first trimester, but slowly returns to pre-pregnancy levels in late gestation. The transplant recipient often experiences a similar, but blunted, pattern of blood pressure variation.[25] Therapeutic targets for mild to moderate hypertension in the CKD population are not known, although recommendations have been made to treat at blood pressure levels $\geq$ 150/90 mmHg.[26] Treatment recommendations in the gravid renal transplant recipient are more aggressive, with advice now to achieve a normotensive state.[26]

The optimal choice of antihypertensive therapy depends on hypertension severity. For mild hypertension, methyldopa was recommended by several consensus studies, since it is well tolerated and does not alter uteroplacental or fetal hemodynamics.[27] Other antihypertensives considered acceptable include labetalol, nifedipine, and thiazide diuretics.[27] For urgent blood pressure control hydralazine, labetalol, and nifedipine are considered the drugs of choice. Angiotensin converting enzyme inhibitors and angiotensin receptor blockers are contraindicated in pregnancy because of adverse fetal effects, and atenolol should be avoided because of concerns about fetal growth.[26,27]

Preeclampsia

Maternal renal transplant patients are at high risk for preeclampsia – an incidence of 15–25% compared with 5% of normotensive pregnancies.[26] Preeclampsia is a syndrome defined by the development of hypertension in association with new-onset proteinuria during the second half of pregnancy. Severe maternal and fetal complications such as renal failure, HELLP syndrome (hemolysis, elevated liver enzymes, and thrombocytopenia), seizures, liver failure, stroke, or death accompany preeclampsia. For the fetus, preeclampsia can result in small-for-gestational-age infants, preterm delivery, hypoxic neurologic injury, or death.[28] Unfortunately, it is difficult to make the diagnosis of preeclampsia in the gravid renal transplant recipient because blood pressure commonly rises late in pregnancy and many patients have preexisting proteinuria.[29] In addition, associated features of hyperuricemia and edema often coexistent in renal transplant patients.[30] Preeclampsia is associated with placental hypoxia and endothelial dysfunction, but the pathogenic mechanisms are yet unknown.[31] Whether markers such as angiogenic or antiangiogenic proteins will provide specific markers for preeclampsia is unknown, but they could provide a very important area for future study.

Graft Rejection

Another significant risk to consider for the mother is graft rejection. Due to changes in blood volume, maintenance of immunosuppressive medication dosing can be difficult and vigilant monitoring of serum immunosuppressive levels is recommended.[16] The recommendation by the AST Consensus Conference is that in order to avoid graft rejection, immunosuppressive dosing should be maintained at pre-pregnancy levels through frequent monitoring of serum drug levels.[21,32] The mother is not immunosuppressed by her pregnancy and therefore allowing immunosuppressive medication levels to fall risks graft rejection.

Pregnancy induces hyperfiltration of transplanted kidneys, as it does in normal kidneys during pregnancy.[33] Therefore, detection of rejection can be very difficult when monitoring for changes in serum creatinine. If rejection is suspected, the kidney can be safely biopsied under ultrasound guidance.[25] If rejection occurs it can be treated with corticosteroids.[16] There is very little data on which to base recommendations for treatment of rejection with other agents, such as OKT3 or anti-thymocyte globulin.[21]

Graft Loss

Generally, the risk of graft loss due to pregnancy is low in transplant recipients with good graft function. Pregnancy has been studied in patients with various levels of CKD and the degree of renal dysfunction appears to predict graft loss. Mild renal impairment (creatinine <1.3 mg/dl) does not risk worsening of kidney function.[34] Patients with moderate kidney disease though (defined as serum creatinine of 1.3–1.9 mg/dl) or severe kidney disease (creatinine >1.9 mg/dl) often experience a decline in kidney function with pregnancy that can proceed to end-stage renal disease (ESRD).[15,35] Registry reports and expert consensus opinion suggest that a serum creatinine >1.5 mg/dl and greater than 500 mg/24 h proteinuria significantly increases the risk of irreversible graft loss due to the pregnancy in the transplant recipient.[16]

Additional Risks

Other risks to be considered for the maternal transplant recipient include gestational diabetes, anemia, and infections such as urinary tract infections.[24,36] Since allograft recipients have increased risk for gestational diabetes, it has been recommended that they should be screened every trimester with a 50 g oral glucose load.[25] Likewise maternal transplant recipients should be screened for urinary tract infections. Urinary tract infections occur in up to 42% of pregnant renal transplant patients,[37] although pyelonephritis is rare.[25] Anemia is common during pregnancy and should be treated with erythropoietin if necessary to maintain adequate fetal oxygen delivery.

The maternal transplant recipient is placed at increased risk of infection due the use of immunosuppressive medications. Maternal–fetal transmission of infectious agents needs to be considered as a potential risk not only to the mother but also to the fetus. Cytomegalovirus infection is particularly serious as it is associated with hearing/vision loss and mental retardation and can be transmitted from the mother to the fetus through a transplacental route, as well as during delivery or breast-feeding.[38] Unfortunately the presence of maternal immunity does not absolutely protect the fetus although it does reduce the likelihood of transmission.[39] Anti-viral medication prophylaxis has not generally been recommended during pregnancy.[40] Other infections that may pose additional risks in the immunosuppressed mother include toxoplasmosis, primary herpes simplex infection, primary varicella infection, HIV infection, as well as infection with either hepatitis B or C viruses.[41,42] Prenatal screening can detect each of these infections, although in many cases the mother presents before prenatal screening when maternal prophylaxis can no longer be considered.

Fetal Risks

The risks to the fetus include risks commonly associated with pregnancy in a patient with CKD, as well as risks associated with intrauterine exposure to immunosuppressive medications. The risks associated with renal dysfunction are common in transplant recipients and these include a high risk of preterm delivery (<37 weeks) and low birth weight (<2,500 g). The mean gestational age at delivery in kidney transplant recipients is 34 weeks[25] and approximately 50% of infants are delivered with low birth weight.[21] In kidney transplant recipients, most deliveries occur early because of maternal and/or fetal compromise, rather than spontaneous preterm labor.[25] Transplant recipients are also at high risk for premature rupture of membranes, which also contributes to the increased risk for preterm labor, as do pyleonephritis and acute allograft rejection.

All immunosuppressive medications cross the maternal–fetal barrier to variable degrees, but scant information is available regarding fetal bioavailability of commonly used agents. The Food and Drug Administration safety classification is generally not helpful due to limited clinical data on which to determine the safety of many medications during pregnancy.[24]

The incidence of major structural malformations is similar to the general population, except for mycophenolate mofetil, which is associated with significant structural malformations.[43,44] The transplant physician is often confronted with a dilemma – to continue mycophenolate in a stable kidney transplant recipient and risk fetal abnormalities if she becomes pregnant or to switch the immunosuppressive regimen (e.g., to azathioprine) and risk altering the immunosuppressive stability of the patient. Current recommendations are to avoid mycophenolate mofetil and sirolimus (due to limited data) for 6 weeks prior to pregnancy.[16,32]

The risks for more subtle deficits in the fetus are not known, but several studies have suggested that immunologic and neurologic abnormalities are possible.[21] It is advisable therefore that the offspring's pediatrician be informed that the fetus was exposed in utero to immunosuppressive agents so that the pediatrician is altered to any immunologic abnormalities or developmental delays. Prospective evaluations of childhood development have not been conducted in infants born to transplant recipients. Data from the NTPR are limited but suggest that developmental delays have been seen in up to 26% of children after the age of 5 years.[45] The significance of this finding though is not known, as prospective neurocognitive testing has not routinely been performed on children born to maternal transplant recipients. While the long-term outcomes associated with in utero immunosuppressive medication exposure have been poorly studied, the consequences of low and very low birth weight for the fetus are substantial. These include neurologic, endocrine, cardiac, and renal abnormalities.[46–53]

Delivery and Breastfeeding

The presence of the transplanted kidney in the false pelvis does not in itself indicate the need for caesarean delivery. Interestingly though most infants of maternal transplant recipients are delivered by caesarean section for unclear reasons.[23] Expert consensus opinion is that unless there is an obstetrical reason to indicate caesarean delivery, vaginal delivery is preferred.[16]

Breastfeeding is often a concern of the maternal transplant recipient. Immunosuppressive medications have been detected in human breast milk, but little data is available regarding the excreted levels of immunosuppressive medications. The American Association of Pediatrics (AAP) supports breastfeeding in mothers on prednisone and advises against it in those on cyclosporine,[54] yet there are no specific recommendations regarding azathioprine, tacrolimus, mycophenolate mofetil or sirolimus. Until more information is available, the opinion of experts is that breastfeeding is not necessarily contraindicated and the decision should lie with patient and physician preference[16] (Tables 20.1, 20.2, and 20.3).

Table 20.1 Pre-transplant counseling guidelines

1. Begin pregnancy and contraceptive counseling before transplantation in order to
   - Avoid unplanned pregnancy early after transplant
   - Avoid exposure to fetotoxic and teratogenic medications/infections
2. Discuss high prevalence of sexual dysfunction
   - High prevalence with ESRD that may persist after transplantation
3. Early menopause may limit reproductive years
   - Menopause occurs about 4.5 years earlier than in women with normal renal function
4. Optimal contraception
   - Begin *effective* contraception before transplantation in women of reproductive age
   - Barrier methods ineffective
   - Oral contraceptives can be prescribed
5. Optimal timing of pregnancy should coincide with optimal graft function
   - Guidelines of optimal timing: creat <1.5 mg/dl, <500 mg proteinuria/24 h, stable graft function, no rejection, no fetotoxic or teratogenic medications/infections
6. Inform the patient about maternal risks:
   - High risk for hypertension, preeclampsia, preterm birth, infections (especially urinary track infections), gestational diabetes, anemia
   - Graft rejection (risk lowered by maintaining pre-pregnancy immunosuppressive blood levels)
   - Graft loss (unlikely if renal function optimal at time of pregnancy – see No. 5 – and if no graft rejection during pregnancy)
7. Inform the patient about fetal risks
   - High risk of preterm birth, prematurity, structural malformations with mycophenolate mofetil, transmission of acute maternal infections
   - Unknown risks for immunologic and neurologic deficits
   - Transmission of maternal infections (e.g., CMV), unknown risks for sirolomus
8. Inform the patient that she will need to be followed closely during the gestation by her transplant nephrologist and high-risk obstetrician
   - Every 2–3 weeks initially and then every 1–2 weeks after 28 weeks
9. Recommend that offspring's pediatrician be informed that fetus was exposed in utero to immunosuppressive medications
   - Screen for immunologic and developmental problems
10. Breastfeeding recommendations are not clear, although possibly not contraindicated

Table 20.2 Guidelines for follow-up of maternal transplant recipient

Maternal screening	Interval	Purpose
Before pregnancy		
Pre-pregnancy counseling	At pre-transplant evaluation and yearly if on UNOS wait list	See Table 20.1
During pregnancy		
Home blood pressure monitoring	Daily	Early detection of accelerated hypertension or preeclampsia
Clinic visits Q 2–3 weeks[a]	Conception to 28 weeks	Monitor immunosuppressive drug levels, renal function, metabolic function, screen for pathogens (see Table 20.3)
Clinic visits Q 1–2 weeks[a]	28 weeks to deliver	Monitor immunosuppressive drug levels, renal function, proteinuria, metabolic function, preeclampsia
After pregnancy		
Clinic visits Q 2–3 weeks	2–3 months post-partum	Monitor immunosuppressive drug levels, renal function, frequency depends on renal function

[a]Follow-up should be done in conjunction with high-risk obstetrician.

Table 20.3 Guidelines for screening of maternal transplant recipient

Evaluation		Purpose
HBV, HCV, HSV, CMV, HIV, toxoplasmosis, rubella	Pre-transplant	Provides opportunity to counsel regarding risks of fetal transmission. Hepatitis B vaccine can be given, although rubella is contraindicated (live vaccine)
CBC	Each visit	Screen for WBC and anemia – ESA often needed
BUN, creatinine	Every 2–4 weeks	Screen for rejection and preeclampsia
Calcineurin inhibitor levels	Every 2–4 weeks	Levels may vary throughout gestation Expect decrease in second trimester
Liver function tests	Every 6 weeks	Screen for drug toxicities, HELLP, etc.
Glucose tolerance test	Each trimester	Screen for gestational diabetes
IgM to toxoplasmosis	Each trimester if seronegative	Risk of congenital infection
IgM to CMV	Each trimester if seronegative	Risk of congenital infection

References

1. Anantharaman P, Schmidt. RJ. Sexual function in chronic kidney disease. *Adv Chronic Kidney Dis.* 2007;14:119–125.
2. Palmer BF. Sexual dysfunction in uremia. *J Am Soc Nephrol.* 1999;10:1381–1388.
3. Raiz L, Davies EA, Ferguson. RM. Sexual functioning following renal transplantation. *Health Soc Work.* 2003;28:264–272.

4. Schover LR, Novick AC, Steinmuller DR, Goormastic. M. Sexuality, fertility, and renal transplantation: a survey of survivors. *J Sex Marital Ther*. 1990;16:3–13.
5. Saha MT, Saha HH, Niskanen LK, Salmela KT, Pasternack. AI. Time course of serum prolactin and sex hormones following successful renal transplantation. *Nephron*. 2002;92: 735–737.
6. Lim VS, Henriquez C, Sievertsen G, Frohman. LA. Ovarian function in chronic renal failure: evidence suggesting hypothalamic anovulation. *Ann Intern Med*. 1980;93:21–27.
7. Holley JL, Schmidt RJ, Bender FH, Dumler F, Schiff. M. Gynecologic and reproductive issues in women on dialysis. *Am J Kidney Dis*. 1997;29:685–690.
8. Zeyneloglu HB, Oktem M, Durak. T. Male infertility after renal transplantation: achievement of pregnancy after intracytoplasmic sperm injection. *Transplant Proc*. 2005;37:3081–3084.
9. Akbari F, Alavi M, Esteghamati A, Mehrsai A, Djaladat H, Zohrevand R, Pourmand. G. Effect of renal transplantation on sperm quality and sex hormone levels. *BJU Int*. 2003;92:281–283.
10. Tondolo V, Citterio F, Panocchia N, Nanni G, Castagneto. M. Sirolimus impairs improvement of the gonadal function after renal transplantation. *Am J Transplant* 2005;5:197.
11. Tondolo V, Citterio F, Panocchia N, Nanni G, Favi E, Brescia A, Castagneto. M. Gonadal function and immunosuppressive therapy after renal transplantation. *Transplant Proc*. 2005;37:1915–1917.
12. Fritsche L, Budde K, Dragun D, Einecke G, Diekmann F, Neumayer. HH. Testosterone concentrations and sirolimus in male renal transplant patients. *Am J Transplant*. 2004;4:130–131.
13. Kaczmarek I, Groetzner J, Adamidis I, Landwehr P, Mueller M, Vogeser M, Gerstorfer M, Uberfuhr P, Meiser B, Reichart. B. Sirolimus impairs gonadal function in heart transplant recipients. *Am J Transplant*. 2004;4:1084–1088.
14. Guazzelli CA, Torloni MR, Sanches TF, Barbieri M, Pestana. JO. Contraceptive counseling and use among 197 female kidney transplant recipients. *Transplantation*. 2008;86:669–672.
15. Fischer MJ, Lehnerz SD, Hebert JR, Parikh. CR. Kidney disease is an independent risk factor for adverse fetal and maternal outcomes in pregnancy. *Am J Kidney Dis*. 2004;43:415–423.
16. McKay D, Josephson. M. Reproduction and Transplantation: report on the AST consensus conference on reproductive issues and transplantation. *Am J Transplantation*. 2005;5:1–8.
17. Josephson MA, McKay. DB. Considerations in the medical management of pregnancy in transplant recipients. *Adv Chronic Kidney Dis*. 2007;14:156–167.
18. Estes CM, Westhoff. C. Contraception for the transplant patient. *Semin Perinatol*. 2007;31:372–377.
19. Davison JM, Bailey. DJ. Pregnancy following renal transplantation. *J Obstet Gynaecol Res*. 2003;29:227–233.
20. Reddy SS, Holley. JL. Management of the pregnant chronic dialysis patient. *Adv Chronic Kidney Dis*. 2007;14:146–155.
21. McKay DB, Josephson. MA. Pregnancy in recipients of solid organs – effects on mother and child. *N Engl J Med*. 2006;354:1281–1293.
22. Coscia LA, Constantinescu S, Moritz MJ, Radomski JS, Gaughan WJ, McGrory CH, Armenti. VT. Report from the National Transplantation Pregnancy Registry (NTPR): outcomes of pregnancy after transplantation. *Clin Transpl* 2007;29–42.
23. Sibanda N, Briggs JD, Davison JM, Johnson RJ, Rudge. CJ. Pregnancy after organ transplantation: a report from the UK Transplant pregnancy registry. *Transplantation*. 2007;83:1301–1307.
24. McKay DB, Josephson. MA. Pregnancy after kidney transplantation. *Clin J Am Soc Nephrol* 2008;3(Suppl 2):S117-S125.
25. del Mar Colon M, Hibbard. JU. Obstetric considerations in the management of pregnancy in kidney transplant recipients. *Adv Chronic Kidney Dis*. 2007;14:168–177.
26. Podymow T, August. P. Hypertension in pregnancy. *Adv Chronic Kidney Dis*. 2007;14:178–190.
27. Umans JG. Medications during pregnancy: antihypertensives and immunosuppressives. *Adv Chronic Kidney Dis*. 2007;14:191–198.

28. Baumwell S, Karumanchi. SA. Pre-eclampsia: clinical manifestations and molecular mechanisms. *Nephron Clin Pract*. 2007;106:c72-c81.
29. Stratta P, Canavese C, Giacchino F, Mesiano P, Quaglia M, Rossetti. M. Pregnancy in kidney transplantation: satisfactory outcomes and harsh realities. *J Nephrol*. 2003;16:792–806.
30. Morales J, Hernandez Poblete G, Andres A, Prieto C, Hernandez E, Rodicio. J. Uric acid handling, pregnancy and cyclosporin in renal transplant women. *Nephron*. 1990;56:97–98.
31. Mutter WP, Karumanchi. SA. Molecular mechanisms of preeclampsia. *Microvasc Res* 2008 Jan;75(1):1–8.
32. EBPG Expert group in renal transplantation. European best practice guidelines for renal transplantation. Section IV. Long-term management of the transplant recipient. IV.10. Pregnancy in renal transplant recipients. *Nephrol Dial Transplant* 2002;17(Suppl 4):50–55.
33. Davison JM. Changes in renal function in early pregnancy in women with one kidney. *Yale J Biol Med*. 1978;51:347–349.
34. Katz AI, Davison JM, Hayslett JP, Singson E, Lindheimer. MD. Pregnancy in women with kidney disease. *Kidney Int*. 1980;18:192–206.
35. Fischer MJ. Chronic kidney disease and pregnancy: maternal and fetal outcomes. *Adv Chronic Kidney Dis*. 2007;14:132–145.
36. Ghanem ME, El-Baghdadi LA, Badawy AM, Bakr MA, Sobhe MA, Ghoneim MA. Pregnancy outcome after renal allograft transplantation: 15 years experience. *Reprod Biol*. 2005;121:178–181.
37. Oliveira LG, Sass N, Sato JL, Ozaki KS, Medina Pestana. JO. Pregnancy after renal transplantation – a five-yr single-center experience. *Clin Transplant*. 2007;21:301–304.
38. Ross DS, Dollard SC, Victor M, Sumartojo E, Cannon. MJ. The epidemiology and prevention of congenital cytomegalovirus infection and disease: activities of the Centers for Disease Control and Prevention Workgroup. *J Womens Health (Larchmt)*. 2006;15:224–229.
39. Ornoy A, Diav-Citrin. O. Fetal effects of primary and secondary cytomegalovirus infection in pregnancy. *Reprod Toxicol*. 2006;21:399–409.
40. Michaels MG. Treatment of congenital cytomegalovirus: where are we now?. *Expert Rev Anti Infect Ther*. 2007;5:441–448.
41. Gardella C, Brown. ZA. Managing varicella zoster infection in pregnancy. *Cleve Clin J Med*. 2007;74:290–296.
42. Shiono Y, Mun HS, He N, Nakazaki Y, Fang H, Furuya M, Aosai F, Yano. A. Maternal-fetal transmission of Toxoplasma gondii in interferon-gamma deficient pregnant mice. *Parasitol Int*. 2007;56:141–148.
43. Sifontis NM, Coscia LA, Constantinescu S, Lavelanet AF, Moritz MJ, Armenti. VT. Pregnancy outcomes in solid organ transplant recipients with exposure to mycophenolate mofetil or sirolimus. *Transplantation*. 2006;82:1698–1702.
44. LeRay C, Coulomb A, Elefant E, Frydman R, Audibert. F. Mycophenolate mofetil in pregnancy after renal transplantation: a case of major fetal malformations. *Obstet Gynecol*. 2004;103:1091–1094.
45. Stanley CW, Gottlieb R, Zager R, Eisenberg J, Richmond R, Moritz MJ, Armenti. VT. Developmental well-being in offspring of women receiving cyclosporine post-renal transplant. *Transplant Proc*. 1999;31:241–242.
46. Phillips DI. Programming of the stress response: a fundamental mechanism underlying the long-term effects of the fetal environment?. *J Intern Med*. 2007;261:453–460.
47. Neubauer AP, Voss W, Kattner. E. Outcome of extremely low birth weight survivors at school age: the influence of perinatal parameters on neurodevelopment. *Eur J Pediatr* 2008 Jan;167(1):87–95.
48. Phillips DI. External influences on the fetus and their long-term consequences. *Lupus*. 2006;15:794–800.
49. Saenger P, Czernichow P, Hughes I, Reiter. EO. Small for gestational age: short stature and beyond. *Endocr Rev*. 2007;28:219–251.

50. Schreuder M, Delemarre-van de Waal H, van Wijk A. Consequences of intrauterine growth restriction for the kidney. *Kidney Blood Press Res*. 2006;29:108–125.
51. Reyes L, Manalich. R. Long-term consequences of low birth weight. *Kidney Int* 2005;97(Suppl):s68–s77
52. Taylor HG, Minich N, Bangert B, Filipek PA, Hack. M. Long-term neuropsychological outcomes of very low birth weight: associations with early risks for periventricular brain insults. *J Int Neuropsychol Soc*. 2004;10:987–1004.
53. Gluckman PD, Hanson. MA. The consequences of being born small - an adaptive perspective. *Horm Res* 2006;65(Suppl 3):5–14.
54. American Academy of Pediatrics. Committee on Drugs the transfer of drugs and other chemicals into human milk. *Pediatrics*1994;93:137–150.

Chapter 21
Socioeconomic Issues and the Transplant Recipient

Mary Beth Callahan and Connie L. Davis

Introduction

Socioeconomic status (SES), a composite variable based on education, income, and occupation, has long been a prime predictive variable of clinical outcomes. SES determines access to care and can contribute to non-adherence when people have to make choices between health care and basic needs. Lower life expectancy and higher mortality rates are linked with SES.

SES is interrelated with several variables, including geography, demographic characteristics, ethnicity, and cultural considerations. When statistically controlling for SES, the effects of many other variables are often statistically insignificant and clinically unimportant.[1] It is generally accepted that life stress associated with SES is experienced more often and to a greater degree by individuals of low SES and may, therefore, be considered a risk factor for adherence to medical recommendations[2] as discussed in Chapter 22.

Widely Accepted Socioeconomic Issues: Age, Gender, Education, and Ethnicity

Demographic variables significantly impact transplant outcomes. Age, gender, education level, socioeconomic status, and ethnicity are but a few of the characteristics that influence how a transplant recipient fares. Age determines attitudes toward medication adherence as well as the status of the immune system. It also represents a general outlook on other health issues that will intersect with transplant procedures and medications. The gender of the donor and that of the recipient influence kidney transplant outcomes. Gender disparity between donor and recipient leads to immunological responses against gender-specific proteins.[3] Size differences between the donor and the recipient can lead to hyperfiltration of a small kidney in

M.B. Callahan (✉)
Dallas Transplant Institute, Dallas, TX, USA
e-mail: mbcallahan@sbcglobal.net

D.B. McKay, S.M. Steinberg (eds.), *Kidney Transplantation: A Guide to the Care of Kidney Transplant Recipients*, DOI 10.1007/978-1-4419-1690-7_21, © Springer Science+Business Media, LLC 2010

a large recipient and lack of recognition of transplant damage in a large kidney in a small recipient.[4]

Higher education level and socioeconomic status often impact patient or family resources that influence early or preemptive transplant and medical coverage following transplant. Ethnicity may be associated with different socioeconomic status, language other than English, and variable pharmacogenomics or other genetically determined pathways that impact the risk for rejection, the development of posttransplant diabetes, or transplant scarring.[5,6] Thus, who a person is sets the stage for transplant outcome and needs to be taken into consideration to optimize transplant success and limit toxic outcomes (Table 21.1).

Table 21.1 Average cost of medications after transplant

	Total cost (cost is decreased by insurance; however, co-pays and deductibles apply)
Anti-rejection medications	$1,500/month
Prophylactic anti-viral medication	$2,500/month for 3–6 months
Clotrimazole (4–6 weeks), antihypertensives, Bactrim, PPIs	Approximately $400/month
Insulin, diabetes supplies	Approximately $400/month

Access to Health Care and Its Impact on the Transplant Recipient

When assessing access to health care, it is important to try to understand the experiences of people living on the margins of our healthcare system. When insurance is limited, money is pinched and food is not on the shelves; whether it is due to high insurance premiums, deductibles, medication co-pays, or non-existent insurance, living with chronic illness can pauperize those who thought they had financial security. Moreover, preemptive transplant may not be available to those with lower SES. In a 10-year (1996–2005) review using United States Renal Data System (USRDS) data, access to kidney transplantation varied markedly by state. Even with adjustment for patient case mix and for insurance, there remained statistically significant differences in access by state to the kidney transplant waiting list and to either a living or deceased donor kidney transplant.[7]

Additionally, medical status and age can impact access to kidney transplantation. Patients without diabetes and under age 39 have been shown to undergo preemptive referral more often, while minority patients are less likely than white patients to undergo early referral and transplantation.[7] Only 2.5% of incident patients ("new cases accepted for treatment," as defined by USRDS) receive kidney transplants preemptively.[8]

Most people with kidney failure have access to Medicare under ESRD. Once a person has Medicare under ESRD, it covers any health problem that Medicare covers, not just kidney disease. However, according to current Medicare regulations, if a person has Medicare only based on kidney disease, coverage will *end* 3 years after transplant. The rationale for Medicare having a specified time benefit for people entitled to it based on ESRD was because it was thought that people post kidney transplant would be able to return to vocational activities and achieve insurance. In reality, access to employer group health insurance is scarcer than anticipated for many reasons. Some reasons are as follows:

1. Transplant age has increased, thus, patients get transplanted and lose Medicare in their 50s and early 60s before they are eligible for Medicare based on age, but when reentry into the workforce is difficult.
2. Waiting time on transplant lists has increased, often decreasing functional status of the dialysis patient while they wait, again, making reentry into a tightening and very competitive job market difficult.
3. Since waiting time on transplant lists has increased, time on dialysis has increased which makes continuance in current employment more difficult. Sometimes employers begin to see problems with work schedule, missed days due to illness, etc., when a person remains on dialysis for a long period of time while awaiting transplant. Often a dialysis patient will need to have dialysis access revisions, develop an infection, be overly fatigued, or develop a vascular issue that results in diminished work attendance or performance
4. Today's ESRD population is not the same as the population of ESRD patients served prior to the inception of Medicare coverage for ESRD (1973). Prior to Medicare coverage for ESRD, during the 1960s and early 1970s, "Life and Death Committees" were required due to extremely limited access to dialysis. Admission to dialysis programs was restricted to those who were "young" (21–45 years old), "responsible" (employed, housewives, full-time students), and "involved" (participating in their care).[9]
5. Individuals with ESRD are more often from the lowest SES class and therefore have often not had prior employment or access to healthcare benefits.[10]

Medicare Coverage

During the time a person has Medicare, it will pay 80% of an allowed amount. If a person has Medicare only, this can still be problematic for the following reasons:

1. Twenty percent of anti-rejection medications, costs approximately $300 a month (2009)
2. Twenty percent of co-pays for physician visits and tests
3. Hospital deductibles, in 2009, are nearly $1,100 for each possible admission every 61st day period

These financial barriers are many and often without resolution.

In 2006, Medicare Part D (prescription drug) plans began helping people with only Medicare to pay for medications other than immunosuppressants. Prior to this time Medicare covered only immunosuppressant medications. However, even with Medicare Part D today, patients often must rely on pharmaceutical assistance programs to supplement their Medicare Part D plans, due to the complicated structure of Medicare Part D plans. Because of these issues, assessment of cognitive capacity and support systems to manage multiple programs to access medications to remain adherent to one aspect of medical recommendations should be a component of the pre-transplant evaluation. Back-up financial support within the family or social network should also be assessed.

Lack of adequate insurance coverage can greatly impact transplant outcome. Three years after a transplant, when Medicare coverage often lapses, a person may be unable to continue their access to health care and may have problems accessing medications. Even though a nephrologist may have a financial assessment process that can deem someone eligible for an indigent fee waiver in their office, the cost of other medical care, such as for cancer and diabetes, often cannot be waived by other medical providers.

An additional gap in insurance coverage is demonstrated by rules surrounding disability benefits. Should a person become disabled by Social Security after he has returned to employment, Medicare will become effective *after* the 24th SSDI check (*24 months*) has been received. This, of course, means that a person can be without adequate access to health care for 2 years, even when deemed disabled by Social Security if the disability is not related to ESRD. It is only the narrowest minority of patients that would be able to afford testing such as an MRI or other procedures at cash pay amounts. Often county hospital districts accept only the poorest of the poor. Those not in this category are, thus, without a home for healthcare provision when Medicare ends. Despite the best plans for rehabilitation pre- and post-transplant, being without insurance is often the reality.

A comprehensive psychosocial assessment can often predict psychosocial barriers, particularly financial, to positive transplant outcome. Often lack of a previous history of employer group health plan (EGHP) may predict problems in accessing future EGHP. A person may have been able to get by without medical coverage prior to ESRD and transplant, but once a person has ESRD, dialysis, and transplant, specialized medical care and medications will always be needed. Thus, an EGHP will be needed if a person is not eligible for Medicare or Medicaid and does not have an individual coverage plan in place. The potential for someone to access EGHP post-transplant at age 35 when they have never had EGHP pre-transplant is less likely than someone who has had a history of employment with EGHP. In many cases, the potential for vocational rehabilitation leading to EGHP may not be viable due to the ability to learn, motivation, life skills, and/or social support. It may be difficult for the transplant team to see a healthy person from a medical standpoint and accept that there are no quick answers to the overwhelming psychosocial barriers that will ultimately impact treatment outcome. Each transplant committee grapples with placing someone on a waiting list for transplantation who can't afford medications or testing and who will likely not have access to health care 3 years after transplant.

Insurance, Co-pays, Deductibles, and Premiums

Many years ago, it was less complicated for those with insurance, those who had only small co-pays and deductibles to worry about, to pay for care associated with chronic kidney disease. Today, there are ever-increasing costs associated with the continuum of care for a patient with chronic kidney disease. Deductibles can be thousands of dollars each year and co-pays for medications can easily be 30%. Adding together just the immunosuppressant and anti-viral medications for the first 3–6 months post-transplant equals a monthly cost of over $4,000 in 2009. Thirty percent of that is, of course, $1,200. Most patients seeking kidney transplant cannot afford 3–6 months with these co-pays. Middle-income families, with insurance and high co-pays and deductibles may fall through the cracks of pharmaceutical companies that offer assistance programs for patients who cannot afford their medications. Alternatively, fundraising (raising money specifically to pay for post-transplant needs) prior to and following transplant may be required to meet the medication cost needs. Even the first 30 days of medications after transplant may require savings beyond what insurance companies or Medicare provide because of deductibles and co-pays.

Because of the complexities and risks of inadequate resources and savings that are needed in addition to insurance coverage for transplant, patients must be assessed before transplant for the cognitive capacity to manage access to medications through pharmaceutical assistance programs (PAPs) and/or to have the social support available to help them with this tedious process. Each pharmaceutical assistance program has a different application form, timeline, requirements for participation, method of shipping, and amount of medication they will provide as well as location they will ship to. If a patient with lower SES is using seven pharmaceutical assistance programs (PAPs) and has low cognitive capacity, problems with literacy, and no social support, this patient has a high level of psychosocial risk factors that will contribute to a negative transplant outcome.

Young adults may have special issues as they may have limited access to their parents' insurance. Sometimes this is based on an age cut-off. Sometimes young adults' access to parents' insurance is based on how much support the parent provides the young adult each year. Additionally, the parents often have been taking care of all the insurance and medical communication; however, when the child turns 18 this responsibility often falls directly and quickly onto the child. Early preparation for this transition to adulthood by the young with chronic illness is very important in long-term successful outcomes with chronic kidney disease (CKD). The parents, child, healthcare workers, and social worker need to work in concert to optimize ongoing coverage.

The Importance of Fundraising

There is also the cost of insurance. Many families cannot afford the cost of the insurance premiums. Many believe that having the insurance just long enough to *get* the transplant will be enough. Education by the social worker is important in helping the patient understand the need for planning to maintain insurance. Support and education on methods of fundraising in order to pay the co-pays, deductibles, and premiums for the long term may also be of benefit. Allowing the patient time to raise funds before transplant allows the patient to preserve their dignity and way of life and can be empowering. To support the idea of fundraising, it is helpful to the patient for the healthcare team to understand the extreme costs associated with transplant and to realize that resources in agency and community systems are limited. False hope that there is money and resources to pay for the many expenses post-transplant is misleading and can be very discouraging for the patient who is living on the margins of financial ruin.

Insurance opportunities vary state by state for people with a chronic illness. However, consistently, young adults between the ages of 18 and 21 are among the most uninsured and underinsured in the United States.[11]

Transportation, Lodging, and Food

Patients who live away from a transplant center must prepare for additional costs:

(1) Lodging immediately post-transplant and for follow-up visits
(2) Food while away from home
(3) Transportation to and from the transplant center

These costs are significant. If a person has an employer group health plan, transportation, lodging, and food costs are occasionally covered. If the person has Medicare and/or Medicaid, these costs *are not* covered. Most often, the person, who is not working, has a difficult time saving for even the most discounted lodging and food for a period of 6 weeks post-transplant. Fundraising is essential for these patients. In pre-transplant evaluation they should be provided with an accurate perception of an amount they will need for lodging, food, and transportation (for the surgery and for the first 3 months of medical follow-up).

Making It Work (Employment Maintenance or Initiation)

Providing encouragement to dialysis and transplant recipients to maintain their current employment is the best way to avoid work disincentives. While preemptive transplant is increasing and numbers of those working while on dialysis are improving, the majority of transplant recipients have been on dialysis for a period of time. Based on 2004 CMS data, only 18.9% of prevalent dialysis patients aged 18–54 were employed. Several factors were found to impact employment rates. These were

– availability of peritoneal dialysis or home hemodialysis
– provision of frequent hemodialysis
– patient/social work staffing ratio

– rural setting
– unit size
– availability of vocational rehabilitation services[12]

Dialysis, whether hemodialysis or peritoneal dialysis, can take a toll on a person through deconditioning and lower energy levels which often leads to multiple psychosocial barriers that impact employment status and insurance. From a socioeconomic perspective, planning for income, insurance, and family security is worrisome yet, imperative and unfortunately, it is not always possible.

If a person stops employment once they have started dialysis, they may be eligible for Social Security Disability Insurance (SSDI) based on the initiation of dialysis or transplant and not working, if, they have worked enough work quarters in 5 of the last 10 years. Social Security deems kidney transplantation "a disability for 12 months following surgery." This, of course, is dependent upon whether a person returns to *substantial gainful activity* (www.ssa.gov) or not during this period.

A plan for returning to gainful employment, if possible, should begin during the pre-transplant social work assessment and include

1. Referral to vocational rehabilitation services if the patient is not employed
2. Careful partnering with the current employer if the patient is working
3. Review of short-term and long-term disability through current employment if possible
4. Review of the patient's perception of fatigue and encourage increased physical activity and a plan to improve activity as increased fatigue is associated with lower rates of employment.[13]

Many times people with chronic kidney disease are not able to pay the extra premiums for short-term and long-term disability through their employer. This ultimately leaves them in a precarious socioeconomic position throughout the course of their illness. Encouraging people to try to pay at least short-term disability premiums is worthwhile, as there is a 5-month waiting period before Social Security Disability can begin on the sixth month.

Ease of Communication Between Patient and Healthcare Provider

The ability to communicate one's condition, concerns, and worries to the care provider has a tremendous impact on transplant outcome. Language barriers and the social/cultural issues often associated with different languages often determine adherence with treatment. The basis of trust of the care providers is determined by one's ethnicity, language, gender, and age. Trust is key to believing in the care provider's plan for the patient and, thus, adherence with the appropriate medication regimen.[14–17] It also impacts behaviors that can lead to post-transplant infection such as travel, managing animals, certain types of employment and avocations (gardening, hunting). Completely open communication without fear of retribution or being rebuked needs to be the norm for the transplant clinic.

Language barriers are becoming more common as the diversity of our population grows. No matter the geographical location, if a patient does not have the same primary language as their care providers, important information can be lost in translation. Translators can help, but it is not the same as being able to talk one on one with a patient from the same level of language usage and cultural basis. There are hidden meanings in conversations between native speakers. Thus, it is preferable to have native speakers provide patient care. Lacking that, non-family member translators are preferred. This decreases the possibility of mistakes or guilt should something unforeseen occur.

The frequency of follow-up visits post-transplant helps to determine how often a patient thinks about their health issues. The more frequent the follow-up visit, the more expensive; but the more distant, the more risk for non-compliance. Thus, setting a certain expectation for laboratory and clinical visit follow-up is important. Instilling the sense that the provider is always overseeing and concerned may help in maintaining the connection that fosters adherence and the recognition that timely communication of changes in condition will improve outcome.[18,19]

Each patient should be assessed to determine the optimal way to communicate medical information. Some are better with oral instruction, some with written, and some with pictorial visual means. Additionally, it is optimal to have family or friends hear the key instructions in order to make sure that recipients complete the needed tasks. The post-transplant time period can be very overwhelming to most patients and therefore care needs to be taken in communicating important instructions.

Medication Side Effects

Remembering to take a pill is difficult enough but if it causes unwanted side effects that may increase the possibility of non-adherence with the medication.[20] The question is a balance between life and quality of life. All medications have side effects. The most problematic are those that cause external physical changes and those that impair important functional abilities. Specific side effects associated with immunosuppressive medications are discussed in Chapter 9.

Living Donation

Relationship of Donor to Recipient

The relationship of the donor to the recipient has changed over time. Previously, the donors were family members, especially siblings or parents. This is now changing with an increasing number of donors being unrelated to the recipient. There is also an increase in children donating to parents. Spousal donors are a special group as are altruistic donors. Altruistic donors are infrequent but increasing and often demonstrate generous behaviors in other parts of their lives more so than the general population.[21]

Social Status of Donors

Living donors are most often from the middle socioeconomic group of society.[22,23] The average educational level and income level of living donors is comparable with the national census.[24] Thus, for years living donors have been paying out of pocket to the best of their ability for the right to donate. They have paid for travel expenses, lodging, childcare costs and have lost wages in the process of donating. The Donor Nephrectomy Outcomes Research (DONOR) Network study, done by the Division of Nephrology, University of Western Ontario, Canada, showed the following: total out of pocket expenses for donors is on average $400–800; the average number of days of unpaid leave needed by living donors is 12; the average lost wages is between $600.00 and 3,400.00.[25]

Costs Related to Living Donation

If the transplant candidate is covered by a private insurance plan, most insurance companies pay for the donor's evaluation expenses. They may not provide coverage for extensive follow-up should the living donor experience medical problems related to the donation. If Medicare covers the transplant candidate, Medicare Part A pays for donor testing, surgery, and hospitalization. Medicare Part B pays for donor physician services during the hospital stay. Medicare covers *limited* follow-up care for living donors. This coverage may be extended for a further limited time if complications arise following donation. Medicare does not cover transportation expenses, lodging, food, lost wages, or childcare or adult care. Some insurance plans may cover transportation and lodging expenses for the donor.

The National Living Donor Assistance Center was established to assist living donors who need financial assistance to help defray travel and subsistence expenses. It was authorized by the Organ Donation and Recovery Improvement Act (P.L. 108–216; http://www.livingdonorassistance.org).

The South-Eastern Organ Procurement Foundation (SEOPF), an association of transplant-related professional organizations, maintains and operates the Living Organ Donor Network (LODN), which became operational in October 2000. Through this network, donors can be provided with a safety net of protection in the form of life, disability, and medical insurance for complications that might arise from being a living related or unrelated kidney donor. The insurance is optional for transplant centers that participate in the program as well as for individuals that may wish to benefit from this protection. SEOPF secured coverage for LODN through AIG Insurance, which currently underwrites the coverage for donors in the National Bone Marrow Donor Program upon which LODN is modeled. SEOPF offers LODN to all kidney transplant centers in the country and there is no cost to the donor or the recipient to participate in the registry. However, the transplant center has to participate in order for the donors to be enrolled. There is a one-time fee of $550 per donor for the optional insurance protection. The lifetime follow-up of the donor, the coordination with the donation center, research and data analysis are provided at no fee to SEOPF members (www.seopf.org/lodn_info.htm; 1/7/09).

Specialty Focus

Transplantation provides the best outcome for those with kidney failure. However, waiting times for those without living donors can be over 10 years in some areas of the United States. Thus, those waiting have sought innovative approaches over the last several years. Transplant tourism, where an individual goes to another country and purchases a transplant, has recently increased.[26,27] The problem with traveling abroad to receive a transplant is that many of the donors are *paid* unrelated donors and thus have not been optimally evaluated. Furthermore, the recipients of such transplants have been shown to develop more post-transplant problems.[28,29] The outcome of the donors is also less than optimal because their medical evaluation may not be rigorous.[30] Additionally, Medicare will not cover the anti-rejection medications under Part B for people who have their transplant at a non-Medicare-approved facility creating financial hardships for the duration of the transplant.

International Perspective

Transplant tourism has been discussed and defined by the Istanbul Declaration.[31] The international community made the decision to support this declaration as has the World Health Organization and almost all international and national transplant societies. The definitions surrounding transplant tourism as taken from the declaration are as follows:

> **Organ trafficking** is the recruitment, transport, transfer, harboring, or receipt of living or deceased persons or their organs by means of the threat or use of force of other forms of coercion, of abduction, or fraud of deception, of the abuse of power or of a position of vulnerability, of or giving to, or the receiving by, a third party of payments or benefits to achieve the transfer of control over the potential donor, for the purpose of exploitation by the removal of organs for transplantation.

> **Transplant commercialism** is a policy or practice in which an organ is treated as a commodity, including by being bought or sold or sued for material gain.

> **Travel for transplantation** is the movement of organs, donors, recipients, or transplant professionals across jurisdictional borders for transplantation purposes. Travel for transplantation becomes **transplant tourism** if it involves organ trafficking and/or transplant commercialism or if the resources (organs, professionals, and transplant centers) devoted to providing transplants to patients from outside a country undermine the country's ability to provide transplant services for its own population.

In order to prevent organ trafficking and transplant commercialism the declaration recommends that governments commit to: support research to decrease the development of end-stage organ disease, support ways to optimize deceased organ donation, pass legislation that clearly defines the rules of organ donation, ban payment for organs, and prohibit advertisements for transplant commercialism. These principles are easy to understand; however, the difficulty is in the details of implementation. Many activities go undetected and legislative prohibitions on payment or exchange of some commodities are not tightly defined. What constitutes valuable consideration for an organ may be interpreted differently in different societies.

What is known about the transfer of cash between donor and recipient in living organ donation is that those who donate are from the financially disadvantaged part of society, the money they receive has often been diminished by brokers, the money does not have a long-term positive impact on their financial state or that of their family, if indeed, they receive it at all, the health of the donor is diminished after donation, and the recipient more often has infectious and other complications.[22,30,32,33] Importantly, payment for organs leads to a decrease in voluntary donation by family members and friends leading to an overall decrease in organ donation.[34]

Provider and Patient Factors: Culture and Ethnicity

Culture, ethnicity, and race, which all have different meanings, factor into the patient and provider's socioeconomic gestalt and, as such, relate to the patient's ability to adhere to medical recommendations in many different ways. The World Health Organization's (WHO) *Adherence to Long-term Therapies Project*, a global initiative launched in 2001, states, "Adherence is a multidimensional phenomenon determined by the interplay of five sets of factors:

- Social and economic factors
- Health care team and system-related factors
- Condition-related factors
- Therapy-related factors
- Patient-related factors"[2]

Social and economic factors include considerations that may be indicative of a wide range of socioeconomic variables including education, income, environment, social cohesion, family dysfunction, social and family support, health literacy, and beliefs about medication, disease, and treatment. Culture, ethnicity, and race, regardless of whether its members are living in their country of origin or elsewhere as immigrants, can be important in helping a patient understand medical recommendations and can have a bearing on SES. Each person involved in a patient's care brings a preconceived notion about culture, ethnicity, and race to that interaction. Awareness of this concept is important for effective interactions with the patient.

High-Risk Behaviors

Abuse of illicit drugs or alcohol can negatively impact transplant outcome. Chronic alcohol use can lead to decreased immunosuppressive drug absorption and forgetfulness when it comes to taking immunosuppressive medications. The use of illicit drugs can result in vasoconstriction (amphetamines, cocaine), infection (aspergillus – marijuana), or other toxicities due to impurities contained in the preparations. Additionally, intravenous drug use leads to increased rates of viral infections such as hepatitis B, hepatitis C, and HIV. These infections can also impact drug metabolism, increase the risk for other infections, and impair the ability to use certain types of drugs in the transplant recipient.

Most transplant programs require that anyone with a substance abuse problem undergo rehabilitation prior to transplant. Patients with past histories of drug abuse need continued surveillance to avoid unnecessary risk to transplant failure. The rate of recidivism[35] is usually between 20 and 30% but decreased by intervention.[35,36]

Non-adherence is a problem for all medical therapies. Past problems with adherence can certainly be more prominent in those that have problems after transplant but even those who are very compliant will have problems. It is known that almost all patients will miss drug doses sometime after transplant and that this increases with time from transplant and with increasing times between provider visits. However, predicting non-adherence can be very difficult.

Lifestyle Choices and Impact on the Transplant Recipient

Lifestyle choices that lead to obesity and smoking lead to a poorer outcome following transplant.[37] Obesity is associated with increased wound infections, lung problems, venous thrombosis, and overall decreased kidney transplant function after surgery. Patients develop more transplant diabetes with the downstream risk of cardiovascular disease and graft diabetic nephropathy and fibrosis. Smoking is associated with vascular disease and cancer. A sedentary lifestyle independent of weight or weight gain is also associated with a transplant outcome.[38,39]

Emotional and Cognitive Status and Its Relationship to Socioeconomic Status

Stress is a concomitant of chronic illness and is compounded by long-term costs of care and unpredictability of kidney failure and its treatment. Additionally, depression has been found in a large percentage of people with kidney failure[40] and can be exacerbated by immunosuppressive medications. Depression and stress lead to unemployment, which in turn leads to loss of insurance. Life stress associated with SES is experienced more often and to a greater degree by individuals of low SES and may impact their management of the disease process. The assessment of emotional health and cognitive status is important for short-term and long-term outcomes of transplant. The emotional health and stable cognitive status of a person impacts their management of tasks needed to manage illness.

Evidence exists that social support, particularly from the family, profoundly influences overall morbidity and mortality and the course of chronic illness[41,42] Additionally, family stress and multiple family losses related to the illness may play an important role in mediating treatment outcome. ESRD often impacts marital role and marital adjustment as well as changes in other relationships by impacting the functioning of the family system. In preparing for transplant, social support is additionally important in planning and fundraising. As stated earlier, the cost of transplant can be overwhelming, not only in the immediate post-transplant period but throughout the course of the transplant.

Patients with a history of psychiatric illness require specialized assessment during the evaluation process. Consideration should be given to the impact that a rejection episode and treatment will have upon the mental state of the individual, i.e., bipolar disease. Additionally, the family support system for pediatric transplant candidates should be assessed to determine the same areas as mentioned for the adult candidate, with additional emphasis on the impact of illness on the caregivers and their ability to maintain their normal roles and how this impacts the SES of the family. For patients who are mentally challenged, the extended support system should be assessed to determine primary and secondary support, should primary supports of adult patients become incapacitated or die. The question needs to be answered: How will the patient be able to manage access to health care and medications and what will the psychosocial barriers be? Is there a plan?

Summary

Providing the best care for kidney transplant recipients may not mean always using the newest, most expensive medications. If patients have working transplants, but can't buy bread for their tables and lose their cars or can't pay their rent, are we truly providing the assistance they need? Patients won't always tell us they don't have money, don't have a job, or haven't taken their medications because they can't afford them. For every patient that tells us, how many have not? It is prime time to move the discussion of medical coverage after transplant and for chronic disease care in general, to the front page. Public policy makers need to consider what the fair and right approach to care is. Will we remain one of the wealthiest countries in the world that has some of the worst access to what citizens need to maintain their health? Or will steps be taken to rectify this situation? Patient and professional organizations have started this process for transplant recipients by encouraging legislation that maintains insurance coverage for the lifetime of the transplant. This legislation is a start, hopefully of a more all-inclusive correction of healthcare financing.

References

1. Evans R. Non-Adherence in the Transplant Patient. National Institutes of Health conference, January 2008, Tampa, FL, 2008.
2. World Health Organization, . *Adherence to Long-Term Therapies*. World Health Organization, Geneva, 2001.
3. Gratwohl A, Dohler B, Stern M, Opelz G. H-Y as a minor histocompatibility antigen in kidney transplantation: a retrospective cohort study. *Lancet* 2008 July 5;372(9632):49–53.
4. Oh CK, Jeon KO, Kim HJ, Kim SI, Kim YS, Pelletier SJ. Metabolic demand and renal mass supply affecting the early graft function after living donor kidney transplantation. *Kidney Int* 2005 Feb;67(2):744–749.

5. Kasiske BL, Snyder JJ, Gilbertson D, Matas AJ. Diabetes mellitus after kidney transplantation in the United States. *Am J Transplant* 2003 Feb;3(2):178–185.
6. Keith DS, Cantarovich M, Paraskevas S, Tchervenkov J. Recipient age and risk of chronic allograft nephropathy in primary deceased donor kidney transplant. *Transpl Int* 2006 Aug;19(8):649–656.
7. Ashby VB, Kalbfleisch JD, Wolfe RA, Lin MJ, Port FK, Leichtman AB. Geographic variability in access to primary kidney transplantation in the United States, 1996–2005. *Am J Transplant* 2007;7(Suppl 1):1412–1423.
8. Abecassis M, Bartlett ST, Collins AJ et al. Kidney transplantation as primary therapy for end stage renal disease: Proceedings of a National Kidney Foundation/Kidney Disease Outcomes Quality Initiative Conference. *Clin J Am Soc Nephrol* 2008;3(2):471–480.
9. *aakpRENALIFE*. She focuses on the present and remembers the past. *aakpRENALIFE* 2002 May;17(6).
10. White SL, McGeechan K, Jones M, Cass A, Chadban SJ, Polkinghorne KR, Perkovic V, Roderick PJ. Socioeconomic disadvantage and kidney disease in the United States, Australia, and Thailand. *Am J Public Health* 2008 Jul;98(7)1306–1313. E-pub 2008.
11. National Kidney Foundation/Council of Nephrology Social Workers Pediatric Toolkit, 2008.
12. Kutner N, Bowles T, Zhang R, Huang Y, Pastan S. Dialysis facility characteristics and variation in employment rates: A National Study. *Clin J Am Soc Nephrol* 2008 Jan;3(1):111–116.
13. O'Sullivan D, McCarthy G. An exploration of the relationship between fatigue and physical functioning in patients with end stage renal disease receiving haemodialysis. *J Clin Nurs* 2007 Nov;16(11C):276–284.
14. Navaneethan SD, Singh S. A systematic review of barriers in access to renal transplantation among African Americans in the United States. *Clin Transplant* 2006 Nov–Dec;20(6): 769–775.
15. Shilling LM, Norman ML, Chavin KD, Hildebrand LG, Lunsford SL, Martin MS, Milton JE, Smalls GR, Baliga PK. Healthcare professionals' perceptions of the barriers to living donor kidney transplantation among African Americans. *J Natl Med Assoc* 2006 Jun;98(6):834–840.
16. Ayanian JZ, Cleary PD, Weissman JS, Epstein AM. The effect of patients' preferences on racial differences in access to renal transplantation. *N Engl J Med* 1999 Nov 25;341(22): 1661–1669.
17. Russell CL. Culturally responsive interventions to enhance immunosuppressive medication adherence in older African American kidney transplant recipients. *Prog Transplant* 2006 Sep;16(3)187–195. quiz 196.
18. Shemesh E, Annunziato RA, Shneider BL, Dugan CA, Warshaw J, Kerkar N, Emre S. Improving adherence to medications in pediatric liver transplant recipients. *Pediatr Transplant* 2008 May;12(3):316–323.
19. Berquist RK, Berquist WE, Esquivel CO, Cox KL, Wayman KI, Litt IF. Non-adherence to post-transplant care: prevalence, risk factors and outcomes in adolescent liver transplant recipients. *Pediatr Transplant* 2008 Mar;12(2):194–200.
20. Orr A, Orr D, Willis S, Holmes M, Britton P. Patient perceptions of factors influencing adherence to medication following kidney transplant. *Psychol Health Med* 2007 Aug;12(4):509–517.
21. Henderson AJ, Landolt MA, McDonald MF, Barrable WM, Soos JG, Gourlay W, Allison CJ, Landsberg DN. The living anonymous kidney donor: lunatic or saint? *Am J Transplant* 2003 Feb;3(2):203–213.
22. Manauis MN, Pilar KA, Lesaca R, de Belen Uriarte R, Danguilan R, Ona E. A national program for nondirected kidney donation from living unrelated donors: the Philippine experience. *Transplant Proc* 2008 Sep;40(7):2100–2103.
23. Reimer J, Rensing A, Haasen C, Philipp T, Pietruck F, Franke GH. The impact of living-related kidney transplantation on the donor's life. *Transplantation* 2006 May 15;81(9):1268–1273.
24. McCune TR, Armata T, Mendez-Picon G, Yium J, Zabari GB, Crandall B, Spicer HG, Blanton J, Thacker LR. The living organ donor network: a model registry for living kidney donors. *Clin Transplant* 2004;18(Suppl 12):33–38.

25. Clarke KS, Klarenbach S, Vlaicu S, Yang RC, Garg AX. The direct and indirect economic costs incurred by living kidney donors—a systematic review. *Nephrol Dial Transplant* 2006 July;21(7)1952–1960. E-pub 2006 Mar 22.

26. Gill J, Madhira BR, Gjertson D, Lipshutz G, Cecka JM, Pham PT, Wilkinson A, Bunnapradist S, Danovitch GM. Transplant tourism in the United States: a single-center experience. *Clin J Am Soc Nephrol* 2008 Nov;3(6)1820–1828. E-pub 2008 Oct 1.

27. Budiani-Saberi DA, Delmonico FL. Organ trafficking and transplant tourism: a commentary on the global realities. *Am J Transplant* 2008 May;8(5):925–929.

28. Rizvi SA, Naqvi SA, Zafar MN, Mazhar F, Muzaffar R, Naqvi R, Akhtar F, Ahmed E. Commercial transplants in local Pakistanis from vended kidneys: a socio-economic and outcome study. *Transpl Int* 2009 Jan 31;22(6):615–621.

29. Naqvi SA, Rizvi SA, Zafar MN, Ahmed E, Ali B, Mehmood K, Awan MJ, Mubarak B, Mazhar F. Health status and renal function evaluation of kidney vendors: a report from Pakistan. *Am J Transplant* 2008 Jul;8(7):1444–1450.

30. Steering Committee of the Istanbul Summit. Organ trafficking and transplant tourism and commercialism: the Declaration of Istanbul. *Lancet* 2008 Jul;5(372):963.

31. Nejatisafa AA, Mortaz-Hedjri S, Malakoutian T, Arbabi M, Hakemi MS, Haghighi AN, Mohammadi MR, Fazel I. Quality of life and life events of living unrelated kidney donors in Iran: a multicenter study. *Transplantation* 2008 Oct 15;86(7):937–940.

32. Barsoum RS. Trends in unrelated-donor kidney transplantation in the developing world. *Pediatr Nephrol* 2008 Nov;23(11)1925–1929. E-pub 2008 Jun 7.

33. Einollahi B, Taheri S. Renal transplantation practice in Iran and the Middle East: report from Iran and a review of the literature. *Ann Transplant* 2008;13(1)5–14. PMID: 18344938 PubMed.

34. Ghods AJ, Savaj S. Iranian model of paid and regulated living-unrelated kidney donation. *Clin J Am Soc Nephrol* 2006 Nov;1(6)1136–1145. E-pub 2006 Oct 11.

35. Björnsson E, Olsson J, Rydell A, Fredriksson K, Eriksson C, Sjöberg C, Olausson M, Bäckman L, Castedal M, Friman S. Long-term follow-up of patients with alcoholic liver disease after liver transplantation in Sweden: impact of structured management on recidivism. *Scand J Gastroenterol* 2005 Feb;40(2):206–216.

36. Nickels M, Jain A, Sharma R, Orloff M, Tsoulfas G, Kashyap R, Bozorgzadeh A. Polysubstance abuse in liver transplant patients and its impact on survival outcome. *Exp Clin Transplant* 2007 Dec;5(2):680–685.

37. Lentine KL, Rocca-Rey LA, Bacchi G, Wasi N, Schmitz L, Salvalaggio PR, Abbott KC, Schnitzler MA, Neri L, Brennan DC. Obesity and cardiac risk after kidney transplantation: experience at one center and comprehensive literature review. *Transplantation* 2008 Jul 27;86(2):303–312.

38. Painter PL, Topp KS, Krasnoff JB, Adey D, Strasner A, Tomlanovich S, Stock P. Health-related fitness and quality of life following steroid withdrawal in renal transplant recipients. *Kidney Int* 2003 Jun;63(6):2309–2316.

39. Ibels LS, Stewart JH, Mahony JF, Neale FC, Sheil AG. Occlusive arterial disease in uraemic and haemodialysis patients and renal transplant recipients. A study of the incidence of arterial disease and of the prevalence of risk factors implicated in the pathogenesis of arteriosclerosis. *Q J Med* 1977 Apr;46(182):197–214.

40. Watnick S, Kirwin P, Mahnensmith R, Concato J. The prevalence and treatment of depression among patients starting dialysis. *Am J. Kidney Dis* 2003;41(1):105–110.

41. McClellan W, Stanwyck D, Anson C. Social support and subsequent mortality among patients with end-stage renal disease. *J Am Soc Nephrol* 1993;4:1028–1034.

42. Cohen, S & Syme, S (eds). *Social Support and Health*. Academic Press, Orlando, FL, 1985.

Chapter 22
Adherence to the Immunosuppressive Regimen in Adult and Pediatric Kidney Transplant Recipients

Fabienne Dobbels and Richard N. Fine

Introduction

Although kidney transplantation (KTx) prolongs life and improves quality of life, it remains a chronic illness, in which patients require continued medical follow-up to monitor graft function and lifelong medication intake. *Adherence* (also called compliance or concordance) can be defined as the extent to which a person's behavior (taking medications, following a recommended diet, and/or executing lifestyle changes) corresponds with the *agreed* recommendations of a healthcare provider.[1] For kidney transplantation, non-adherence to the immunosuppressive regimen is common and is increasingly recognized as an important predictor of poor long-term posttransplant outcomes.[2,3] Non-adherence is defined as "any deviation from the prescribed medication regimen sufficient to influence adversely the regimen's intended effect."[4]

Non-adherence is very common in adult and pediatric kidney transplant recipients and accounts for a quarter of graft losses. The purpose of this review is to summarize the state-of-the-art evidence of non-adherence to the immunosuppressive regimen, its associated factors, and its impact on posttransplant outcomes in adult and pediatric kidney transplant patients. Potential interventions will also be discussed.

Prevalence of Non-adherence to the Immunosuppressive Regimen

One cannot ignore that non-adherence to the immunosuppressive regimen is a significant problem in kidney transplant patients, with one out of four to one out of

F. Dobbels (✉)
Center for Health Services and Nursing Research, Katholieke Universiteit Leuven, Leuven, Belgium
e-mail: fabienne.dobbels@med.kuleuven.be

D.B. McKay, S.M. Steinberg (eds.), *Kidney Transplantation: A Guide to the Care of Kidney Transplant Recipients*, DOI 10.1007/978-1-4419-1690-7_22,
© Springer Science+Business Media, LLC 2010

three adult patients being non-adherent.[5,12] A recent meta-analysis of Dew et al. reported a prevalence of non-adherence of 36 cases per 100 patient-years for adult kidney transplant patients, which is much higher compared to prevalences found in other organ transplant domains.[13] It is possible that kidney transplant patients feel less vulnerable as they always can return to dialysis in case of graft failure. This hypothesis, however, needs to be further explored.

In pediatric patients, non-adherence seems to be higher compared to adult kidney transplant patients, particularly in adolescents. We discovered a prevalence of about 40–60% in this age group, which is significantly higher compared to the numbers found in studies investigating adherence in pediatric patients in general, indicating that adolescents are at a higher risk for non-adherence.[14]

When interpreting these findings both in the adult and pediatric population, one should be cautious, as different measurement methods have been used. Self-report still is the most popular measurement option as it is cheap and easy to use, although it underestimates non-adherence. Most authors developed a questionnaire for the purpose of the study, using varying cut-offs to classify patients into adherers and non-adherers. Two self-report instruments were published for adherence assessment in transplant populations specifically, but these instruments are suboptimal, since (1) evidence demonstrating their reliability and validity is limited; (2) they only assess medication taking, and not timing; (3) the recall period is too long; or (4) the answering options are too broad (e.g., 21–50% of the drugs taken).[15,16]

Electronic monitoring (EM) is often promoted as the gold standard, as it allows measurement of adherence on a continuous basis, providing information on both the taking and timing of medication intake. However, unbiased electronic monitoring assessment requires fulfillment of the following assumptions: (1) EM equipment functions correctly; (2) all EM registrations correspond to the actual medication intake; (3) EM does not influence a patient's normal medication intake behavior; and (4) EM should not affect sample representativeness. A recent study of Denhaerynck et al. in 250 adult kidney transplant patients revealed that one EM device showed malfunctioning (0.4%), that self-reported mismatches between EM bottle openings and actual drug intake occurred in 62% of the patients, and that adherence decreased over the first 5 weeks of monitoring, indicating that EM has a waning intervention effect.[17] Moreover, a tendency toward non-adherent patients refusing to participate in the adherence observation study was observed, which may affect the generalizability of the results. These results show that all these assumptions should be tested when using existing and newly developed electronic monitoring tools in future adherence studies.

Moreover, using electronic monitoring can be challenging in pediatric populations. Based on their inclusion criteria, Schellmer and colleagues[18] deemed 59 pediatric kidney transplant patients eligible to participate in their electronic monitoring adherence observation study. Thirty patients (51%) could not be included for the following reasons: (a) not wanting to disrupt their medication-taking routine or use of pillboxes by introducing the Medication Event Monitoring System (MEMS) into it; (b) being on liquid medications making it impossible to use the MEMS system; and (c) refusing to use the MEMS system. Of the final sample of

29 patients, 41% found transferring medication into the bottle difficult, and 27% reported that the MEMS bottle was a burden or difficult to transport. Another 22% reported that using MEMS changed their routine, and 10% worried about missing their immunosuppressive medications.

Because of the above-mentioned problems with electronic monitoring, transplant centers should be cautious about using electronic monitoring as the sole measure of non-adherence. Indeed, all measurement techniques have advantages and disadvantages.[19] Consequently, it is recommended to combine measurement techniques to increase the accuracy to detect non-adherence behavior.[4,19] Recently, Schäfer-Keller et al.[12] explored different combinations in a study of 249 adult kidney transplant patients. Using electronic monitoring as the reference value, she found that the following algorithm yielded the best diagnostic accuracy: self-reported non-adherence and/or at least 1 clinician reporting non-adherence and/or subtherapeutic blood levels, yielded a sensitivity of 72% and a specificity of 43%, respectively. Future research in adult and pediatric transplant populations, however, is needed to investigate which combinations of assessment methods yield the best diagnostic accuracy.

Consequences of Non-adherence to the Immunosuppressive Regimen

In adult kidney transplant patients, about one out of four graft losses and 20–25% of the late acute rejections are due to non-adherence,[5,7,11,20,21] although large differences across studies exist (i.e., 1–69.2% for graft loss and 2.5–37% for late acute rejections).[7,22–24] Similarly, on average 44.4% of the graft losses in pediatric kidney transplant patients (range 13–75%) and 23.2% of late acute rejections are associated with non-adherence (range 13–31.8%).[25–28]

Other outcomes, besides graft loss and late acute rejection, which seem to be associated with non-adherence are worse serum creatinine[21] and a poorer perceived health status in children and adults,[29–31] although these outcomes have been less frequently explored. Future studies should pay attention to the impact of transitioning from pediatric to adult care with respect to adherence and its impact on clinical outcomes, as anecdotal evidence shows that health deteriorates after the transition.[32,33]

Despite the above-mentioned striking numbers, these results cannot automatically be generalized to more recently implemented immunosuppressive regimens, as the majority of studies investigated the relationship between non-adherence to the older generation immunosuppressive drugs and clinical outcomes. Newer immunosuppressive regimens may be more forgiving for adherence problems.

It should also be noted that the majority of studies are retrospective in nature, only studying non-adherence as a potential explanation in case a clinical outcome occurs. If one wants to know the natural history of non-adherence and its predictive capacity of poor clinical outcomes, prospective studies are needed. Surprisingly, however, only two prospective studies on adult patients have been published in kidney transplantation, both confirming that non-adherence is a risk factor for poor outcome.[7,21] Further prospective research is mandatory to identify how much adherence is enough to prevent poor clinical outcomes. Until now, different operational definitions or cut-offs are used to classify patients into adherers or non-adherers, but a clinically meaningful definition of non-adherence is currently lacking. A recent large study showed that minor deviations from the prescribed regimen, i.e., taking less than 98% mycophenolate mofetil, are already sufficient to be associated with graft loss.[11]

Besides clinical consequences, the economic impact of non-adherence has received more attention in the last 5 years. Cleemput et al.[34] in her landmark study modeled costs over a lifetime and surprisingly found that long-term costs of treatment in non-adherent patients are lower compared to the costs in adherent kidney transplant patients. Yet, the difference in costs was attributable to the fact that adherent patients live longer and hence generate additional treatment costs in the additional years of life (median 16 years versus 12 years, respectively). In addition, by living longer, adherent patients experienced better long-term outcomes in view of quality adjusted life years (QALYs) relative to dialysis than non-adherent patients (5.2 versus 4.0 QALYs, respectively). Several studies suggest that $150 million could be saved annually, if one is able to prevent poor outcomes caused by non-adherence to the immunosuppressive regimen.[35]

Factors Associated with Non-adherence to the Immunosuppressive Regimen

Given the known adverse impact of non-adherence on outcomes, it is crucial to implement adherence-enhancing interventions early. Using the World Health Organization (WHO) taxonomy, identified determinants or correlates of non-adherence are *patient-related, socio-economic, treatment-related, condition-related,* and *healthcare system- and healthcare team-related factors.*[1] The determinants seem to be quite similar between pediatric and adult kidney transplant patients (see Table 22.1 for an overview).

Table 22.1 Factors associated with non-adherence to the immunosuppressive regimen in adult and pediatric kidney transplant patients

Factors in adult patients	Factors in pediatric patients
Socio-economic factors	
Younger age[11,15,36,37]/older age[38]	
Non-white ethnicity[11,36,38]	Non-white ethnicity or cultural factors[39,40]
Poor socio-economic status[41,42,44]/better income[43]	Poor socio-economic status[39]
Conflicts within the family[44]	Family conflicts[25]
Female gender[41]/male gender[10,15,38]	

Table 22.1   (continued)

Factors in adult patients	Factors in pediatric patients
Higher education[11]/lower education[42]	
Being married[41]/being divorced or single[6,8]	
Marital problems[45]	
Lower perceived social support[21]	Lack of social support from the parents[47,48]/poor communication between patient and parents[47]
	Limited parent supervision or having the sole responsibility for medication taking[25,48]
	High parental distress[29]
Condition-related factors	
Depression/psychological distress/feeling bothered by parts of the Tx experience[42,44,49]	Depressive symptoms[50,51]
Longer time since Tx[11,38,42,43,57,58]	Longer time since Tx; chronicity of illness and treatment[52]
Addiction (smoking/alcohol)[42,49]	
Having received a kidney from a living donor[53]	Having received a kidney from a living donor[54]/having received an organ from a cadaveric donor[47]
Better perceived health[55]	Feeling of good health; lower perception of vulnerability[51,52]
Having more physical limitations or having had a rejection or infection during the first year post-Tx[11]	
	Lack of experience with dialysis[54]
Treatment-related factors	
Higher number of tablets[56]	Total number of medications[25,39,52]
High occurrence and distress related to side effects[11,56]/fear concerning adverse reactions[57]	Cosmetic side effects[33,39,51]
Use of non-prescribed drugs[58]	
Increasing dosing frequency[9]	Higher number of doses per day[51,52]
Having to take an evening dose[57]	Having to take a morning dose[48]
	Taste of medication[40,51]
	Size of tablets/difficulty to swallow the tablets[40,51]
Patient-related factors	
Poor knowledge[6,38]	Poor knowledge[39,52]
Low self-efficacy[6,10]	
Low self-care agency[6]	
Pretransplant non-adherence[59]	
Wrong health beliefs[15,53]	
External locus of control[56]	
Non-adherence to other medications[58]	
Lower feeling of indebtedness[49]	
Not using a pill box[10]	
Perception of less autonomy[60]	Striving toward independence/attempts to be normal[46,48]

Table 22.1 (continued)

Factors in adult patients	Factors in pediatric patients
Interference with lifestyle (work-related barriers or being away from home)[57,60,62]	Busy lifestyle or hectic daily schemes[25,48,52]
Having an active coping style[60]	
High levels of hostility[56]	Anger[61]
Higher stress levels[49,55]/denial of disease and its associated emotions[45]	Feeling overwhelmed about Tx and treatment[51]/denial[47]
Lack of motivation[37]	
Sleeping/slept in[62]	Medication schedule interfering with their sleep[51]
Forgetfulness[58,62]	Forgetfulness[48,51,52]
	Low self-esteem or poor body image[25,29,46]
	Attention problems[29]
	Not liking to carry medications with them[51]
	To receive more attention from family and doctors when messing up with medications[51]
Factors related to the healthcare system	
Transplant center[9]	
Poor patient–provider relationship[38]	Poor communication between parents and medical team[25]
Insurance status/lack of financial resources to pay[15,23,38,43]	
Inability of the provider to deliver optimal care[43,62]	

Socio-economic variables related to medication non-adherence are younger age, living alone, being unmarried, marital or family problems, non-Caucasian race, and perceived lower social support. In pediatric patients, limited parent supervision was also an important determinant. Factors such as gender and education yield inconclusive results, although several studies found poor socio-economic status to be a significant determinant. Insurance, however, might become a significant problem in American patients when being transferred to the adult clinic.

Patient-related factors refer to the resources, knowledge, attitudes, beliefs, and expectancies of the patient. Having a low self-efficacy with medication intake, having high levels of anxiety or hostility, lack of knowledge about the regimen, denial of disease and its associated emotions as coping style, lack of motivation, and pre-transplant non-adherence were all significantly related to non-adherence with the immunosuppressive regimen. Furthermore, believing that the immunosuppressive drugs are not needed to keep the kidney, or that their intake may be delayed, forgetfulness, not using pillboxes, and using an external locus of control (i.e., believing that the evolution of the disease is a matter of chance) were also associated with non-adherence. Indebtedness toward the donor seems to increase adherence in living donor renal recipients.

Condition or disease-related factors refer to depression, psychological distress, addiction and dependency on illicit drugs and smoking. Better self-rated health and less adverse events were also a determinant of medication non-adherence, as well as lack of experience with dialysis and length of time since transplantation. Having received a kidney from a living donor also seems to play a role, as these patients generally have less dialysis exposure.

Important therapy or treatment-related factors to be considered when examining the patient's risk profile for medication non-adherence are complexity of medication regimen in view of number of medications and daily doses and experiencing distressing symptoms of side effects of immunosuppressive medication. Interestingly, adult patients report more adherence problems when they need to take medication in the evening[57] and express a preference for a once-daily regimen, while pediatric patients report more problems with the morning dose.[48]

Healthcare system- and healthcare team-related factors have seldom been taken into account when explaining adherence behavior. Insurance status or availability of free immunosuppressive drugs, a poor patient–healthcare provider relationship, and inability of the provider to deliver optimal care were the only factors explored thus far. This reflects that research until now mirrors the fact that the patient is seen as the defaulter. One study rightfully pointed toward the fact that the healthcare provider and setting often give the impression that strict adherence is not that important by scheduling tests or follow-up appointments at times that interfere with a patient's medication-taking routines.[63] This "gatekeeper" healthcare system mentality places the patient at risk of non-adherance by separating the patient from self-responsibility. Further research should aim at unraveling the dynamics at the healthcare provider, setting, and system level, as factors at the patient level only explain a limited portion of the variance in adherence.[13]

Interventions to Improve Adherence

It might be clear from the above-mentioned evidence that adherence-enhancing interventions, as part of state-of-the-art clinical management to improve outcomes, should gain momentum in transplantation. Yet, scarce evidence exists on interventions aiming to improving medication adherence in renal transplant populations, as well as in other transplant populations. Only five adherence-enhancing intervention studies have been published in the kidney transplant literature since 1990: four on adult[63–66] and one on pediatric kidney transplant patients.[67] Only three used a randomized controlled trial design,[64–66] yet, with the exception of the study of De Geest et al.,[65] all showed poor methodological quality according to the Consolidated Standards of Reporting Trials (CONSORT) guidelines and were not sufficiently powered. Only two used electronic monitoring,[65,67] while the others heavily relied on suboptimal measurement tools such as pill count.

Proposed interventions refer to education,[63,64,67] financial support programs for drugs,[63] the use of clinical pharmacy support services,[64] and feedback based on electronic monitoring outprints.[65,66] Only the study of Chisholm et al.,[64] however, found a significant improvement in adherence. She randomized 24 patients to a clinical pharmacy service intervention or usual care clinic services. In the intervention group, the pharmacist gave information on patient's medications and how to take them, revised the patient's drug regimens, and encouraged patients to call in case of questions related to their medical regimen. All patients showed decreasing adherence during the 12-month study period, but patients in the intervention group showed a longer duration of adherence to their immunosuppressive drugs compared to patients in the control group.

Because of the methodology and interventions used, the pilot study of De Geest et al. holds promise to yield significant results when being repeated in a fully powered study.[65] More specifically, the authors randomly assigned 18 patients to a multidimensional, individualized intervention ($N= 6$) and an enhanced usual care group ($N= 12$). More specifically, the 3-months intervention (1 home visit and 2 follow-up calls) aimed at increasing patients' self-efficacy in taking their medication. To accomplish this, electronic monitoring printouts for problem detection, proxy goal setting (i.e., definition of short-term goals), and regular targeted feedback were used, in combination with individualized educational, behavioral, and social support interventions. Being included in this study resulted in a significant decrease in non-adherence in both groups during the 3-months intervention period. In addition, the intervention group showed the greatest decrease in non-adherence at 3 months, albeit in a non-significant way due to the small sample size. Non-adherence increased gradually in both groups during the 6-months follow-up period and was comparable between both groups at 9 months. This waning effect indicates the need for sustained intervention over a longer period of time.

Several other interventions have been suggested in the literature to improve adherence in kidney transplant patients, but have not been formally tested, such as financial incentives for being adherent,[68] or extended daclizumab monotherapy to prolong rejection-free survival in non-adherent adolescent kidney transplant recipients.[69] A cost modeling study showed that once-daily tacrolimus might save nearly $10,000 over a 5-year period relative to twice-daily tacrolimus, due to an increased graft survival.[70] It can be hypothesized, but again needs further tested that a less complex regimen may improve adherence and subsequently clinical outcomes. Tolerance induction has been suggested as a possible solution for non-adherence in the future, but, until now, attempts to generate tolerance in man have failed.[71] Even if tolerance would be possible in the future, one might not forget that other non-immunosuppressive medication regimens, behavior modifications, and follow-up schedules still require strict adherence.

All of the above-suggested or -tested interventions heavily focus on the patient level and ignore the increasing evidence that factors at the healthcare provider, healthcare team, and policy level also contribute to medication non-adherence. Based on evidence from systematic reviews on the efficacy of adherence-enhancing interventions across all chronic illness populations,[72] it is recommended that future intervention studies in transplantation are multilevel and multidimensional, targeting more than one risk factor over a sustained period of time, combining educational/counseling, cognitive-behavioral and social support interventions at the patient level, with interventions targeting risk factors at the various levels of the healthcare system.

Recommendations for Future Research

The adherence literature in renal transplantation is predominantly focused on medication non-adherence. The prevalence consequences and determinants of non-adherence with various aspects of the treatment regimen, including adherence to non-immunosuppressive medications, should be further explored in prospective descriptive studies. Furthermore, studies investigating determinants of non-adherence almost exclusively focus on socio-economic, patient-related, treatment-related, and condition-related factors, while the impact of the healthcare provider, the transplant team, and the healthcare setting remains largely unaddressed. This dimension should be further scrutinized in future studies, also taking cultural differences in posttransplant care into account. Finally, given the detrimental impact of medication non-adherence on posttransplant outcome, researchers should invest more in testing the effectiveness and determine the costs of adherence-enhancing interventions. Moreover, interventions targeting on non-adherence with other aspects of the treatment regimen should be developed and tested both in renal transplant, and in other transplant populations.

References

1. Sabaté E. *Adherence to Long-Term Therapies: Evidence for Action.* World Health Organisation, Geneva, 2003.
2. Matas AJ, Humar A, Gillingham KJ et al. Five preventable causes of kidney graft loss in the 1990 s: a single-center analysis. *Kidney Int* 2002;62:704–714.
3. Nankivell BJ, Chapman JR. Chronic allograft nephropathy: current concepts and future directions. *Transplantation* 2006;81:643–654.
4. Fine RN, Becker Y, De Geest S. Nonadherence Consensus Summary Conference Report. *Am J Transplant* 2009;9:35–41.
5. Kiley DJ, Lam CS, Pollak R. A study of treatment compliance following kidney transplantation. *Transplantation* 1993;55(1):51–56.
6. De Geest S, Borgermans L, Gemoets H et al. Incidence, determinants, and consequences of subclinical noncompliance with immunosuppressive therapy in renal transplant recipients. *Transplantation* 1995;59(3):340–347.
7. Nevins TE, Kruse L, Skeans MA et al. The natural history of azathioprine compliance after renal transplantation. *Kidney Int* 2001;60(4):1565–1570.
8. Butler JA, Peveler RC, Roderick P et al. Measuring compliance with drug regimens after renal transplantation: comparison of self-report and clinician rating with electronic monitoring. *Transplantation* 2004;77(5):786–789.
9. Weng FL, Israni AK, Joffe MM et al. Race and electronically measured adherence to immunosuppressive medications after deceased donor renal transplantation. *J Am Soc Nephrol* 2005;16(6):1839–1848.

10. Denhaerynck K, Steiger J, Bock A et al. Prevalence and risk factors of non-adherence with immunosuppressive medication in kidney transplant patients. *Am J Transplant* 2007;7: 108–116.
11. Takemoto SK, Pinsky BW, Schnitzler MA et al. A retrospective analysis of immunosuppression compliance, dose reduction and discontinuation in kidney transplant recipients. *Am J Transplant* 2007;7:2704–2711.
12. Schäfer-Keller P, Steiger J, Bock A et al. Diagnostic accuracy of measurement methods to assess non-adherence to immunosuppressive drugs in kidney transplant recipients. *Am J Transplant* 2008;8(3):616–626.
13. Dew MA, DiMartini AF, De Vito Dabbs A et al. Rate and risk factors for nonadherence to the medical regimen after adult solid organ transplantation. *Transplantation* 2007;83(7):858–873.
14. Dobbels F, Van Damme-Lombaerts R, Vanhaecke J, De Geest S. Growing pains: nonadherence with the immunosuppressive regimen in adolescent transplant recipients. *Pediatr Transplant* 2005;9(3):381–390.
15. Siegal BR, Greenstein SM. Postrenal transplant compliance from the perspective of African-Americans, Hispanic-Americans, and Anglo-Americans. *Adv Ren Replace Ther* 1997;4(1):46–54.
16. Chisholm MA, Lance CE, Williamson GM et al. Development and validation of the immunosuppressant therapy adherence instrument (ITAS). *Patient Educ Couns* 2005;59(1):13–20.
17. Denhaerynck K, Schäfer-Keller P, Young J et al. Examining the assumptions regarding valid electronic monitoring of medication therapy: development of a validation framework and its application on a European sample of kidney transplant patients. *BMC Med Res Methodol* 2008;8:E-pub ahead of printing.
18. Schellmer DA, Zelikovsky N. The challenges of using medication event monitoring technology with pediatric transplant patients. *Pediatr Transplant* 2007;11:422–428.
19. Osterberg L, Blaschke T. Adherence to medication. *N Eng J Med* 2005;353(5):487–497.
20. Gaston RS, Hudson SL, Ward M et al. Late renal allograft loss: noncompliance masquerading as chronic rejection. *Transplant Proc* 1999;31(4A):21S–23S.
21. Vlaminck H, Maes B, Evers G et al. Prospective study on late consequences of subclinical non-compliance with immunosuppressive therapy in renal transplant patients. *Am J Transplant* 2004;4(9):1509–1513.
22. Irish W, Sherrill B, Brennan DC et al. Three-year posttransplant graft survival in renal-transplant patients with graft function at 6 months receiving tacrolimus or cyclosporine microemulsion within a triple-drug regimen. *Transplantation* 2003;76(12):1686–1690.
23. Hricik DE, Augustine JJ, Knauss TC et al. Long-term graft outcomes after steroid withdrawal in African American kidney transplant recipients receiving sirolimus and tacrolimus. *Transplantation* 2007;83:277–281.
24. Reinke P, Fietze E, Docke WD et al. Late acute rejection in long-term renal allograft recipients. Diagnostic and predictive value of circulating activated T cells. *Transplantation* 1994;58(1):35–41.
25. Delucchi A, Gutierrez H, Arrellano P et al. Factors that influence nonadherence in immunosuppressant treatment in pediatric transplant recipients: a proposal for an educational strategy. *Transplant Proc* 2008;40:3241–3243.
26. Jarzembowski T, John E, Panaro F et al. Impact of non-compliance on outcome after pediatric kidney transplantation: an analysis in racial subgroups. *Pediatr Transplant* 2004;8(4): 367–371.
27. Cecka JM, Gjertson DW, Terasaki PI. Pediatric renal transplantation; a review of the UNOS data. *Pediatr Transplant* 1997;1:55–64.
28. Brodehl J, Bokenkamp A, Hoyer PF et al. Long-term results of cyclosporin A therapy in children. *J Am Soc Nephrol* 1992;2(12 Suppl):S246–S254.
29. Gerson AC, Furth SL, Neu AM, Fivush BA. Assessing associations between medication adherence and potentially modifiable psychosocial variables in pediatric kidney transplant recipients and their families. *Pediatr Transplant* 2004;8(6):543–550.

30. Rosenberger J, van Dijk JP, Nagyova I et al. Predictors of perceived health status in patients after kidney transplantation. *Transplantation* 2006;81(9):1306–1310.
31. Goetzmann L, Sarac N, Ambühl P et al. Psychological response and quality of life after transplantation: a comparison between heart, lung, liver and kidney recipients. *Swiss Med Wkly* 2008;33–34:477–483.
32. Remorino R, Taylor J. Smoothing things over: the transition from pediatric to adult care for kidney transplant recipients. *Prog Transplant* 2006;16(4):303–308.
33. Watson AR. Non-compliance and transfer from paediatric to adult transplant units. *Pediatr Nephrol* 2000;14(6):469–472.
34. Cleemput I, Kesteloot K, Vanrenterghem Y et al. The economic implications of non-adherence after renal transplantation. *Pharmacoeconomics* 2004;22(18):1217–1234.
35. Hansen R, Seifeldin R, Noe L. Medication adherence in chronic disease: issues in posttransplant immunosuppression. *Transplant Proc* 2007;39:1287–1300.
36. Schweizer RT, Rovelli M, Palmeri D et al. Noncompliance in organ transplant recipients. *Transplantation* 1990;49:374–377.
37. Bittar AE, Keitel E, Garcia CD et al. Patient noncompliance as a cause of late kidney graft failure. *Transplant Proc* 1992;24(6):2720–2721.
38. Chisholm MA, Kwong WJ, Spivey CA. Associations of characteristics of renal transplant recipients with clinicians' perceptions of adherence to immunosuppressant therapy. *Transplantation* 2007;84:1145–1150.
39. Meyers KE, Weiland H, Thomson PD. Paediatric renal transplantation non-compliance. *Pediatr Nephrol* 1995;9(2):189–192.
40. Tucker CM, Petersen S, Herman KC et al. Self-regulation predictors of medication adherence among ethnically different pediatric patients with renal transplants. *J Pediatr Psychol* 2001;26(8):455–464.
41. Frazier PA, Davis-Ali SH, Dahl KE. Correlates of noncompliance among renal transplant recipients. *Clin Transplant* 1994;8(6):550–557.
42. Ghods AJ, Nasrollahzadeh D, Argani H. Risk factors for noncompliance to immunosuppressive medications in renal transplant recipients. *Transplant Proc* 2003;35(7):2609–2611.
43. Chisholm MA, Lance CE, Williamson GM et al. Development and validation of an immunosuppressant therapy adherence barrier instrument. *Nephrol Dial Transplant* 2005;20(1):181–188.
44. Rodriguez A, Diaz M, Colon A et al. Psychosocial profile of noncompliant transplant patients. *Transplant Proc* 1991;23:1807–1809.
45. Rapisarda F, Tarantino A, De Vecchi A et al. Dialysis and kidney transplantation: similarities and differences in the psychological aspects of noncompliance. *Transplant Proc* 2006;38(4):1006–1009.
46. Foulkes LM, Boggs SR, Fennell RS et al. Social support, family variables, and compliance in renal transplant children. *Pediatr Nephrol* 1993;7(2):185–188.
47. Feinstein S, Keich R, Becker-Cohen R et al. Is noncompliance among adolescent renal transplant recipients inevitable? *Pediatrics* 2005;115(4):969–973.
48. Simons LE, McCormick ML, Mee LL et al. Parent and patient perspective on barriers to medication adherence in adolescent transplant recipients. *Pediatr Transplant* 2008;E-pub ahead of printing.
49. Achille MA, Ouellette A, Fournier S et al. Impact of stress, distress and feelings of indebtedness on adherence to immunosuppressants following kidney transplantation. *Clin Transplant* 2006;20(3):301–306.
50. Maikranz JM, Steele RG, Dreyer ML et al. The relationship of hope and illness-related uncertainty to emotional adjustment and adherence among pediatric renal and liver transplant recipients. *J Pediatr Psychol* 2007;32(5):571–581.
51. Bullington P, Pawola L, Walker R et al. Identification of medication non-adherence factors in adolescent transplant patients: the patient's viewpoint. *Pediatr Transplant* 2007;11:914–921.

52. Blowey DL, Hebert D, Arbus GS et al. Compliance with cyclosporine in adolescent renal transplant recipients. *Pediatr Nephrol* 1997;11(5):547–551.
53. Butler JA, Peveler RC, Roderick P et al. Modifiable risk factors for non-adherence to immunosuppressants in renal transplant recipients: a cross-sectional study. *Nephrol Dial Transplant* 2004;19(12):3144–3149.
54. Fennell RS, Tucker C, Pedersen T. Demographic and medical predictors of medication compliance among ethnically different pediatric renal transplant patients. *Pediatr Transplant* 2001;5(5):343–348.
55. Rosenberger J, Geckova AM, van Dijk JP et al. Prevalence and characteristics of noncompliant behaviour and its risk factors in kidney transplant recipients. *Transplant Int* 2005;18(9):1072–1078.
56. Sketris I, Waite N, Grobler K et al. Factors affecting compliance with cyclosporine in adult renal transplant patients. *Transplant Proc* 1994;26(5):2538–2541.
57. Ichimaru N, Kakuta T, Abe M et al. Treatment adherence in renal transplant recipients: A questionnaire survey on immunosuppressants. *Transplant Proc* 2008;40:1362–1365.
58. Liu WJ, Zaki M. Medication compliance among renal transplant patients: a Hospital Kuala Lumpur experience. *Med J Malaysia* 2004;59(5):649–658.
59. Douglas S, Blixen C, Bartucci MR. Relationship between pretransplant noncompliance and posttransplant outcomes in renal transplant recipients. *J Transpl Coord* 1996;6:53–58.
60. Gremigni P, Bacchi F, Turrini C et al. Psychological factors associated with medication adherence following renal transplantation. *Clin Transplant* 2007;21:710–715.
61. Penkower L, Dew MA, Ellis D et al. Psychological distress and adherence to the medical regimen among adolescent renal transplant recipients. *Am J Transplant* 2003;3(11):1418–1425.
62. Gordon EJ, Prohaska TR, Gallant MP et al. Adherence to immunosuppression: a prospective diary study. *Transplant Proc* 2007;39:3081–3085.
63. Chisholm MA, Vollenweider LJ, Mulloy LL et al. Renal transplant patient compliance with free immunosuppressive medications. *Transplantation* 2000;70:1240–1244.
64. Chisholm MA, Mulloy LL, Jagadeesan M et al. Impact of clinical pharmacy services on renal transplant patients' compliance with immunosuppressive medications. *Clin Transplant* 2001;15(5):330–336.
65. De Geest S, Schafer-Keller P, Denhaerynck K et al. Supporting medication adherence in renal transplantation (SMART): a pilot RCT to improve adherence to immunosuppressive regimens. *Clin Transplant* 2006;20(3):359–368.
66. Hardstaff R, Green K, Talbot D. Measurement of compliance posttransplantation – the results of a 12-month study using electronic monitoring. *Transplant Proc* 2003;35(2):796–797.
67. Fennell RS, Foulkes LM, Boggs SR. Family-based program to promote medication compliance in renal transplant children. *Transplant Proc* 1994;26(1):102–103.
68. Henning Beier U. Financial incentives to promote prolonged renal graft survival: potential for patients and public health. *Med Hypotheses* 2008;70:218–220.
69. Chaudhuri A, Salvatierra O Jr, Sarwal MM. Extended daclizumab monotherapy for rejection-free survival in non-adherent adolescent recipients of renal allografts. *Pediatr Transplant* 2008;E-pub ahead of printing.
70. Abecassis MM, Seifeldin R, Riordan ME. Patient outcomes and economics of once-daily tacrolimus in renal transplant patients: results of a modeling analysis. *Transplant Proc* 2008;40:1443–1445.
71. Dhanireddy KK, Maniscalco J, Kirk AD. Is tolerance induction the answer to adolescent non-adherence? *Pediatr Transplant* 2005;9:357–363.
72. Haynes RB, Ackloo E, Sahota N et al. Interventions for enhancing medication adherence. *Cochrane Database Syst Rev* 2008;16(2):CD 000011.

Chapter 23
Transitioning Between Pediatric and Adult Clinics

Elizabeth Ingulli

Introduction

Improved outcomes of children with renal transplants have resulted in a high rate of survivorship among young adults. In 2008, approximately 1,500 late adolescent and young adults with solid organ transplants in the United States have been reported to have graft survival rates of at least 5 years.[1] Teenagers with kidney transplants have the highest rates of graft loss due to acute and chronic rejection and the highest rates of nonadherence.[2,3]

Adolescents experience many transitions as part of the natural course of events as they move toward adulthood. They enter post-secondary education or the workplace. They eventually achieve financial independence, live independent lives, and engage in sexual relationships. Chronic illness such as organ transplantation may complicate this difficult period of time by adding intense healthcare and medication regimens. In some circumstances multiple hospitalizations, post-transplant complications, and/or the original disease can add to both cognitive and social delays.[4] Studies focusing on adults who received kidney transplants as children have shown that these adults were socially immature, were more likely to live with their parents, had less education, had fewer intimate relationships, and were less likely to be employed than their healthy counterparts.[5] These findings have resulted in more focus by the transplant community on the successful transition of these pediatric patients to adulthood.[6]

Transition of care has been defined by the American Society for Adolescent Medicine as the "purposeful, planned movement of adolescents and young adults with chronic physical and medical conditions from child-centered to adult-oriented health care systems."[7,8] Although it is essential to make sure all the necessary medical records are transferred, the challenge for the pediatric transplant community is to develop a comprehensive program that addresses the many unique needs of this patient population. It must be "uninterrupted, coordinated, developmentally

E. Ingulli (✉)
Renal Transplant Program, UCSD and Rady Children's Hospital, Pediatrics, San Diego, CA, USA
e-mail: eingulli@ucsd.edu

D.B. McKay, S.M. Steinberg (eds.), *Kidney Transplantation: A Guide to the Care of Kidney Transplant Recipients*, DOI 10.1007/978-1-4419-1690-7_23,
© Springer Science+Business Media, LLC 2010

appropriate, and psychologically sound."[9] It is understood that many adolescent transplant recipients are poorly equipped to manage the adult healthcare system.[9,10] In addition, financial reasons such as insurance changes and inadequate funding during the transition process can adversely affect graft outcomes.[11] Studies in children with diabetes, cystic fibrosis, and renal failure suggest that successful transition programs improve health outcomes and quality-of-life measures.[12–15] This chapter discusses the essential components of transitioning patients, which focuses on providing teenagers with the skills and knowledge necessary to eventually take primary responsibility for their health and their lives.

Planning for Transition with a Multidisciplinary Approach

It is important to emphasize that the transition of these patients is a dynamic *process* and not a one-time event. Transition planning should begin early. Some suggest that the process can be introduced in the early teenage years or shortly after diagnosis.[16] The early initiation of the process will ensure that by young adulthood, the recipients will be fully prepared to negotiate the adult healthcare system.

In many circumstances, the same pediatric team has cared for the transplant recipient since infancy, and families are often reluctant to transfer to adult centers.[10] Adolescents with chronic illnesses have been reported to be afraid to leave the familiar surroundings and physicians with whom they have developed long-standing personal relationships while "growing up."[17–19] The adult centers are thought to be less personal and fun.[20] The reluctance may also be based on perceptions that the adult providers may be unfamiliar with managing their disease. This is not unlike the cystic fibrosis patient population where patients rarely survived into adulthood and, therefore, adult physicians had very little experience with these patients.[18] The long-standing relationship with and trust of the pediatric team, together with the team's knowledge of the patient's history and disease, can work in the patient's favor to support a successful transition. Adequate preparation, timing, planning, and good communication between the adult and pediatric caregivers will help allay these fears.

The process of transition should engage the entire multidisciplinary team.[21] The team includes transplant physicians, transplant coordinators, social workers, dieticians/nutritionists, financial planners, and child family life specialists/mentors. Each team member must develop the skills and strategies necessary to integrate transition planning into his/her everyday practice.[22] Since the planning should start early, the information discussed and the education provided must be appropriate and tailored to each patient's cognitive and social development.[23] Although the materials need to be geared toward the adolescent, the family should be included in the process not only to provide support but also to learn how to transition primary responsibility from themselves to the young adult.[24]

The pace of transition should be gradual and individualized with the flexibility to adapt to the changing world of the adolescent. Abstract reasoning, as well as higher levels of cognitive function, can be delayed in adolescents with chronic illness and may complicate the learning process.[4] Studies of brain structure and function in adolescents demonstrate significant maturational changes that continue well into adulthood. These can clearly affect impulsivity, delayed gratification, and planning.[25–27] Both pediatric and adult transplant physicians must be aware of the continuing brain development into young adulthood.

Identifying and contacting the adult transplant center early in the transition process will help facilitate collaborative interactions. Knowledge of the procedures at the adult center will help the pediatric team prepare the young adult for the culture of the adult environment.[28] Sharing treatment protocols with the adult centers and minimizing changes to treatment regimens will promote trust between the patient and the adult transplant team.[6]

Components of the Transition Process

Each clinic visit is an opportunity to address each component of the transition process. These components include *knowledge* of the disease process and *self-advocacy*, *independent healthcare behaviors*, *sexual health* (including pregnancy, contraception, sexually transmitted infections, and HPV infection), *education/vocational training and financial planning*, and *health and lifestyle*.[29] Goals need to be set for each component at each stage of development in transition planning. The planning should be future focused to optimize lifelong health and well-being. In general, planning must aim to promote skills in communication, decision making, problem solving, assertiveness, autonomy, self-management, and self-advocacy for the adolescent.[10] For the parent and family, a shift must eventually come to transition from a primary role to a more supportive or secondary role.

Knowledge and Self-Advocacy

The transition process starts with the early teenager learning about the process itself and the expectations at each visit. The role of the family and/or support network in this process must be clearly defined as well as the delineation of expectations and short- and long-term goals. A timeline for transition should be set.

Teenagers must be educated so that they have an understanding of the cause of their kidney failure and the reason for transplantation since in many cases those discussions occurred with parents many years earlier. Eventually young adults should be able to summarize their chronic conditions and the implications a transplant has on their daily lives and the long-term implications on their health. The adolescent should understand the importance of keeping a record of the important events and dates associated with his/her health history.[30] Some healthcare professionals have suggested that a portable summary of the transplant recipient's health history be made available to the adolescent.[9] Recipients need to have a clear understanding of the signs and symptoms that indicate graft dysfunction or complications that may arise. They need to be given clear direction as to whom to call and when to call when problems or questions arise. A dialogue should be established to be able to discuss puberty and the effect of medications and graft dysfunction on pubertal development.

Adolescents need to understand that they need to be proactive in their health care. In order to empower the teenagers to be their best advocate and to care for themselves, they need to be encouraged to ask health-related questions. Peer pressure and medication side effects need to be explored with the understanding of the consequences of nonadherence. In spite of peer pressure, transplant recipients need to remain focused on self-preservation. Historically, focus within the transplant community has been on medication regimens and noncompliance issues, which has been shown to be a significant problem among this patient population. The causes of nonadherence in adolescents are multifactorial and include emotional stress, lack of abstract thinking, impulsivity, social immaturity, and disruptive home situations, to name just a few. Nonadherence can complicate, delay, and/or prevent successful transition to adulthood.

Independent Behaviors

Parents of transplant recipients may be impeding self-sufficiency or, worse, may be expecting more from their teenagers than they are developmentally or emotionally capable of. Healthcare providers need to help design age and developmentally appropriate health-related tasks for which adolescents can be responsible. Eventually, the adolescent should be able to name each of his/her medications, describe any unique features of the pills, the doses, and the schedule. They should choose the method that will best allow them to remember to take medications (alarm clock, pill box, etc.) and assist in setting up the medications. However, young and mid-teens must still be supervised in both setting up and actually taking their medication. When approaching the late teenage years the recipients should call the pharmacy for refills, be able to complete all health records requested, contact health providers when problems or questions arise, and schedule future appointments. These teenagers should begin to participate in treatment plans and decision making. Parents during this time should take on a more supportive role while the adolescent becomes more autonomous.[31] In cases where the disease process results in significant psychosocial and cognitive developmental delays, guardianship issues need to be clarified and documented before transfer.

Sexual Health

The amount of information available addressing sexual activity in adolescent renal transplant patients is extremely limited. Studies of sexual activity in chronically ill adolescents have shown similar rates compared with healthy peers.[32,33] However, these results may be hard to interpret because of the wide variety of clinical conditions included in the sample populations.[34] Studies assessing sexual activity specifically in renal transplant patients indicate that the prevalence of sexual activity and romantic relationships may be lower compared with healthy peers.[35,36] However, a low response rate could potentially mean that the rates of sexual activity were underestimated. In addition, the studies were performed in the late 1980s. Since that time treatment regimens have improved and medication side effects have been minimized. Therefore, it is possible that transplant recipients blend more with their general adolescent peers.

Although chronically ill adolescents are likely to have many encounters with healthcare professionals, most report that they have not been advised about contraception or sexuality.[32,34] This may be due to the fact that chronically ill patients often use subspecialists for their primary care needs who are not necessarily set up for sexual health education. It has been suggested that subspecialty physicians may be likely to dramatically underestimate sexual activity in adolescent female patients.[37] Taken together, these data suggest that chronically ill adolescents demonstrate a low level of knowledge regarding sexual health and a low level of contraceptive use.[34] Yet they demonstrate a higher rate of sexually transmitted diseases.[33] Thus, the transplant provider may need to provide this information.

Experience in the field of sexual health education has shown that large disparities can exist in the information individuals receive based on school and church sexual education programs and information obtained at home. Additionally, many clinics that traditionally provide access to family planning resources may be uncomfortable working with medically complicated patients.[38,39] To complicate matters further, it is not uncommon for parents to be present during all visits with the transplant team,[38,40] a fact that limits the ability of the healthcare professional to address sexual health issues without a concerted effort.

Although numerous factors can complicate the adolescent renal transplant recipient's access to sexual health information and services, this patient population is at the greatest potential risks posed by sexual activity. Thus, a comprehensive understanding of sexual health is essential for renal transplant recipients to maintain their health post-transplant. It is essential that the transplant team speak to adolescent renal transplant recipients regularly, privately, and confidentially about their sexual health before and following transplantation to ensure that they receive all relevant information regarding their sexual health and have access to resources such as contraception and reproductive healthcare services.[34,38,39,41]

Pregnancy and Contraception

It has been noted that transplant recipients may underestimate their own fertility.[39,40] Females, in particular, may not believe that it is possible for them to become pregnant.[42] Genetic counseling under certain circumstances may be warranted.

Furthermore, it is important that they understand that pregnancy after transplant may be *complicated*. There is evidence to suggest that pregnancy in recipients with marginal renal function can potentially lead to graft damage or loss.[42–45] All recommendations emphasize the importance of avoiding pregnancy for at least 6–12 months post-transplantation and even longer in some cases.[38–40,44,45] In addition, patients need to be educated regarding the teratogenic risks of certain medications such as mycophenolate (CellCept® and Myfortic®) and ACE inhibitors.[38,45,46] Based on these risks it is essential that the adolescent renal transplant patient use a highly effective method of contraception.

Condoms should always be recommended; however, the high failure rates of barrier methods observed in adolescents make condoms not suitable as the only form of birth control.[38–40] Combined hormonal contraceptives provide the most effective pregnancy protection. Uncontrolled hypertension is a contraindication to the use of combined oral contraceptives.[38,39] However, when blood pressure is controlled, birth control pills are generally regarded as safe.[38,39] It is essential that the adolescent renal transplant patient understand the possibility of health effects and drug interactions resulting from hormonal contraceptives in case birth control is acquired outside the transplant clinic.

There are also a variety of alternatives to traditional oral contraceptives. Estrogen- and progesterone-combined contraceptives are also available as a vaginal ring. The vaginal ring may be a good option because it is likely to provide a constant level of hormone delivery with fewer side effects.[47] However, there is still only a small amount of data available for this method, and it should, therefore, be regarded as having the same potential side effects and interactions as an orally administered contraceptive. The progesterone shot (DepoProvera) is another option that does not include the estrogen component associated with potential interactions. This method has been previously found to decrease bone density and is also associated with more significant weight gain than other options.[38,39,41] The traditional copper IUD is not advised because the mechanism of pregnancy protection is believed to depend in part on a competent immune system.[38] The newer progesterone IUD is a viable option because it works as a progesterone-based hormonal contraceptive.[38] Although IUDs have been previously discouraged in the transplant population based on the risk of infection, more current literature indicates that these infections are more likely the result of sexually transmitted infections. Furthermore, the possibility of infection can be managed with short-term prophylactic antibiotic treatment at the time of IUD insertion.[38] Based on the variety of potential interactions and side effects associated with various contraceptive choices, it is essential that risks are considered on a case-by-case basis and weighed against the potential detrimental effects of an unplanned pregnancy in the female adolescent renal transplant patient.

Additionally, adolescent renal transplant patients should be educated about the availability of emergency contraception. Although not suitable as a regular form of birth control, emergency contraception is able to prevent up to 85% of pregnancies that would occur following unprotected sexual intercourse.[38,40] There are no contraindications to the use of emergency contraception in transplant recipients even in cases that contraindicate the use of regular hormonal birth control.[38] Emergency contraception can be used for up to 5 days following intercourse but effectiveness decreases as more time is allowed to pass.[40] Therefore, the importance of education regarding the availability of emergency contraception is emphasized to enable timely access when necessary.

Sexually Transmitted Infections

All sexually active adolescents are at high risk of contracting sexually transmitted infections.[38-40] Furthermore, it has been noted that chronically ill adolescents may present higher rates of such infections[34] and that renal transplant recipients specifically may be at a higher risk of contracting these infections. These infections are more likely to result in complications from immunosuppressant medications. Infectious complications are seen as a significant cause of morbidity and mortality in solid organ transplant recipients.[38] Although rare, severe herpes simplex virus (HSV) I and II infections have been reported in renal transplant recipients leading to systemic infection and contributing to death.[48-51] In addition, sexually transmitted infections may be more difficult to eradicate in immunosuppressed patients.[38-40] It is essential that adolescent renal transplant patients understand the risk of acquiring sexually transmitted infections and how to best protect themselves from them. It is essential that they understand the importance of condoms as their only means of protection from sexually transmitted infections and how to properly use condoms to maximize their effectiveness. Additionally, they must understand that condoms can only prevent skin to skin transmission of sexually transmitted infections if the infected genital area is covered.[52] While some sexually transmitted infections can be treated, others have no cure and, therefore, will be carried by the patient for life (or until a treatment is developed).

It is important that healthcare providers specifically address oral sex because experience in the field of sexual education has shown that it is common for adolescents not to consider oral sex to be "sex" and to hold the misconception that there are no potential risks of acquiring sexually transmitted infections when engaging in oral sex. Additionally, the most recent sexual behavior statistics reported by the CDC indicate a significant prevalence of oral sexual activity among teens with approximately 55% of teens aged 15–19 engaging in these activities, a number slightly higher than those engaging in vaginal intercourse in both males and females of this age group.[53] Additionally, the CDC data point out that a significant population of adolescents, up to 15%, may engage in oral sex activities in the absence of vaginal intercourse.[53] This information highlights the importance of acknowledging that teens not involved in vaginal intercourse may still be engaging in activities that expose them to the risk of acquiring sexually transmitted infections. It is important for the adolescent renal transplant patient to understand the potential for passing herpes between oral and genital areas[52] as well as the potential for oral infection of some bacteria and viruses.[54,55] As with vaginal intercourse, barrier methods are the only means of protection from sexually transmitted infections that may be passed during oral sex.

HPV Infection

Human papilloma virus (HPV) presents a serious risk to the renal transplant patient. HPV is a sexually transmitted infection that can result in genital warts and cancer. HPV is an extremely prevalent infection in the general population that often presents no symptoms. Transmission is based on skin to skin contact; therefore, condoms only provide protection when the condom covers the infected area. While spontaneous remission is common in healthy, immunocompetent women, this is rarely seen in the renal transplant population.[56] The literature examining the prevalence of oncogenic HPV subtypes 16 and 18, pre-cancerous neoplasias, and malignancies clearly demonstrates an increased prevalence in renal transplant patients.[38–40,56–58] Furthermore, these lesions are found to progress more rapidly and to be more difficult to cure in this population.[39,56] Of particular relevance are the observations that the incidence of neoplasia increases with time post-transplant and the duration of immuosuppressive therapy.[38,39,56,57,59,60] Recent evidence has also established the connection between oral HPV infection and oropharyngeal cancer.[54] Patients with an established oral HPV infection were found to be 32 times more likely to develop such cancers. This association was most strongly established for HPV-16, one of the subtypes also considered to be the highest risk for women developing cervical cancer.

While adolescent renal transplant patients are a high-risk population with regard to HPV and genital lesions, available literature indicates that female renal transplant patients are likely to be underserved in the area of gynecological/reproductive health.[38,40,57] In spite of the fact that it is recommended they obtain more frequent routine gynecological exams and pap tests (every 6 months), it is common for them to receive no routine exams. Adolescent renal transplant patients and gynecological healthcare providers working with renal transplant patients should understand the importance of routine reproductive health care.[38] Additionally, based on evidence of increased risk for anogenital neoplasias in women, it may be important to recommend anal screening for male renal transplant recipients engaging in anal intercourse.[39]

Although its use and effectiveness has not yet been studied in a transplant population, the HPV vaccine is likely to be the best form of protection from HPV and resulting cancers. The currently approved vaccine, Gardasil, is made from recombinant virus-like particles and protects against four HPV subtypes: 6, 11, 16, and 18. Subtypes 16 and 18 are responsible for approximately 70% of the current cases of cervical cancer in women, and subtypes 6 and 11 result in the vast majority of cases of genital warts.[61] The vaccine is administered in three doses over a 6-month period of time and is believed to be nearly 100% effective in preventing the four subtypes of HPV it includes.[62] The vaccine is currently approved for use in females aged 9–26 with further studies being done to assess the effectiveness of the vaccine in males who may also experience genital warts, genital neoplasias, and oropharyngeal cancers resulting from HPV.

Educational/Vocational/Financial Planning

Reasonable and attainable goals for future education or vocational training post-transplant are essential for young adults to have a sense of self-worth and become contributing members of society. Allowing patients to take on chores at home or part-time work will assist to develop a sense of responsibility. Multiple school absences due to frequent and/or prolonged hospitalizations or chronically feeling unwell can alter future plans. Assessments of the adolescent's aptitudes and opportunities can help facilitate future planning and allow recipients to achieve their full potential.

The challenge for pediatric transplant patients is to maintain insurance coverage after transfer to the adult service. In order to prevent lapses in insurance coverage, patients and healthcare providers need to be aware of the changing insurance issues that arise upon entering adulthood. Prescription medications, laboratory tests, and physician visits can be costly for the adolescent trying to gain financial independence and may lead to nonadherence. Applications for health insurance should be submitted early.

Health and Lifestyle

Pediatric renal transplant patients should be encouraged to adapt a lifestyle that is consistent with promoting good health behaviors such as regular exercise, participation in sports activities, healthy food choices, and consumption in moderation. Healthcare providers must begin a discussion about risky behaviors such as tobacco, alcohol, and drug use; unsafe sex practices; and the consequences of abuse to their health and graft function. Anticipatory guidance should be provided about prevention of post-transplant complications such as infection, cancer, rejection, heart disease, and the consequences of nonadherence.

Conclusion

The transition of pediatric transplant recipients to adult transplant providers can be very difficult for this highly vulnerable group. Although adolescence is a time of tremendous growth, it is also a time of tremendous turmoil causing teenagers to struggle with issues of autonomy, sexuality, career planning, and financial independence. There are many impediments to adolescents assuming adult responsibilities. For the transition to be successful it must encompass all aspects of the teenager's life. A multidisciplinary approach that individualizes the planning to suit the developmental stage of the adolescent will promote skill building and adherence. Parents and family members must learn to assume a more secondary or supportive role. The

Rosen

ultimate goal of the transition process is for the young adult to achieve independence and self-sufficiency while being able to safely and securely negotiate the adult healthcare system. Research is needed to evaluate the various transition programs that will optimally benefit patients and maximize outcomes.

References

1. Data, O.P.T.N. 2008.
2. Dobbels F, Van Damme-Lombaert R, Vanhaecke J, De Geest S. Growing pains: non-adherence with the immunosuppressive regimen in adolescent transplant recipients. *Pediatr Transplant* 2005;9:381–390.
3. Keith DS, Cantarovich M, Paraskevas S, Tchervenkov J. Recipient age and risk of chronic allograft nephropathy in primary deceased donor kidney transplant. *Transpl Int* 2006;19: 649–656.
4. Stam H, Hartman EE, Deurloo JA, Groothoff J, Grootenhuis MA. Young adult patients with a history of pediatric disease: impact on course of life and transition into adulthood. *J Adolesc Health* 2006;39:4–13.
5. Reynolds JM, Morton MJ, Garralda ME, Postlethwaite RJ, Goh D. Psychosocial adjustment of adult survivors of a paediatric dialysis and transplant programme. *Arch Dis Child* 1993;68:104–110.
6. Bell LE, Bartosh SM, Davis CL, Dobbels F, Al-Uzri A, Lotstein D, Reiss J, Dharnidharka VR. Adolescent Transition to Adult Care in Solid Organ Transplantation: a consensus conference report. *Am J Transplant* 2008;8:2230–2242.
7. Blum RW. Transition to adult health care: setting the stage. *J Adolesc Health* 1995;17:3–5.
8. Blum RW, Garell D, Hodgman CH, Jorissen TW, Okinow NA, Orr DP, Slap GB. Transition from child-centered to adult health-care systems for adolescents with chronic conditions. A position paper of the Society for Adolescent Medicine. *J Adolesc Health* 1993;14: 570–576.
9. Rosen DS, Blum RW, Britto M, Sawyer SM, Siegel DM. Transition to adult health care for adolescents and young adults with chronic conditions: position paper of the Society for Adolescent Medicine. *J Adolesc Health* 2003;33:309–311.
10. McDonagh JE. Growing up and moving on: transition from pediatric to adult care. *Pediatr Transplant* 2005;9:364–372.
11. Watson AR. Non-compliance and transfer from paediatric to adult transplant unit. *Pediatr Nephrol (Berlin, Germany)* 2000;14:469–472.
12. Cameron JS. The continued care of children with renal disease into adult life. *Pediatr Nephrol (Berlin, Germany)* 2001;16:680–685.
13. Court JM. Issues of transition to adult care. *J Paediatr Child Health* 1993;29(Suppl 1): S53–S55.
14. Nasr SZ, Campbell C, Howatt W. Transition program from pediatric to adult care for cystic fibrosis patients. *J Adolesc Health* 1992;13:682–685.
15. Watson AR, Shooter M. Transitioning adolescents from pediatric to adult dialysis units. *Adv Perit Dial* 1996;12:176–178.
16. Patterson D, Lanier C. Adolescent health transitions: focus Group Study of Teens and Young Adults with Special Health Care Needs. *Fam Community Health* 1999;22:42–58.
17. Hauser ES, Dorn L. Transitioning adolescents with sickle cell disease to adult-centered care. *Pediatr Nurs* 1999;25:479–488.
18. Landau LI. Cystic fibrosis: transition from paediatric to adult physician's care *Thorax* 1995;50:1031–1032.
19. Shaw KL, Southwood TR, McDonagh JE. User perspectives of transitional care for adolescents with juvenile idiopathic arthritis. *Rheumatology (Oxford, England)* 2004;43:770–778.

20. McCurdy C, DiCenso A, Boblin S, Ludwin D, Bryant-Lukosius D, Bosompra K. There to here: young adult patients' perceptions of the process of transition from pediatric to adult transplant care. *Prog Transplant (Aliso Viejo, Calif)* 2006;16:309–316.

21. Paone MC, Wigle M, Saewyc E. The ON TRAC model for transitional care of adolescents. *Prog Transplant (Aliso Viejo, Calif)* 2006;16:291–302.

22. Geenen SJ, Powers LE, Sells W. Understanding the role of health care providers during the transition of adolescents with disabilities and special health care needs. *J Adolesc Health* 2003;32:225–233.

23. Gutgesell ME, Payne N. Issues of adolescent psychological development in the 21st century. *Pediatr Rev; Am Acad Pediatr* 2004;25:79–85.

24. White PH. Transition to adulthood *Curr Opin Rheumatol* 1999;11:408–411.

25. Giedd JN. The teen brain: insights from neuroimaging. *J Adolesc Health* 2008;42:335–343.

26. Hazen E, Schlozman S, Beresin E. Adolescent psychological development: a review. *Pediatr Rev; Am Acad Pediatr* 2008;29:161–167, quiz 168.

27. Steinberg L. A social neuroscience perspective on adolescent risk-taking. *Dev Rev* 2008;28:78–106.

28. Dovey-Pearce G, Hurrell R, May C, Walker C, Doherty Y. Young adults' (16–25 years) suggestions for providing developmentally appropriate diabetes services: a qualitative study. *Health Soc Care Community* 2005;13:409–419.

29. Reiss J, Gibson R. Health care transition: destinations unknown. *Pediatrics* 2002;110: 1307–1314.

30. Kaufman M. Transition of cognitively delayed adolescent organ transplant recipients to adult care. *Pediatr Transplant* 2006;10:413–417.

31. Kieckhefer GM, Trahms CM. Supporting development of children with chronic conditions: from compliance toward shared management. *Pediatr Nurs* 2000;26:354–363.

32. Carroll G, Massarelli E, Opzoomer A, Pekeles G, Pedneault M, Frappier JY, Onetto N. Adolescents with chronic disease. Are they receiving comprehensive health care? *J Adolesc Health Care* 1983;4:261–265.

33. Suris JC, Resnick MD, Cassuto N, Blum RW. Sexual behavior of adolescents with chronic disease and disability. *J Adolesc Health* 1996;19:124–131.

34. Valencia LS, Cromer BA. Sexual activity and other high-risk behaviors in adolescents with chronic illness: a review. *J Pediatr Adolesc Gynecol* 2000;13:53–64.

35. Henning P, Tomlinson L, Rigden SP, Haycock GB, Chantler C. Long term outcome of treatment of end stage renal failure. *Arch Dis Child* 1988;63:35–40.

36. Melzer SM, Leadbeater B, Reisman L, Jaffe LR, Lieberman KV. Characteristics of social networks in adolescents with end-stage renal disease treated with renal transplantation. *J Adolesc Health Care* 1989;10:308–312.

37. Britto MT, Rosenthal SL, Taylor J, Passo MH. Improving rheumatologists' screening for alcohol use and sexual activity. *Arch Pediatr Adolesc Med* 2000;154:478–483.

38. Sucato GS, Murray PJ. Gynecologic issues of the adolescent female solid organ transplant recipient. *Pediatr Clin North Am* 2003;50:1521–1542.

39. Sucato GS, Murray PJ. Developmental and reproductive health issues in adolescent solid organ transplant recipients. *Semin Pediatr Surg* 2006;15:170–178.

40. Sucato GS, Murray PJ. Gynecologic health care for the adolescent solid organ transplant recipient. *Pediatr Transplant* 2005;9:346–356.

41. Sucato GS, Gerschultz KL. Extended cycle hormonal contraception in adolescents. *Curr Opin Obstetr Gynecol* 2005;17:461–465.

42. McKay DB, Josephson MA, Armenti VT, August P, Coscia LA, Davis Cl, Davison JM, Easterling T, Friedman JE, Hou S, Karlix J, Lake KD, Lindheimer M, Matas AJ, Moritz MJ, Riely CA, Ross LF, Scott JR, Wagoner LE, Wrenshall L, Adams PL, Bumgardner GL, Fine RN, Goral S, Krams SM, Martinez OM, Tolkoff-Rubin N, Pavlakis M, Scantlebury V. Women's Health Committee of the American Society of Transplantation. Reproduction

and transplantation: report on the AST Consensus Conference on Reproductive Issues and Transplantation. *Am J Transplant* 2005;5:1592–1599. Review.

43. Armenti VT, Moritz MJ, Davison JM. Medical management of the pregnant transplant recipient. *Adv Ren Replace Ther* 1998;5:14–23.

44. Armenti VT, Moritz MJ, Davison JM. Pregnancy in female pediatric solid organ transplant recipients. *Pediatr Clin North Am* 2003;50:1543–1560, xi.

45. EBPG. European best practice guidelines for renal transplantation. Section IV: Long-term management of the transplant recipient. IV.10. Pregnancy in renal transplant recipients. *Nephrol Dial Transplant* 2002;17(Suppl 4):50–55.

46. Armenti VT, Moritz MJ, Davison JM. Drug safety issues in pregnancy following transplantation and immunosuppression: effects and outcomes. *Drug Saf* 1998;19:219–232.

47. Sarkar NN. The combined contraceptive vaginal device (Nuvaring): a comprehensive review. *Eur J Contracept Reprod Health Care* 2005;10:73–78. Review.

48. Gomez E, Melon S, de Ona M, Alvarez R, Laures A, Alvarez-Grande J. Disseminated herpes simplex virus infection in a renal transplant patient as possible cause of repeated urinary extravasations. *Nephron* 1999;82:59–64.

49. Kang YN, Oh HK, Chang YC, Kim HC, Lee SL, Hwang M, Park KK. Systemic herpes simplex virus infection following cadaveric renal transplantation: a case report. *Transplant Proc* 2006;38:1346–1347.

50. Montgomerie JZ, Becroft DM, Croxson MC, Doak PB, North JD. Herpes-simplex-virus infection after renal transplantation. *Lancet* 1969;2:867–871.

51. Nebbia G, Mattes FM, Ramaswamy M, Quaglia A, Verghese G, Griffiths PD, Burroughs A, Geretti AM. Primary herpes simplex virus type-2 infection as a cause of liver failure after liver transplantation. *Transpl Infect Dis* 2006;8:229–232.

52. UNOS. 2007. Staying healthy with your new transplant.

53. Mosher WD, Chandra A, Jones J. Sexual behavior and selected health measures: men and women 15–44 years of age, United States, 2002. *Adv Data* 2005;15(362):1–55.

54. D'Souza G, Kreimer AR, Viscidi R, Pawlita M, Fakhry C, Koch WM, Westra WH, Gillison ML. Case-control study of human papillomavirus and oropharyngeal cancer. *New Engl J Med* 2007;356:1944–1956.

55. Youth, A.f.

56. Petry KU, Scheffel D, Bode U, Gabrysiak T, Kochel H, Kupsch E, Glaubitz M, Niesert S, Kuhnle H, Schedel I. Cellular immunodeficiency enhances the progression of human papillomavirus-associated cervical lesions. *Int J Cancer* 1994;57:836–840.

57. Alloub MI, Barr BB, McLaren KM, Smith IW, Bunney MH, Smart GE. Human papillomavirus infection and cervical intraepithelial neoplasia in women with renal allografts. *BMJ* (Clinical research ed) 1989;298:153–156.

58. Fairley CK, Chen S, Tabrizi SN, McNeil J, Becker G, Walker R, Atkins RC, Thomson N, Allan P, Woodburn C et al. Prevalence of HPV DNA in cervical specimens in women with renal transplants: a comparison with dialysis-dependent patients and patients with renal impairment. *Nephrol Dial Transplant* 1994;9:416–420.

59. Brown MR, Noffsinger A, First MR, Penn I, Husseinzadeh N. HPV subtype analysis in lower genital tract neoplasms of female renal transplant recipients. *Gynecol Oncol* 2000;79:220–224.

60. Morrison EA, Dole P, Sun XW, Stern L, Wright TC Jr. Low prevalence of human papillomavirus infection of the cervix in renal transplant recipients. *Nephrol Dial Transplant* 1996;11:1603–1606.

61. Siddiqui MA, Perry CM. Human papillomavirus quadrivalent (types 6, 11, 16, 18) recombinant vaccine (Gardasil). *Drugs* 2006;66:1263–1271, discussion 1272–1263.

62. FDA. New vaccine prevents cervical cancer. *FDA Consum* 2006;40:37.

Index

Note: Locators followed by 'f' and 't' refer to figures and tables respectively.

Socioeconomic issues and transplant (*cont.*)
culture, 365
education, 356
emotional and cognitive status, 366–367
employment maintenance or initiation, 360–361
ethnicity, 356, 365
food, 360
fundraising, importance of, 359–360
gender, 355–356
high-risk behaviors, 365–366
insurance, co-pays, deductibles, and premiums, 359
international perspective, 364–365
introduction, 355
lifestyle choices, 366
living donation, 362–364
  costs related to, 363–364
  relationship of donor to recipient, 362
  social status of donors, 363
lodging, 360
Medicare coverage, 357–358
medication side effects, 362
race, 365
summary, 367
transportation, 360
Solid organ tumors, other, 321–322
South-eastern Organ Procurement Organization (SEOPF), 57, 363
Special situations of candidate for kidney transplant, 195–200, 196t
advancing age, 198
cardiovascular disease, 196–197
combined and sequential multi-organ transplantation, 199–200
liver disease, 197–198
malignancy, 196
obesity, 195–196
pulmonary disease, 197
recurrence of native kidney disease, 198–199
urological issues, 198
Standard criteria donor (SCD), 62–64, 204
Steroid withdrawal
early, 142–143
late, 141–142
Strongyloidiasis, 304–305
Surgical site infections, 284
Surgical techniques and complications, 15–23
kidney transplantation, 15–18
  history, 16–18
  introduction, 15–16
  organ implantation, 18–23

closing, 21
complications, 21–22
exposure, 19–20
preparation, 18–19
summary, 22–23
ureteral anastomoses, 20–21
vascular anastomoses, 20
Synapse, formation of immunologic, 30–31

T
Tacrolimus, 261–262
Target of rapamycin, *see* TOR inhibitors
T cells
activation of, 32
division of, 32–33
effectors of rejection and adaptive immune system, 33–34
interaction of donor dendritic cells with, 29–30
mediated rejection, 178–180
  acute, 178–180
  chronic, 180
receptor-mediated signaling events, 31–32
Teriparatide, 336
Thrombotic microangiopathy, 217–218
T lymphocytes and cytotoxic crossmatch, 48t
TOR inhibitors, 131–132
dosing, 131
drug interactions, 131
mechanisms of action, 131
side effects, 132
Transaminitis, 230–231
Transition of care, 383
components of transition process, 385
  educational/vocational/financial planning, 391
  health and lifestyle, 391
  human papilloma virus (HPV), 390
  independent behaviors, 386
  knowledge and self-advocacy, 385–386
  pregnancy and contraception, 387–389
  sexual health, 386–387
  sexually transmitted infections, 389
conclusion, 391–392
defined by American Society for Adolescent Medicine, 383–384
introduction, 383–384
multidisciplinary approach to, 384–385
Transplant center, 57–60
Transplant immunology and allograft rejection, 25–37
acute allograft rejection, 221
after transplantation, later phase months to years later, 36–37